Arrhythmogenic Cardiomyopathy

Guest Editors

DOMENICO CORRADO, MD, PhD, FESC
CRISTINA BASSO, MD, PhD, FESC
GAETANO THIENE, MD, FRCP, FESC

CARDIAC ELECTROPHYSIOLOGY CLINICS

www.cardiacEP.theclinics.com

Consulting Editors
RANJAN K. THAKUR, MD, MPH, MBA, FHRS
ANDREA NATALE, MD, FACC, FHRS

June 2011 • Volume 3 • Number 2

SAUNDERS an imprint of ELSEVIER, Inc.

W.B. SAUNDERS COMPANY
A Division of Elsevier Inc.

1600 John F. Kennedy Boulevard • Suite 1800 • Philadelphia, Pennsylvania 19103-2899

http://www.theclinics.com

CARDIAC ELECTROPHYSIOLOGY CLINICS Volume 3, Number 2
June 2011 ISSN 1877-9182, ISBN-13: 978-1-4377-2428-8

Editor: Barbara Cohen-Kligerman
Developmental Editor: Teia Stone

Cardiac Electrophysiology Clinics (ISSN 1877-9182) is published quarterly by Elsevier Inc., 360 Park Avenue South, New York, NY 10010-1710. Months of issue are March, June, September, and December. Subscription prices are $167.00 per year for US individuals, $250.00 per year for US institutions, $88.00 per year for US students and residents, $187.00 per year for Canadian individuals, $279.00 per year for Canadian institutions, $239.00 per year for international individuals, $299.00 per year for international institutions and $126.00 per year for Canadian and foreign students/residents. To receive student/resident rate, orders must be accompanied by name of affilliated institution, date of term, and the signature of program/residency coordinator on institution letterhead. Orders will be billed at individual rate until proof of status is received. Foreign air speed delivery is included in all Clinics subscription prices. All prices are subject to change without notice. **POSTMASTER:** Send address changes to Cardiac Electrophysiology Clinics, Elsevier Health Sciences Division, Subscription Customer Service, 3251 Riverport Lane, Maryland Heights, MO 63043. **Customer Service: 1-800-654-2452 (US and Canada). From outside of the US and Canada, call 314-477-8871. Fax: 314-447-8029. E-mail: JournalsCustomerService-usa@elsevier.com (for print support); JournalsOnlineSupport-usa@elsevier.com (for online support).**

Reprints. For copies of 100 or more of articles in this publication, please contact the Commercial Reprints Department, Elsevier Inc., 360 Park Avenue South, New York, NY 10010-1710. Tel.: 212-633-3812; Fax: 212-462-1935; E-mail: reprints@elsevier.com.

Cover illustration: ECG abnormalities of arrhythmogenic cardiomyopathy: low QRS voltages in frontal leads, T-wave inversion in right precordial leads and ventricular arrhythmias with a left bundle branch block morphology.

Printed and bound by CPI Group (UK) Ltd, Croydon, CR0 4YY

Transferred to Digital Print 2011

Contributors

CONSULTING EDITORS

RANJAN K. THAKUR, MD, MPH, MBA, FHRS
Professor of Medicine, and Director, Arrhythmia Service, Thoracic and Cardiovascular Institute, Sparrow Health System, Michigan State University, Lansing, Michigan

ANDREA NATALE, MD, FACC, FHRS
Executive Medical Director of the Texas Cardiac Arrhythmia Institute at St David's Medical Center, Austin, Texas; Consulting Professor, Division of Cardiology, Stanford University, Palo Alto, California; Clinical Associate Professor of Medicine, Case Western Reserve University, Cleveland, Ohio; Senior Clinical Director, EP Services, California Pacific Medical Center, San Francisco, California; Department of Biomedical Engineering, University of Texas, Austin, Texas

GUEST EDITORS

DOMENICO CORRADO, MD, PhD, FESC
Division of Cardiology, Department of Cardiac, Thoracic and Vascular Sciences, University of Padua Medical School, Padua, Italy

CRISTINA BASSO, MD, PhD, FESC
Cardiovascular Pathology, Department of Medical-Diagnostic Sciences and Special Therapies, University of Padua Medical School, Padua, Italy

GAETANO THIENE, MD, FRCP(Hon), FESC
Cardiovascular Pathology, Department of Medical-Diagnostic Sciences and Special Therapies, University of Padua Medical School, Padua, Italy

AUTHORS

ANNA BARITUSSIO, MD
Division of Cardiology, Department of Cardiac, Thoracic and Vascular Sciences, University of Padua Medical School, Padua, Italy

CRISTINA BASSO, MD, PhD, FESC
Cardiovascular Pathology, Department of Medical-Diagnostic Sciences and Special Therapies, University of Padua Medical School, Padua, Italy

BARBARA BAUCE, MD, PhD
Division of Cardiology, Department of Cardiac, Thoracic and Vascular Sciences, University of Padua Medical School, Padua, Italy

GIANFRANCO BUJA, MD
Division of Cardiology, Department of Cardiac, Thoracic and Vascular Sciences, University of Padua Medical School, Padua, Italy

HUGH CALKINS, MD
Division of Cardiology, The Johns Hopkins University, Baltimore, Maryland

ELISA CARTURAN, PhD
Department of Medical-Diagnostic Sciences and Special Therapies, University of Padua Medical School, Padua, Italy

DOMENICO CORRADO, MD, PhD, FESC
Division of Cardiology, Department of Cardiac, Thoracic and Vascular Sciences, University of Padua Medical School, Padua, Italy

MONIEK G.P.J. COX, MD
Research Physician, Department of Cardiology, University Medical Center Utrecht; Interuniversity Cardiology Institute of the Netherlands, Utrecht, The Netherlands

N.A. MARK ESTES III, MD
Professor of Medicine, Cardiac Arrhythmia Center, Tufts Medical Center, Tufts University School of Medicine, Boston, Massachusetts

HARIS M. HAQQANI, MBBS (Hons), PhD
Senior Lecturer, School of Medicine, The University of Queensland; Electrophysiologist, Department of Cardiology, The Prince Charles Hospital, Brisbane, Australia

RICHARD N.W. HAUER, MD, PhD
Professor of Clinical Electrophysiology, Department of Cardiology, University Medical Center Utrecht; Interuniversity Cardiology Institute of the Netherlands, Utrecht, The Netherlands

SABINO ILICETO, MD
Division of Cardiology, Department of Cardiac, Thoracic and Vascular Sciences, University of Padua Medical School, Padua, Italy

JULIA H. INDIK, MD, PhD
Associate Professor of Medicine, Section of Cardiology, Sarver Heart Center, University of Arizona College of Medicine, Tucson, Arizona

LOIRA LEONI, MD, PhD
Division of Cardiology, Department of Cardiac, Thoracic and Vascular Sciences, University of Padua Medical School, Padua, Italy

MARK S. LINK, MD
Professor of Medicine, Cardiac Arrhythmia Center, Tufts Medical Center, Tufts University School of Medicine, Boston, Massachusetts

FRANCIS E. MARCHLINSKI, MD
Professor of Medicine, Cardiovascular Division, Department of Medicine, University of Pennsylvania Health System, Philadelphia, Pennsylvania

FRANK I. MARCUS, MD
Professor Emeritus, Division of Internal Medicine, University of Arizona and Sarver Heart Center, Tucson, Arizona

ALESSIO MARINELLI, MD
Division of Cardiology, Department of Cardiac, Thoracic and Vascular Sciences, University of Padua Medical School, Padua, Italy

WILLIAM J. MCKENNA, MD, DSc, FACC
Professor of Cardiology, Department of Cardiovascular Medicine, University College; The Heart Hospital, University College London Hospitals Trust, London, United Kingdom

FEDERICO MIGLIORE, MD
Division of Cardiology, Department of Cardiac, Thoracic and Vascular Sciences, University of Padua Medical School, Padua, Italy

MATTHIAS PAUL, MD
Assistant Professor of Medicine, Department of Cardiology and Angiology, Medizinische Klinik und Poliklinik C (Kardiologie und Angiologie), Universitätsklinikum Münster, Osnabrück, Germany

ANTONIO PELLICCIA, MD
Institute of Sports Medicine and Science, Rome, Italy

MARTINA PERAZZOLO MARRA, MD, PhD
Division of Cardiology, Department of Cardiac, Thoracic and Vascular Sciences, University of Padua Medical School, Padua, Italy

MICHAEL H. PICARD, MD
Director, Cardiac Ultrasound Laboratory, Massachusetts General Hospital; Associate Professor of Medicine, Harvard Medical School, Boston, Massachusetts

KALLIOPI PILICHOU, PhD
Department of Medical-Diagnostic Sciences and Special Therapies, University of Padua Medical School, Padua, Italy

NIKOS PROTONOTARIOS, MD, FESC
Yannis Protonotarios Medical Centre, Hora Naxos, Naxos, Greece

GIOVANNI QUARTA, MD
Cardiology Research Fellow, The Heart Hospital, University College London Hospitals Trust, London, United Kingdom; Department of Cardiology, S. Andrea Hospital, University "La Sapienza", Rome, Italy

ILARIA RIGATO, MD, PhD
Division of Cardiology, Department of Cardiac, Thoracic and Vascular Sciences, University of Padua Medical School, Padua, Italy

STEFANIA RIZZO, MD
Department of Medical-Diagnostic Sciences and Special Therapies, University of Padua Medical School, Padua, Italy

DANITA M.Y. SANBORN, MD
Medical Director, Paul Dudley White Associates, Cardiology Division, Massachusetts General Hospital; Instructor in Medicine, Harvard Medical School, Boston, Massachusetts

MAURIZIO SCHIAVON, MD
Department of Social Health, Center for Sports Medicine and Physical Activity, Padua, Italy

SRIJITA SEN-CHOWDHRY, MBBS, MD (Cantab), FESC
BHF Intermediate Clinical Research Fellow, Department of Cardiovascular Medicine, University College London; Department of Epidemiology, Imperial College, London, United Kingdom

MARIA SILVANO, MD
Division of Cardiology, Department of Cardiac, Thoracic and Vascular Sciences, University of Padua Medical School, Padua, Italy

PETROS SYRRIS, PhD
Director, Cardiovascular Genetics Laboratory, Department of Cardiovascular Medicine, University College London, United Kingdom

HARIKRISHNA TANDRI, MD
Division of Cardiology, The Johns Hopkins University, Baltimore, Maryland

GAETANO THIENE, MD, FRCP(Hon), FESC
Cardiovascular Pathology, Department of Medical-Diagnostic Sciences and Special Therapies, University of Padua Medical School, Padua, Italy

ADALENA TSATSOPOULOU, MD
Yannis Protonotarios Medical Centre, Hora Naxos, Naxos, Greece

THOMAS WICHTER, MD, FESC
Professor of Medicine and Director, Department of Internal Medicine and Cardiology, Heart Center Osnabrück–Bad Rothenfelde, Niels Stensen Kliniken, Marienhospital Osnabrück, Osnabrück, Germany

ALESSANDRO ZORZI, MD
Division of Cardiology, Department of Cardiac, Thoracic and Vascular Sciences, University of Padua Medical School, Padua, Italy

Contents

Foreword: From "Right Ventricular Dysplasia" to "Arrhythmogenic Cardiomyopathy" **xiii**

Ranjan K. Thakur and Andrea Natale

Preface: Arrhythmogenic Cardiomyopathy **xv**

Domenico Corrado, Cristina Basso, and Gaetano Thiene

Arrhythmogenic Cardiomyopathy: A Historical Overview **179**

Gaetano Thiene, Domenico Corrado, Barbara Bauce, and Cristina Basso

This article gives a historical overview of arrhythmogenic cardiomyopathy (AC). First discovered in Italy in the eighteenth century, AC was extensively studied over the years by numerous pioneering investigators, until in 1994 the first international task force published definitive diagnostic criteria. These criteria have been revised recently, taking into account more novel directions in research such as genotype-phenotype correlations, new diagnostic tools, risk stratification and genetic testing.

Pathobiology of Arrhythmogenic Cardiomyopathy **193**

Cristina Basso, Kalliopi Pilichou, Elisa Carturan, Stefania Rizzo, Barbara Bauce, and Gaetano Thiene

Cellular and transgenic animal models with mutant desmosomal genes may help to elucidate the cascade of cellular and molecular events involved in arrhythmogenic cardiomyopathy phenotype development and the clinical relevance of different desmosomal gene variants, either isolated or together. Knowledge of the mechanisms leading from the mutant protein to the clinical phenotype, and the search for genetic or environmental factors that influence the expression of these defective proteins, will allow identification of potential molecular targets for therapeutic intervention to stop disease onset and progression.

Clinical Impact of Genetics in Arrhythmogenic Cardiomyopathy **205**

Srijita Sen-Chowdhry, Petros Syrris, Giovanni Quarta, and William J. McKenna

In the past decade, elucidation of the genetic etiology of arrhythmogenic cardiomyopathy (AC) has shed light on the cellular and molecular mechanisms underlying the disease. In addition to its diagnostic utility, genetic testing has provided a more stringent benchmark for analysis of heterogeneous disease expression. Genotype-phenotype correlation has built on earlier familial studies to redefine the natural history of the disease and its pleiomorphic manifestations. This review provides an up-to-date summary of the genetics of AC as a prelude to discussion of its impact on clinical diagnosis, prognostication, and therapy.

Arrhythmogenic Cardiomyopathy Diagnostic Criteria: An Update **217**

Frank I. Marcus

Multiple criteria are needed to diagnose arrhythmogenic cardiomyopathy (AC) because there is no single criterion that is sufficiently specific to reliably establish the diagnosis. Modified diagnostic criteria have recently been published that improve the sensitivity for detecting AC. In about 50% of patients a desmosomal genetic abnormality can be identified. However, even the presence of a desmosomal abnormality does not indicate that the individual is or will be affected, because the penetrance is so variable. In the early stages the disease may be difficult to differentiate from normal, and in the advanced stage the diagnosis may be obvious.

Arrhythmogenic Cardiomyopathy: Clinical Presentation **227**

Nikos Protonotarios and Adalena Tsatsopoulou

The clinical presentation of arrhythmogenic cardiomyopathy is broad, varying from a concealed phase mainly with electrical abnormalities to overt disease with obvious structural/functional alterations on conventional imaging. Structural presentation ranges from right-dominant to left-dominant disease, while ventricular arrhythmias remain the clinical hallmark of this cardiomyopathy. Thus, the term "arrhythmogenic cardiomyopathy" might be more appropriate than "arrhythmogenic right ventricular cardiomyopathy".

Twelve-Lead ECG in Arrhythmogenic Cardiomyopathy **237**

Richard N.W. Hauer and Moniek G.P.J. Cox

Arrhythmogenic cardiomyopathy (AC) is a disorder characterized histopathologically by fibrofatty replacement of the myocardium, primarily of the right ventricle, and clinically by ventricular tachyarrhythmias, sudden death, and progressive heart failure. The 12-lead electrocardiogram is one of the most important tools for diagnosis of AC, contributing to evaluation of progression of disease during follow-up. Because in AC ventricular arrhythmias and sudden death are caused by reentrant mechanisms, activation delay is a critical component. Recently, a new parameter of activation delay, prolonged terminal activation duration, appeared to be superior in sensitivity to previously defined criteria, without loss of specificity.

Echocardiography in Arrhythmogenic Cardiomyopathy **245**

Danita M.Y. Sanborn and Michael H. Picard

Echocardiography is a useful tool for clinicians treating an individual suspected of having arrhythmogenic cardiomyopathy (AC). Dilatation of the right ventricle (RV) is the most frequently observed echocardiographic abnormality. RV dilatation (parasternal long axis $\geq$32 mm or parasternal short axis $\geq$36 mm) coupled with localized aneurysm (akinesia or dyskinesia) or global RV dysfunction (fractional area change $\leq$33%) is now considered a major criterion for the diagnosis of AC. Morphologic abnormalities are also often noted in individuals with AC and may provide useful supporting evidence when AC is suspected. Echocardiography has a high diagnostic accuracy for the disease compared with magnetic resonance imaging.

Ventricular Angiography in Arrhythmogenic Cardiomyopathy **255**

Thomas Wichter, Julia H. Indik, and Matthias Paul

Arrhythmogenic cardiomyopathy (AC) is characterized by regional or global abnormalities of right ventricular structure and function and ventricular tachyarrhythmias. The structural abnormalities of the right ventricular myocardium provide the basis for the main clinical and diagnostic features of AC. However, the clinical diagnosis of AC may be difficult to make because there is no easily obtained single test or finding with high diagnostic accuracy. This article discusses the role of ventricular angiography in AC and its features.

Magnetic Resonance and Computed Tomographic Imaging in Arrhythmogenic Cardiomyopathy 269

Harikrishna Tandri and Hugh Calkins

Right ventricular (RV) structure and functional alterations are important criteria for the diagnosis of arrhythmogenic cardiomyopathy (AC). Magnetic resonance imaging (MRI) and computed tomography (CT) have emerged as robust tools to evaluate the RV in patients with suspected AC. The noninvasive nature of these investigations, multiplanar capability, and unique ability to provide tissue characterization are ideal for the assessment of AC. Both imaging modalities have the ability to provide direct evidence of fatty infiltration and structural alterations of the RV. This article discusses the current status, strengths, and limitations of MRI and cardiac CT in the evaluation of AC.

Arrhythmogenic Cardiomyopathy: Natural History and Risk Stratification 281

Federico Migliore, Anna Baritussio, Ilaria Rigato, Martina Perazzolo Marra, Barbara Bauce, Cristina Basso, Sabino Iliceto, and Domenico Corrado

Arrhythmogenic cardiomyopathy (AC) is an inherited heart muscle disease whose clinical manifestations are related to ventricular electrical instability, which may lead to sudden cardiac death, mostly in young people. Later in the disease history, the right ventricle becomes more diffusely affected and the involvement of the left ventricle may result in biventricular heart failure. This article addresses the disease natural history and analyzes the clinical predictors of sudden arrhythmic death and clinical outcome of patients with AC.

Pharmacologic Management in Arrhythmogenic Cardiomyopathy 293

Mark S. Link and N.A. Mark Estes III

Pharmacologic management of disease is performed for specific reasons, which include reducing symptoms, preventing disease progression, and preventing mortality. In arrhythmogenic cardiomyopathy (AC), there are no randomized clinical trial data on pharmacologic management, and little data overall on the use of drugs in this condition. This article discusses the role of pharmacology in AC to prevent symptoms, limit progression of disease, and prolong life.

Electroanatomic Mapping and Catheter Ablation of Ventricular Tachycardia in Arrhythmogenic Cardiomyopathy 299

Haris M. Haqqani and Francis E. Marchlinski

Monomorphic ventricular tachycardia (VT) is a natural consequence of the unique fibrotic process seen in arrhythmogenic cardiomyopathy. The fibrosis is confluent and is centered around the epicardium of the right ventricle in most cases, progressing inwards towards the endocardium. This has important implications for the mechanism, surface morphology, size and location of the reentrant VT circuits seen in this disease. This article examines the electrophysiologic substrate underlying monomorphic VT in arrhythmogenic cardiomyopathy. It also explores the current role and technique of endocardial and epicardial catheter ablation of VT in this condition.

Implantable Cardioverter Defibrillator in Arrhythmogenic Cardiomyopathy 311

Domenico Corrado, Maria Silvano, Federico Migliore, Alessio Marinelli, Loira Leoni, Gaetano Thiene, Sabino Iliceto, and Gianfranco Buja

Arrhythmogenic cardiomyopathy (AC) has become an emerging indication for implantable defibrillator (ICD) implantation because its natural history is more strongly related to ventricular electrical instability, which can precipitate sudden cardiac death (SCD) mostly in young people. This article reviews the studies that have become available in the last decade on the efficacy and safety of ICD therapy in patients with AC. Particular reference is reserved for DARVIN studies, which have addressed the clinical impact of ICD therapy in changing the natural history of AC in a large patient population treated for secondary and primary prevention of SCD.

Arrhythmogenic Cardiomyopathy and Sports-Related Sudden Death **323**

Maurizio Schiavon, Alessandro Zorzi, Cristina Basso, Antonio Pelliccia, Gaetano Thiene, and Domenico Corrado

Arrhythmogenic cardiomyopathy (AC) is an inherited heart muscle disease characterized by ventricular electrical instability, which may lead to cardiac arrest from ventricular fibrillation, mostly in young people. AC shows a propensity for life-threatening ventricular arrhythmias during physical exercise, and participation in competitive athletics has been associated with an increased risk for sudden cardiac death (SCD). This article examines the role of AC in causing SCD in young competitive athletes and addresses prevention strategy based on identification of affected athletes at preparticipation screening.

Index **333**

Cardiac Electrophysiology Clinics

FORTHCOMING ISSUES

September 2011

Advances in ICD Therapy
Paul J. Wang, MD, and
Amin Al-Ahmad, MD, *Guest Editors*

December 2011

Contemporary Debates and Controversies in Cardiac Electrophysiology, Part I
Ranjan K. Thakur, MD, MPH, MBA, and Andrea Natale, MD, *Guest Editors*

March 2012

Long QT Syndrome
Silvia G. Priori, MD, PhD, *Guest Editor*

RECENT ISSUES

March 2010

Basic Science for the Clinical Electrophysiologist
Charles Antzelevitch, PhD, *Guest Editor*

December 2010

Genetics of Cardiac Arrhythmias
Silvia G. Priori, MD, PhD, *Guest Editor*

September 2010

Advances in Antiarrhythmic Drug Therapy
Peter R. Kowey, MD, and
Gerald V. Naccarelli, MD, *Guest Editors*

ISSUES OF RELATED INTEREST

Cardiology Clinics May 2011 (Vol. 29, No. 2)
Catheterization Hemodynamics
Michael J. Lim, MD, *Guest Editor*
Available at: http://www.cardiology.theclinics.com/

Heart Failure Clinics April 2011 (Vol. 7, No. 2)
Sudden Cardiac Death
Raul Weiss, MD, and Emile G. Daoud, MD, *Guest Editors*
Available at: http://www.heartfailure.theclinics.com/

Foreword
From "Right Ventricular Dysplasia" to "Arrhythmogenic Cardiomyopathy"

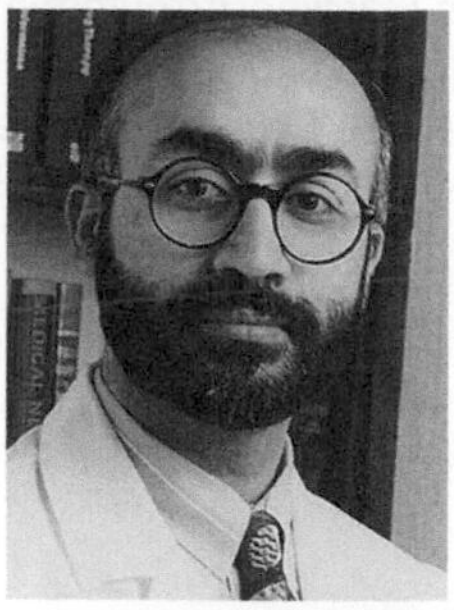

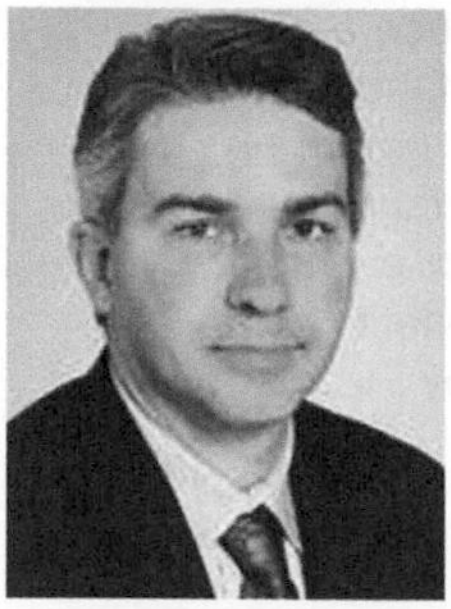

Ranjan K. Thakur, MD, MPH, MBA, FHRS   Andrea Natale, MD, FHRS
Consulting Editors

Our current understanding of the spectrum of right ventricular dysplasia illustrates two important realities of modern medicine. First, like Moor's law—which predicts that the number of transistors that can be placed on an integrated circuit doubles every 18–24 months, leading to ever faster computing capabilities—clinical knowledge is also doubling every 2 years. Second, while clinical knowledge is expanding "horizontally" at the phenotype level, the real growth in knowledge is actually growing "vertically," into the genetic and molecular realms.

When we were medical students, all we knew about "right ventricular dysplasia" was some of its clinical and pathological features, namely, right ventricular enlargement and fatty infiltration ranging from patchy involvement, particularly at characteristic locations in the right ventricle, all the way to Uhl's anomaly, with a "parchment-like" right ventricle. It was only relatively recently (in 1982) that Marcus and colleagues described detailed clinical features of supposed right ventricular dysplasia in 24 patients.

Since then, our understanding of this condition has expanded at the phenotype level, to the point where it may be more prudent to call this syndrome an "arrhythmogenic cardiomyopathy" as the editors of this issue of the *Cardiac Electrophysiology Clinics* have done. Diagnosis of this condition in the past was particularly difficult, especially in milder cases. Diagnosis is now facilitated by the new diagnostic criteria, magnetic resonance imaging, and electroanatomic mapping to demonstrate the characteristic ventricular scars. Recent developments also led to the realization that previously thought benign right ventricular outflow tract ventricular tachycardia (RVOT-VT) might actually be a forme fruste of the same pathogenetic process.

In the "vertical dimension," the disease has been attributed to genes responsible for desmosomal

Card Electrophysiol Clin 3 (2011) xiii–xiv
doi:10.1016/j.ccep.2011.03.001
1877-9182/11/$ – see front matter

proteins, which facilitate cell coupling, and animal models and mechanisms of apoptosis leading to fibro-fatty infiltration have been identified.

This issue of *Cardiac Electrophysiology Clinics* is edited by some of the leaders in this field. They have assembled a group of contributors from both sides of the "pond" to produce a clinically relevant state-of-the-art understanding of this important condition that every practicing electrophysiologist should know. We thank and congratulate the editors for their achievement and hope that the readers will benefit from these thoughtful reviews written by leading researchers.

Ranjan K. Thakur, MD, MPH, MBA, FHRS
Thoracic and Cardiovascular Institute
405 West Greenlawn, Suite 400
Lansing, MI 48910, USA

Andrea Natale, MD, FHRS
Texas Cardiac Arrhythmia Institute
Center for Atrial Fibrillation at
St David's Medical Center
1015 East 32nd Street, Suite 516
Austin, TX 78705, USA

E-mail addresses:
thakur@msu.edu (R.K. Thakur)
andrea.natale@stdavids.com (A. Natale)

Preface
Arrhythmogenic Cardiomyopathy

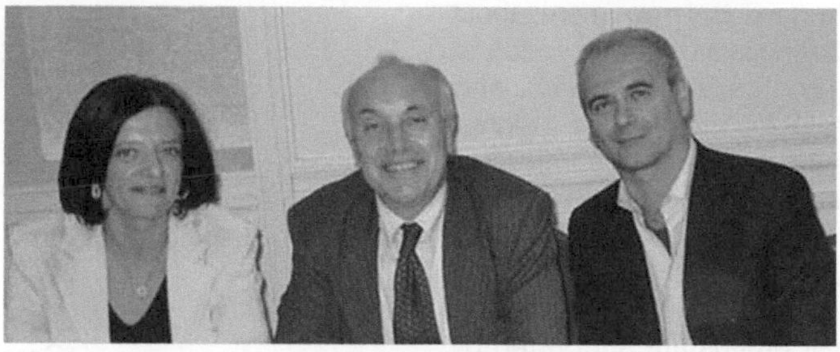

Cristina Basso, MD, PhD, FESC, Gaetano Thiene, MD, FRCP, FESC, Domenico Corrado, MD, PhD, FESC
Guest Editors

In this first decade of the 2000s an impressive increase of knowledge took place in the field of arrhythmogenic right ventricular cardiomyopathy, a disease that was discovered as a clinical entity only 30 years ago. A panel of international experts from both sides of the Ocean contributed to this issue of *Cardiac Electrophysiology Clinics*.

Molecular genetic investigations established that this hereditable cardiac disorder is a cell junction disease, due to mutations of genes encoding desmosomal proteins in charge of the mechanical coupling. Transgenic mice have been generated to elucidate the pathogenetic mechanism of the cell injury, namely, genetically determined cell death followed by fibro-fatty replacement and ventricular electrical instability.

New diagnostic criteria have been put forward, including quantitative parameters and T-wave inversion in right precordial leads, ventricular tachycardia of left bundle branch block morphology with superior axis, and daily frequency of more than 500 ventricular extra-systoles as major criteria. Identification of pathogenetic mutations is considered as an additional instrument of diagnosis.

The employment of cardiac magnetic resonance imaging has become a widespread tool, for both morphofunctional analysis and tissue characterization.

The implantable cardioverter defibrillator has been revealed to be an extraordinary lifesaving therapy, not only for secondary prevention after aborted cardiac arrest but also for primary prevention following syncopal episodes.

Electroanatomic mapping may be considered an in vivo virtual histology, with low-voltage areas corresponding to fibro-fatty myocardial atrophy, and may be accomplished from either the endocardial or the epicardial side, as to be fundamental to guide catheter ablation.

Cardiac arrest in this disease may be precipitated by effort. It has been proven that sudden death in athletes can be prevented mostly by recognition of cardiomyopathies, such as arrhythmogenic and hypertrophic, during preparticipation screening followed by disqualification from sports activity.

By reading the title and the various articles in this issue, the reader will see that we intentionally introduced a new terminology, namely arrhythmogenic cardiomyopathy "tout court," ruling out the label "right ventricular" to underlie the evolving concept of a genetically determined heart muscle disease extending across the entire heart.

Card Electrophysiol Clin 3 (2011) xv–xvi
doi:10.1016/j.ccep.2011.02.015

Even though we are excited about the terrific advances achieved, we have to admit that only symptomatic therapy is still available. Although the genetic causes of the disease are now well known, we do not understand yet how mutations of genes encoding desmosomal proteins are responsible for cell suicide/death. We need to know more about intracellular signaling linking intercalated disc to cell function and viability, and certainly the transgenic mouse models will help for mechanistic insights, with the hope that the discoveries will be translated soon to the clinical setting for a curative therapy.

ACKNOWLEDGMENTS

The Editors and their groups are supported by the Fondazione Cariparo, Padova and Rovigo; and by the Registry of Cardio-Cerebro-Vascular Pathology, Veneto Region, Venice, Italy.

The research was carried out within a grant from the European Commission, Brussels, Belgium (QLG1-CT-2000-01091).

They also acknowledge the Association for Research of Arrhythmic Cardiac Diseases (ARCA, via Gabelli, 61, 35121 Padua-Italy) and Chiara Carturan for the assistance in preparing this book.

Domenico Corrado, MD, PhD, FESC
Division of Cardiology, Department of Cardiac
Thoracic and Vascular Sciences
University of Padua Medical School
Via Giustiniani, 2
35121 Padua, Italy

Cristina Basso, MD, PhD, FESC
Cardiovascular Pathology
Department of Medical Diagnostic Sciences
and Special Therapies
University of Padua Medical School
Via A. Gabelli, 61
35121 Padua, Italy

Gaetano Thiene, MD, FRCP, FESC
Cardiovascular Pathology
Department of Medical Diagnostic Sciences
and Special Therapies
University of Padua Medical School
Via A. Gabelli, 61
35121 Padua, Italy

E-mail addresses:
domenico.corrado@unipd.it (D. Corrado)
cristina.basso@unipd.it (C. Basso)
gaetano.thiene@unipd.it (G. Thiene)

Arrhythmogenic Cardiomyopathy: A Historical Overview

Gaetano Thiene, MD[a,*], Domenico Corrado, MD, PhD[b], Barbara Bauce, MD, PhD[b], Cristina Basso, MD, PhD[a]

KEYWORDS

- Arrhythmogenic right ventricular cardiomyopathy/dysplasia
- Historical context

Italy may rightly claim the discovery of arrhythmogenic cardiomyopathy (AC) as a distinct heredofamilial morbid entity. In 1738 Giovanni Maria Lancisi posthumously published in Naples the book *De Motu Cordis et Aneurysmatibus*.[1] Lancisi was Professor of Anatomy at the University "La Sapienza" in Rome and personal doctor (archiater) of the Pope. In Chapter V of the book entitled *De Hereditaria ad Cordis Aneurysmata Constitutione: De Cordis Prolapsu* (On the Hereditary Predisposition to Cardiac Aneurysms: Cardiac Prolapse), he reported some examples of such morbid entities and described the history of a family with disease recurrence in 4 generations, all featuring signs and symptoms that were in keeping with what nowadays we call AC: palpitations, dilatation and aneurysms of the right ventricle (RV), heart failure, and sudden death (**Fig. 1**). Thus, the first description of AC dates back nearly two and a half centuries earlier than modern observations.

The first recent pathologic description was made by Laennec, as reported in his bibliography by Saintignon in 1904.[2] In Middlemarch, published in 1871 by George Eliot, the protagonist Dr Lydgate, talking to his patient, says "you are suffering from what is called fatty degeneration of the heart, a disease which was first described by Laennec… it is my duty to tell you that death from the disease is often sudden…."[3]

In 1905 Sir William Osler reported a case of a nearly 40-year-old man who died suddenly while climbing a hill.[4] Postmortem disclosed a biventricular myocardial atrophy, with a thinning and translucency of the ventricular free walls, which Osler immortalized with the name "parchment heart." The heart specimen was part of the Maude Abbot collection.[5] In 1950 Segall reviewed the specimen and republished the case with unequivocal drawings showing paper-thin walls (**Fig. 2**).[6]

A controversial case, which was the source of subsequent misconceptions, was reported by Uhl at the Johns Hopkins Hospital in Baltimore in 1952.[7] He published "A previously undescribed congenital malformation of the heart: almost total absence of myocardium of the right ventricle" in an 8-month-old female infant who died of congestive heart failure and with no arrhythmias at electrocardiography (ECG). The description of the heart at autopsy reads (**Fig. 3**):

> *Externally the heart appears greatly enlarged… almost the entire dilated chamber (RV) was occupied by a large laminated mural thrombosis which adhered firmly to the endocardium along the anterior wall of the ventricle. Examination of the cut edge of the ventricle wall revealed it to be paper-thin with no myocardium visible… In the RV wall epicardium and endocardium lie adjacent to each other with no intervening cardiac muscle… no fibro-fatty tissue in the RV free wall was observed.*

[a] Cardiovascular Pathology, Department of Medical-Diagnostic Sciences and Special Therapies, University of Padua Medical School, Via A. Gabelli, 35121 Padua, Italy
[b] Division of Cardiology, Department of Cardiac, Thoracic and Vascular Sciences, University of Padua Medical School, Via Giustiniani, 2-35121 Padua, Italy
* Corresponding author.
E-mail address: gaetano.thiene@unipd.it

Card Electrophysiol Clin 3 (2011) 179–191
doi:10.1016/j.ccep.2011.02.006

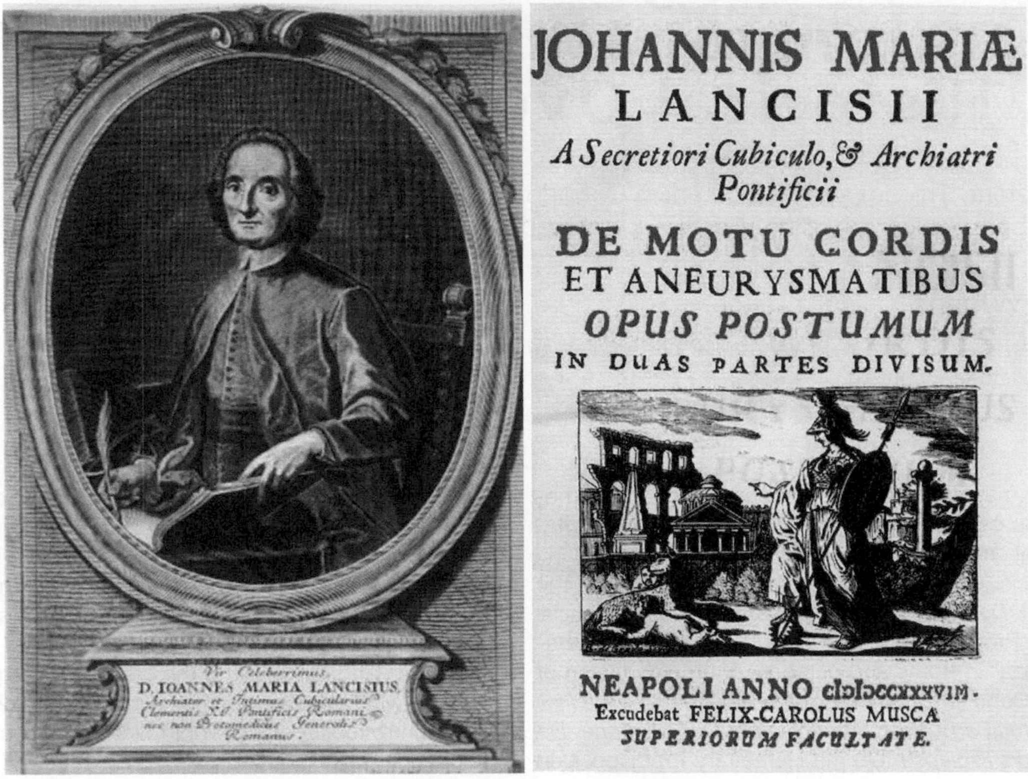

Fig. 1. The book by Giovanni Maria Lancisi published in Naples in 1738.

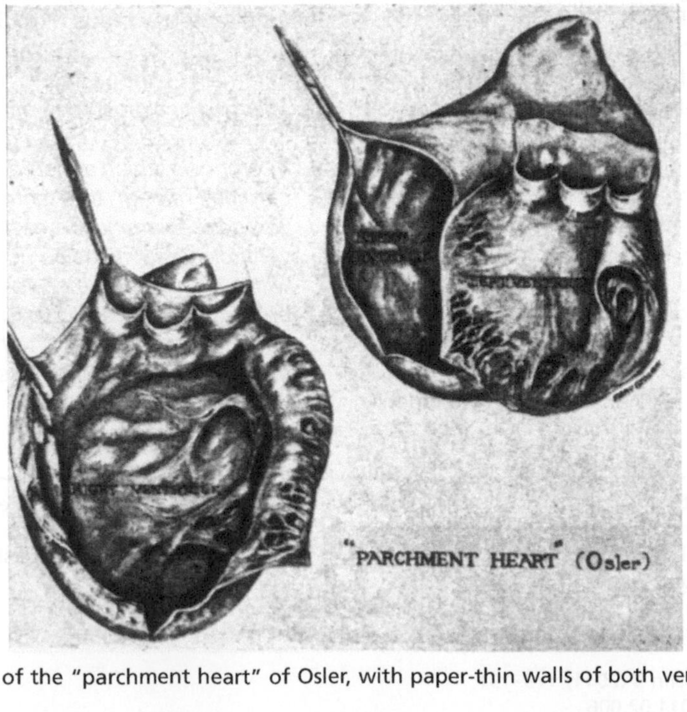

Fig. 2. The drawings of the "parchment heart" of Osler, with paper-thin walls of both ventricles.

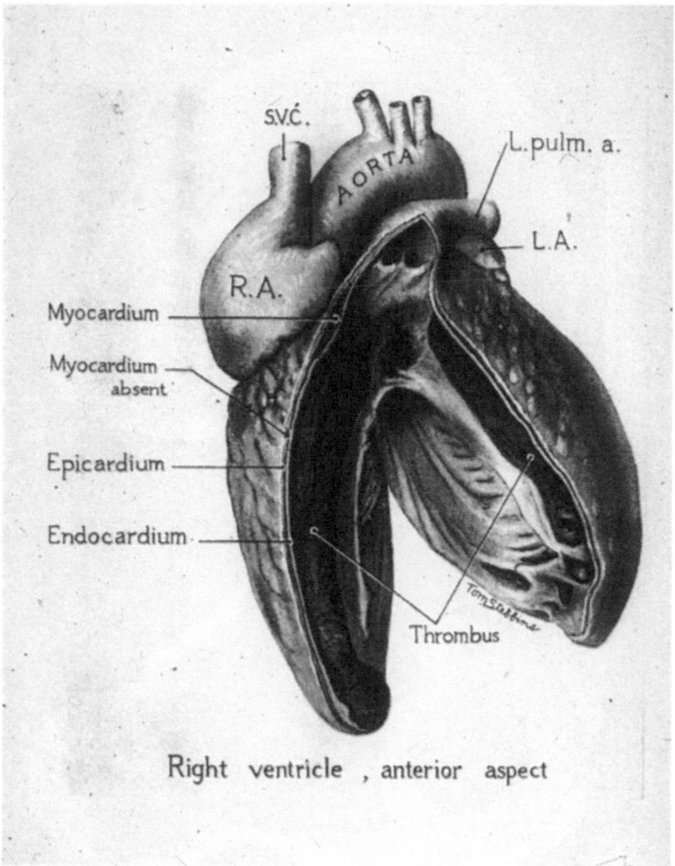

Fig. 3. The original picture of the Uhl's anomaly.

The early age and the peculiar pathologic description pointed to a structural heart disease present at birth (congenital malformation), as emphasized in the title itself. Clinical presentation was characterized neither by cardiac arrhythmias nor by a family history of heart disease. Thereafter, cases in adults with paper-thin ventricular walls have been published with the eponym of Uhl's anomaly, clearly a misnomer because the parchment heart in adult is the end stage of a late progressive loss of the myocardium followed by fibro-fatty replacement. By contrast, the cases reported in the literature in infants under the age of 15 months with the eponym of Uhl's anomaly all featured heart failure and isolated RV involvement (whether segmental or diffuse) without arrhythmias, all in keeping with the original description.[8–15] The parchment heart cases reported in adults (including the Osler heart)[6] varied in age from 17 to 81 years and died either of congestive heart failure or electrical cardiac arrest.[16–26]

The University of Padua published literature that sets milestones in the history of the disease.[27] In 1961 and 1965 Sergio Dalla Volta first reported similar cases under the name of "auricularization of the RV pressure" to emphasize the behavior of the RV chamber without an effective systolic contraction, with the blood being pushed to the pulmonary artery mainly due to the right atrial systole.[28,29] Although the patients presented also with ventricular arrhythmias, Dalla Volta pointed more to the hemodynamic features rather than to the arrhythmogenicity of the RV. One of the original patients reported by Dalla Volta underwent cardiac transplantation 30 years later in 1995 at the age of 65 because of congestive RV failure. The left ventricle was normal, whereas the RV was hugely dilated with diffuse paper-thin free wall and complete disappearance of the myocardium (**Fig. 4**).[30]

At the same University of Padua, in 1972 the pathologist Vito Terribile performed the autopsy of a woman with a history of palpitations and congestive heart failure, who died of pulmonary embolism. The heart showed an extreme dilatation, mural thrombosis, and "adipositas cordis"

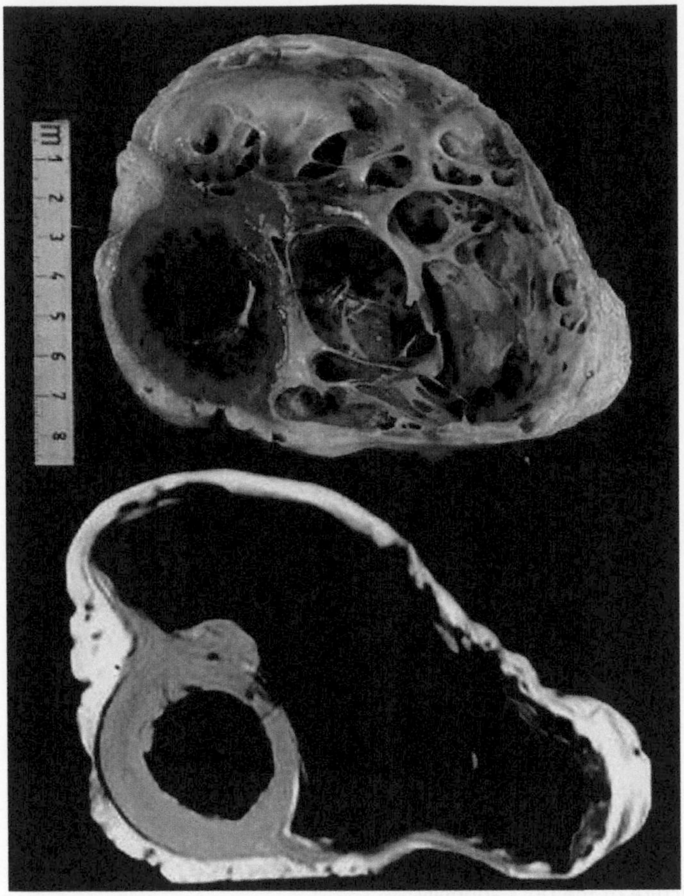

Fig. 4. The heart at cardiac transplantation of one of the patients published by Dalla Volta in 1965. Note the huge dilatation of the RV, both at gross and in vitro magnetic resonance, with paper-thin free wall.

of the RV, and the left ventricular myocardium exhibited areas of "myocardiosclerosis," all structural findings in keeping with AC (**Fig. 5**).[31]

Interest on the arrhythmic aspects of the disease was attracted by Guy Fontaine from Paris in the 1970s with the report of nonischemic ventricular tachyarrhythmias with left bundle branch block morphology originating from the RV.[32] Moreover, he observed in the basal ECG delayed repolarization ("postexcitation syndrome") at the end of the QRS complex, a feature that he named epsilon wave.[33]

Frank Marcus from the University of Arizona, Tucson, fascinated by this new field of RV electrophysiology, decided to spend a sabbatical year in Paris with Fontaine at the Jean Rostand Hospital.[34] He had the time and opportunity to review the adult cases with clinical manifestation of primary RV disease studied by Fontaine. The result was a milestone article, which was published in *Circulation* in 1982.[35] The disease was named "RV dysplasia" because the histology of the myocardial specimens, resected at surgery for removal of arrhythmic foci, showed anomalous histologic features of the RV myocardium consisting of fibro-fatty tissue, which were believed to be the consequence of an embryonic maldevelopment. By observing the presence of aneurysms in the inflow, apex, and outflow of RV, the investigators coined the term "triangle of dysplasia," a pathognomonic landmark of the disease. The same group, with the help of the surgeon Guiraudon, perceived the idea of total disconnection of the RV free wall as surgical treatment of RV tachycardia, by interrupting the reentry into the left ventricle.[36]

The early pioneering contributions of Marcus and Fontaine stimulated the interest of the electrophysiologists. Andrea Nava in Padua, by analyzing the study of families with sudden death and autopsy evidence of AC from Piazzola sul Brenta (a small village close to Padua in the Veneto Region), discovered the heredofamilial nature of the disease, a monogenic disorder with a Mendelian

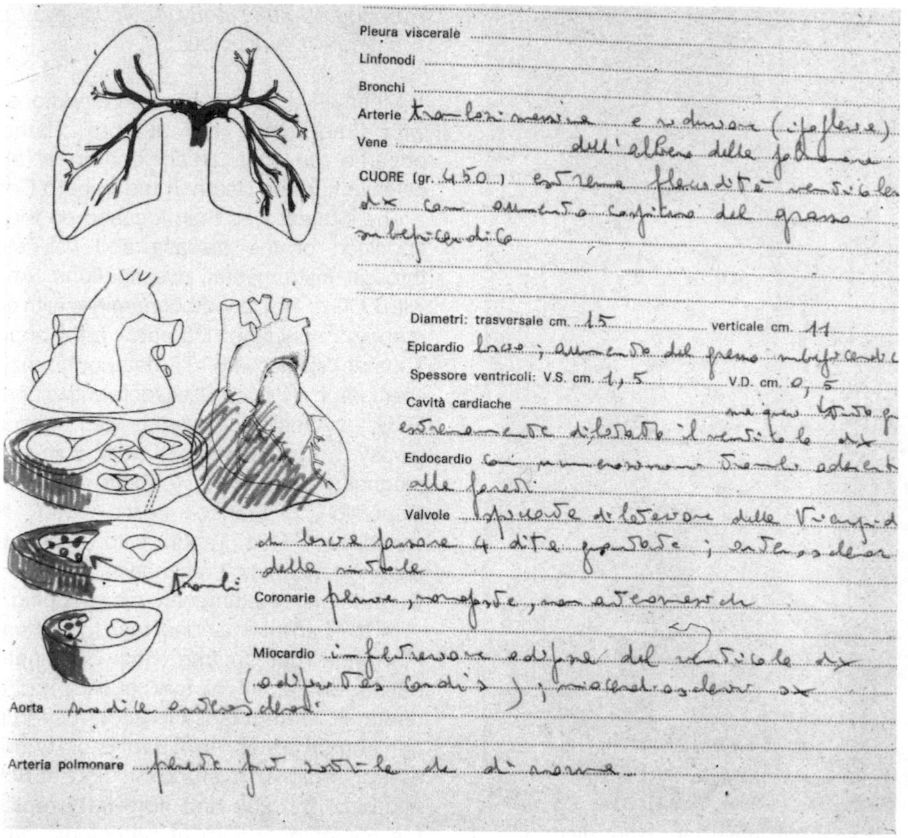

Fig. 5. The 1972 autopsy report of a case of AC of a patient who died of pulmonary embolism with adipositas cordis in the RV and foci of myocardial sclerosis in the left ventricle.

autosomal dominant transmission.[37,38] Gianfranco Buja reported the occurrence of the disease both in homozygous and heterozygous twins.[39]

The risk of sudden death as first manifestation of the disease was proved by the postmortem study of a series of young victims, in the setting of a project supported by the Veneto Region and performed by Gaetano Thiene.

The first observation concerned a young doctor, formerly cycle champion, who died suddenly on a tennis court during a hot afternoon of May 1979 (**Fig. 6**). Fifteen minutes after the starting of the game he stopped, took his pulse, walked back to the border of the tennis court, and suddenly fainted. In his diary, written on October 4, 1978, during preparation of the Internal Medicine examination, the phrase "ventricular tachycardia of left bundle branch block morphology" was found, which retrospectively can refer to his own ECG. His girlfriend related that on that day he had suffered palpitations and had an ECG. It took years to understand that the explanation of cardiac arrest and ventricular fibrillation was the fibro-fatty tissue that had been observed at autopsy in the RV free wall and at apex of the left ventricle, and not conduction system abnormalities as first hypothesized.[40] This experience confirmed an old concept in Medicine, namely that you see only what you look for and you recognize only what you know.

Among the first 60 consecutive cases of sudden death in the young (<35 years) collected in the Veneto Region project, 12 (20%) were found to be affected by AC. Most deaths had occurred during effort and had presented inverted T-wave in the right precordial leads at the basal ECG. The novel findings were promptly submitted to the *New England Journal of Medicine*, which was reluctant to believe that the disease could be a so frequent cause of juvenile sudden death. Eventually, by providing all the data and illustrations case by case, the paper was accepted for publication[41] and was accompanied by a rewarding editorial, signed by Barry Maron, entitled "Right ventricular cardiomyopathy: another cause of sudden death in the young."[42]

A letter to the Editor was then forwarded to the *New England Journal of Medicine* by a group of Greek doctors,[43] claiming that a very similar cardiac malignant disease was observed in Naxos in the

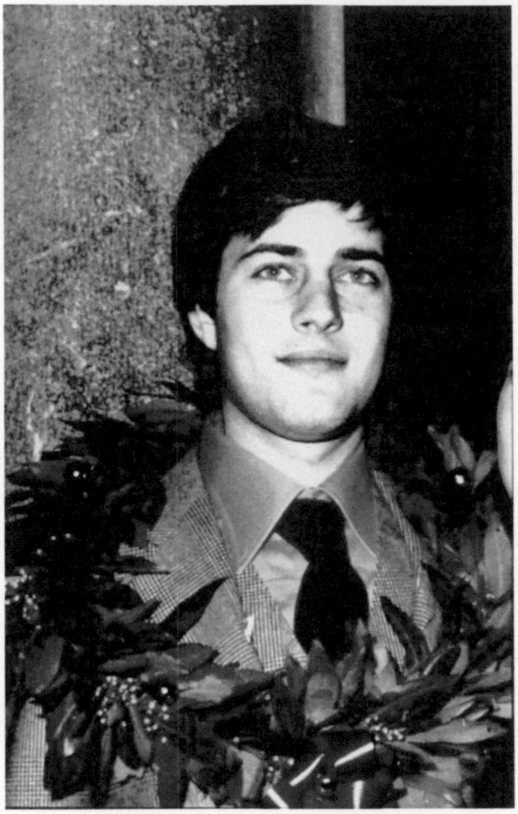

Fig. 6. A 26-year-old physician who died during a tennis game in May 1979. A ventricular tachycardia, left bundle branch block morphology, had been recorded at the ECG during palpitations. The autopsy disclosed for the first time AC as a cause of sudden death in the young.

setting of cardiocutaneous syndrome, consisting of AC, palmoplantar keratosis, and woolly hair (Naxos disease).[44] The Greek group postulated that those patients might belong to families descended from Venetians, who had landed in Naxos in 1207 (**Fig. 7**). Soon after, Domenico Corrado demonstrated that AC was a killer among athletes, accounting for about 25% of fatalities in the Veneto Region,[45] differing from the United States where hypertrophic cardiomyopathy ranked first.

The report of AC as a major cause of sudden death in the young aroused skepticism among the scientific community. Many scientists came to Padua to examine the heart specimens of this morbid entity. The statement of Sir James Mackenzie is quite relevant:

> *There are three stages in the history of every medical discovery. When it is first announced, people say that it is not true. Then, a little later, when its truth has been borne in on them, so that it can no longer be denied, they say it is not important. After that, if its importance becomes sufficiently obvious, they say that anyhow it is not new.*[46]

Meanwhile postmortem observations increased with time, since the authors' Pathology Unit became the only tertiary center for all cases of juvenile sudden death in the Veneto Region.

The interest was then focused on the in vivo recognition of the disease and risk stratification, through instrumental investigations: Andrea Nava with ECG,[47] Roldano Scognamiglio with echocardiography,[48] Luciano Daliento with angiography,[49] Thomas Wichter with ^{123}I-meta-iodobenzylguanidine scintigraphy,[50] Luca Oselladore with signal-averaged ECG,[51] Annalisa Angelini with endomyocardial biopsy,[52] Luigi Menghetti with spin-echo cardiac magnetic resonance,[53] Pietro Turrini with QT dispersion,[54] Franco Folino with heart rate variability,[55] Hari Tandri with contrast-enhanced cardiac magnetic resonance,[56] and Domenico Corrado with electroanatomic mapping.[57]

In 1994 an international task force headed by Bill McKenna put forward the diagnostic criteria, based on family history of AC and/or sudden death, ECG depolarization/conduction/repolarization abnormalities, arrhythmias of RV origin, global and/or regional dysfunction and structural alterations of the RV, and fibro-fatty replacement of the RV myocardium at pathologic analysis.[58] In the absence of a single gold standard, the diagnosis was achieved by major or minor criteria (2 major, or 1 major and 3 minor, or 4 minor).

A revision of the diagnostic criteria was recently accomplished by introducing quantitative other than qualitative diagnostic parameters, including cardiac magnetic resonance and genetic testing.[59] The application of the diagnostic criteria greatly contributed to the early detection in young subjects affected by silent AC at the screening for sport eligibility, thus resulting in a sharp decline (nearly 90%) of sudden death during sport activity.[60]

Regarding the treatment, while curative therapy is still far distant in the absence of precise knowledge of the pathogenesis of cardiomyocyte injury, an algorithm for antiarrhythmic drug therapy in AC patients was first introduced by Thomas Wichter.[61] Endocardial catheter ablation was performed by the group of Hugh Calkins, although of limited value due to a high rate of arrhythmia recurrence during the follow-up.[62] More recently, the group of Francis Marchlinski demonstrated the superiority of epicardial catheter ablation over the endocardial approach.[63]

Prevention of sudden death is now feasible with the introduction of implantable cardioverter-defibrillator (ICD) device. Up to 25% of patients survived from cardiac arrest in a follow-up of 48

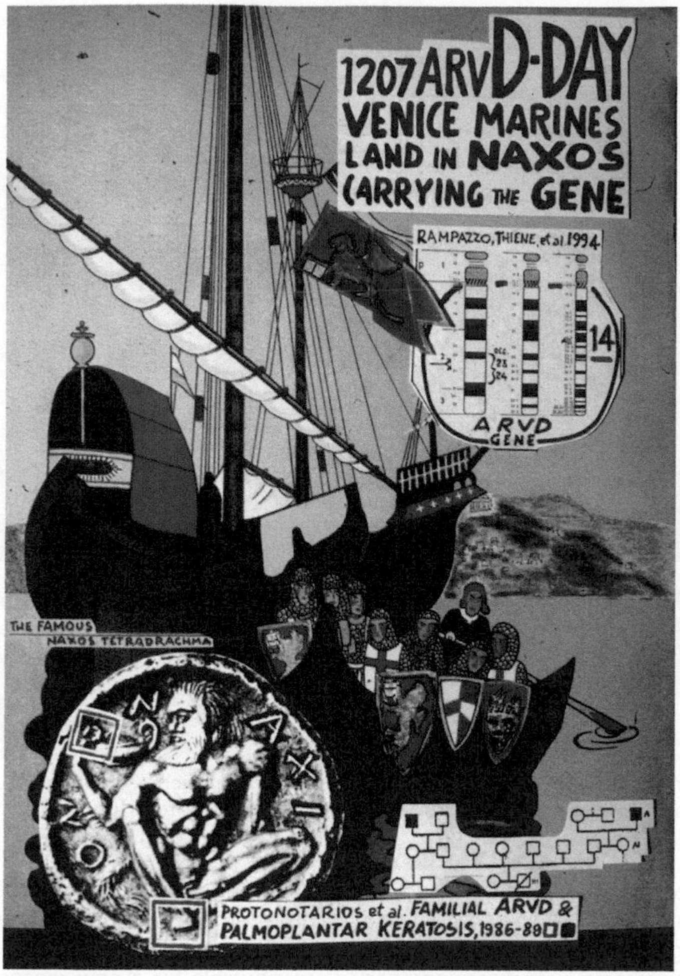
1207 ARV D-DAY
VENICE MARINES
LAND IN NAXOS
CARRYING THE GENE
RAMPAZZO, THIENE, et al. 1994
14
ARVD GENE
THE FAMOUS NAXOS TETRADRACHMA
PROTONOTARIOS et al. FAMILIAL ARVD &
PALMOPLANTAR KERATOSIS, 1986-89

Fig. 7. Cartoon by the late Professor Lino Rossi stressing the connection between Venice and Naxos history.

months, thanks to appropriate electric shocks with cardioversion of ventricular fibrillation to sinus rhythm. ICD implantation is indicated for both secondary[64] and primary[65] prevention.

Other fascinating contributions came from pathobiology and genetics. Cristina Basso, on studying a large series of heart specimens, disclosed that AC is not a congenital heart disorder (ie, lesion present at birth). Rather, it is a genetically determined myocardial dystrophy with acquired cell death occurring with time, mostly during adolescence.[66] It was considered a sort of cell suicide, due to apoptosis, as demonstrated through TUNEL and electron microscopy studies by Marialuisa Valente.[67] Focal myocardial inflammation was found in nearly 75% of cases; however, Fiorella Calabrese ruled out viral infections by enterovirus.[68] Thereafter, AC was added to the list of cardiomyopathies in the World Health Organization classification.[69] Meanwhile the disease was reported to spontaneously occur also in animals, both in cats[70] and dogs.[71]

In 1994, linkage analysis studies in families with AC, performed by Alessandra Rampazzo and Gian Antonio Danieli, led to the identification of the first gene locus in chromosome 14.[72] Thereafter, several loci were demonstrated in other chromosomal sites,[73] suggesting genetic heterogeneity (multiple genes, similar phenotypic expression). The candidate genes were first searched for in the cytoskeleton, as in Duchenne and Becker muscular dystrophies.

The enlightening inspiration to solve the genetic puzzle came to the scholars of the Naxos disease (Nikos Protonotarios and Adalena Tsatsopoulou), who perceived that desmosomes are common to heart and skin and that a cell junction defect might explain their cardiocutaneous syndrome. Other researchers, in previous investigations, by studying mice with targeted mutation of

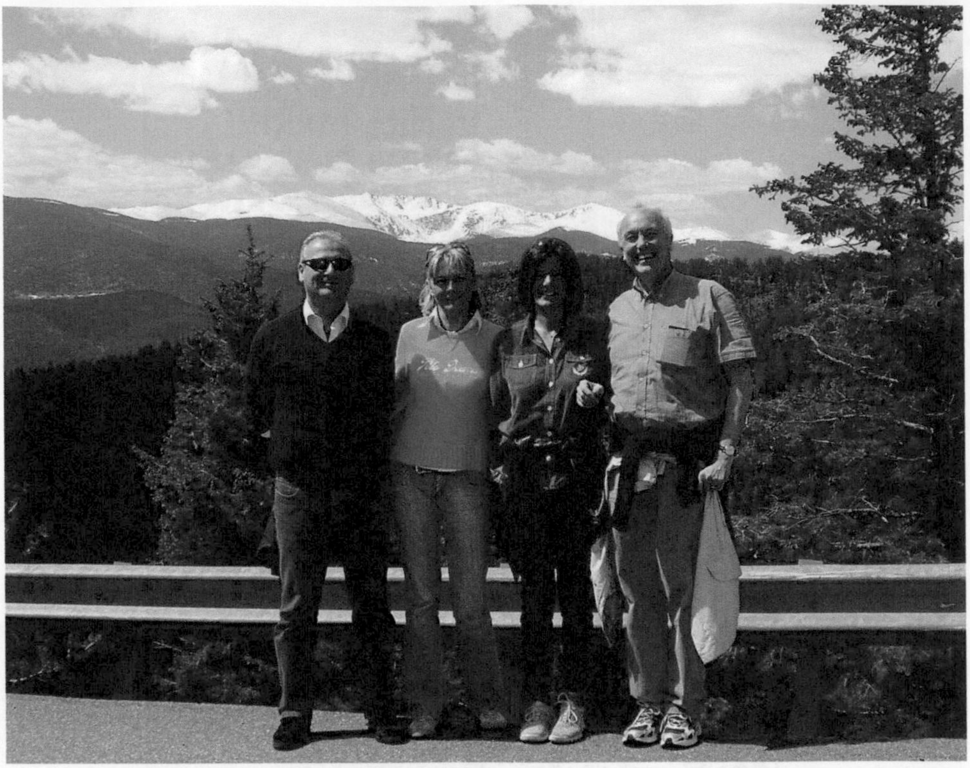

Fig. 8. Domenico Corrado, Barbara Bauce, Cristina Basso and Gaetano Thiene "on the road", in the occasion of one of the International Task Force meetings for updating the AC diagnostic criteria (Denver, Colorado, USA, May 2007).

plakoglobin, a γ-catenin of the desmosome localized in chromosome 17q21, showed that the knock-out of this gene resulted in devastating cardiac lesions in the embryos, with disappearance of the desmosomes and spontaneous cardiac rupture.[74] Based on these observations, the Naxos group performed linkage analysis in their families and identified the Naxos disease locus exactly in the same chromosome 17q21.[75] Thereafter, gene sequencing proved that the molecular defect was a deletion of plakoglobin gene.[76]

At the same time, in Ecuador, Luis Carvajal Huerta reported another recessive cardiocutaneous disease characterized by dilated cardiomyopathy, wooly hair, and palmoplantar keratosis.[77] The gene defect was proved to be a mutation of desmoplakin, another protein of the desmosome.[78] A child of the affected family died suddenly, due to arrhythmic cardiac arrest, and the heart specimen was sent by the wife of Dr Carvajal (who meanwhile passed away) to Jeffrey Saffitz in St Louis for pathologic study. Gaetano Thiene was asked by Dr Saffitz to go to St Louis and examine the heart. It revealed a biventricular cardiomyopathy, with extensive left ventricular dilatation and mural thrombosis. The RV disclosed the typical aneurysms in the triangle of dysplasia with translucent thin wall, and the histology showed mostly fibrous replacement.[79] Thus, another defective gene of desmosome (desmoplakin) was found to be responsible for a new recessive cardiocutaneous syndrome.

Desmoplakin immediately became a candidate gene also for the dominant variant of AC. The genetic screening in Padua in some of Nava's families led to the identification by Alessandra Rampazzo of desmoplakin as the disease-causing gene, in the form of missense mutations.[80] Genotype-phenotype correlations, performed by Barbara Bauce, disclosed that the desmoplakin variant of the disease featured extensive left ventricular involvement so as to suggest that the disease, being biventricular, should be better called AC.[81] By performing contrast-enhanced cardiac magnetic resonance in genotyped AC patients, Sen Chowdhry confirmed that the disease is more broad-based than previously thought, with predominant left ventricular and biventricular forms besides the classic AC with RV involvement.[82]

A missense mutation of the gene encoding ryanodine receptor 2, in charge of the Ca^{2+} release from smooth sarcoplasmic reticulum, was discovered by Natascia Tiso to be associated with a variant of AC with polymorphic ventricular tachyarrhythmias.[83] Because the same defective gene was proved by Silvia Priori[84] to be related to catecholaminergic polymorphic ventricular tachycardia first described by Philip Coumel in 1978,[85] the nosographic entity reported by Tiso was then considered the same as the one reported by Coumel.

All the other genes that encode for desmosomal proteins were subsequently investigated in patients affected by familial dominant (nonsyndromic) AC, and were found to be responsible for the same phenotype: plakophillin-2 by Brenda Gerull,[86] desmoglein-2 by Kalliopi Pilichou,[87] and desmocollin-2 by Petros Syrris,[88] the latter confirmed soon after by Giorgia Beffagna.[89] Thus, both dominant and recessive variants of AC were eventually nosographically identified as cell junction (desmosome) diseases.[90,91]

Electron microscopy studies, performed by Cristina Basso in genotyped patients with AC, revealed abnormalities of the desmosomes. Desmosomes appeared less numerous, short, pale, and fragmented, suggesting that disruption of intercalated discs was the final common pathway of a genetically determined, progressive cell death.[92]

The discovery of the defective genes, although limited to 50% of affected families, opened new avenues. Genetic screening, for early diagnosis and detection of healthy carriers as well as reassurance of noncarriers, entails a tremendous impact on primary prevention of arrhythmic complications and lifestyle, including disqualification from sport activity and genetic counseling for disease recurrence in siblings and offspring, alongside the dilemma of procreation.[93]

Experimental animal models (knock-out, overexpression, knock-in mice) are opening new avenues to understanding disease pathogenesis and identifying targets for therapy.[94–97] After plakoglobin, desmoplakin, and plakophilin transgenic mice, Kalliopi Pilichou recently generated transgenic mice with overexpression of mutated desmoglein-2,[97] the same defective gene previously detected in an AC Italian proband.[87] The recapitulation of the disease in the mice was quite convincing: dilatation and aneurysms at echo of both ventricles, tachyarrhythmias, sudden death, and fibrous replacement of the ventricular myocardium at histology. Interestingly enough, the animals were normal at birth and cell death occurred with time after a few weeks, in the shape of cell necrosis (oncosis) at electron microscopy, thus confirming that the disorder is a genetically determined cardiomyopathy and not a congenital heart disease.[98]

Depletion of a plakoglobin signal at intercellular junctions was found by Angeliki Asimaki in AC patients, whatever the defective gene, and may be considered a biomarker for the diagnosis at endomyocardial biopsy.[99]

Generation of knock-in transgenic mice will contribute to the understanding of the mechanistic events in the effort to find etiologic (not merely symptomatic) therapeutic interventions. Prevention of disease onset and progression will be possible only when the underlying biological and molecular phenomena will be better understood.

European and American teams continue to be committed in the study of the disease. At the turn of the last millennium, following a series of meetings of experts from both sides of the Atlantic Ocean, it became evident that the expertise of scientists and clinicians should merge into an "army" for the fight against the calamity of sudden death due to AC. An International Registry was considered mandatory to collect study material and concentrate efforts on this rare disorder.[100]

It was then decided to apply for grants from the European Commission and the National Institutes of Health (NIH). Two teams were created, one in Europe coordinated by Gaetano Thiene and one in North America coordinated by Frank Marcus. The two projects started by using a similar database and sharing some Core Labs. The method was somewhat different: the European Registry enrolled patients who were previously diagnosed as well as new entries,[101] whereas the North American Registry enrolled only newly diagnosed patients.[102] Previously published diagnostic criteria were employed and protocols implemented accordingly. Genetic investigation was an integral part of both studies. Both projects were approved and funded by the European Commission and the NIH for 5 years, thus allowing the commencement of a major interdisciplinary study of AC. The results exceeded the best expectations, culminating in the discovery of 5 disease genes, numerous publications in highly ranking cardiovascular journals, and new diagnostic criteria. A monograph collected all these achievements.[103]

The progress in the knowledge of AC was possible thanks to a tight international collaboration and loyal competition. The authors (**Fig. 8**) wish to quote here the late Lino Rossi's words[104]:

> *All of them share the unique merit of a skillful and dedicated engagement in a scientific contest of vital importance which is not comparable to any sports competition; as such, the present overview concludes with the popular saying – who cares who came second? – here intended in an entirely positive, even laudative sense.*

SUMMARY

The historical milestones of AC discovery, diagnosis, treatment and pathogenesis are summarized. Starting with the first description of the familial background by Lancisi in 1736, the major contributions of both European and American investigators are reported, coming across the original clinical and autopsy series in the 80ies, the identification of the genetic background in the late 90ies and early 2000, the updated diagnostic criteria and the new cardiac imaging and therapeutic tools in the most recent years. Transgenic animal models are currently developed to elucidate the disease pathogenesis, with the final aim to elaborate targeted therapies to stop or delay disease onset and progression.

REFERENCES

1. Lancisi GM. De motu cordis et aneurysmatibus. Caput V. Neapoli (Italy): Musca; 1738.
2. Saintignon H. Laennec, sa vie et son oeuvre. Paris: Baillière; 1904.
3. Eliot G. Middlemarch. 1st edition. New York, 1871.
4. Osler W. The principles and practice of medicine. 6th edition. New York: D. Appleton & Co; 1905. p. 20.
5. McDermott HE, Abbot M. A memoir. Toronto: The Macmillan Company of Canada, Ltd; 1941. p. 90.
6. Segall HN. Parchment heart (Osler). Am Heart J 1950;40:948–50.
7. UHL HS. A previously undescribed congenital malformation of the heart: almost total absence of the myocardium of the right ventricle. Bull Johns Hopkins Hosp 1952;91:197–209.
8. Castleman B, Sprague HB. Case records of the Massachusetts General Hospital. Weekly clinicopathological exercises. N Engl J Med 1952;246:785–90.
9. Novak G, Szanto PB, Gasul B, et al. Congenital aplasia of the myocardium of the right ventricle. Proc Inst Med Chic 1957;21:334–9.
10. Arcilia RA, Gasul BM. Congenital aplasia or marked hypoplasia of the myocardium. J Pediatr 1961;58:381–8.
11. Sherman FE. An atlas of congenital heart disease. Philadelphia: Lea & Febiger; 1963. p. 270, 290–1.
12. Reeve R, MacDonald D. Partial absence of the right ventricular musculature—partial parchment heart. Am J Cardiol 1964;14:415–9.
13. Cumming GR, Bowman JM, Whytehead L. Congenital aplasia of the myocardium of the right ventricle (Uhl's anomaly). Am Heart J 1965;70:671–6.
14. Perrin EV, Mehrizi A. Isolated free-wall hypoplasia of the right ventricle. Am J Dis Child 1965;109:558–66.
15. Gould K, Guttman AB, Carrasco J, et al. Partial absence of the right ventricular musculature. A congenital lesion. Am J Med 1967;42:636–41.
16. Froment R, Perrin A, Loire R, et al. Ventricule droit papyrace du jeune adultre par dystrophie congenitale. Arch Mal Coeur Vaiss 1968;61:477–503 [in French].
17. Sugiura M, Hayashi T, Ueno K. Partial absence of the right ventricular muscle in an aged. Jpn Heart J 1970;11:582–5.
18. Forssman O, Bjorkman G. Absence of the solid part of the right ventricular musculature. Acta Pathol Microbiol Scand A 1972;80:263–70.
19. Abe T, Kuribayashi R, Sato M, et al. Congenital hypoplasia of the right ventricular myocardium (Uhl's anomaly). A case report and review of literature. J Cardiovasc Surg 1973;14:431–8.
20. Aherne WA. Uhl's anomaly [abstract]. Arch Dis Child 1973;48:160.
21. Diaz LP, Jimenez MQ, Granados FM, et al. Congenital absence of myocardium of right ventricle: Uhl's anomaly. Br Heart J 1973;35:570–2.
22. Haworth SG, Shinebourne EA, Miller GA. Right to left interatrial shunting with normal right ventricular pressure. Br Heart J 1975;37:386–91.
23. Murata K, Matsuo H, Yoshitake Y, et al. Functionally atrialized parchment-like right ventricle with extensive myocardial fibrosis of left ventricle. Jpn Heart J 1976;17:428–35.
24. Bharati S, Ciraulo DA, Bilitch M, et al. Inexcitable right ventricle and bilateral bundle branch block in Uhl's disease. Circulation 1978;57:636–44.
25. Vecht RJ, Carmichael JS, Gopal R, et al. Uhl's anomaly. Br Heart J 1979;41:676–82.
26. Roberts WC, Ko JM, Kuiper JJ, et al. Some previously neglected examples of arrhythmogenic right ventricular dysplasia/cardiomyopathy and frequency of its various reported manifestations. Am J Cardiol 2010;106:268–74.
27. Basso C, Thiene G, Nava A, et al. Arrhythmogenic right ventricular cardiomyopathy: a survey of the investigations at the University of Padua. Clin Cardiol 1997;20:333–6.
28. Dalla Volta S, Battaglia G, Zerbini E. Auricularization of right ventricular pressure curve. Am Heart J 1961;61:25–33.
29. Dalla Volta S, Fameli O, Maschio G. Le sindrome clinique et hemodynamique de l'auricularisation du ventricule droit. Arch Mal Coeur Vaiss 1965; 58:1129–43 [in French].
30. Thiene G, Nava A, Marcus FI. Introduction: arrhythmogenic right ventricular cardiomyopathy/dysplasia clarified. In: Marcus FI, Nava A, Thiene G, editors. Arrhythmogenic right ventricular cardiomyopathy/dysplasia—recent advances. Milano (Italy): Springer; 2007. p. 1–6.
31. Thiene G. Storia di una malattia. In: Basso C, Nava A, Thiene G, editors. La cardiomiopatia aritmogena. Milano (Italy): Arti Grafiche Color Black; 2001. p. 1–7 [in Italian].

32. Fontaine G, Guiraudon G, Frank R, et al. Stimulation studies and epicardial mapping in ventricular tachycardia: study of mechanisms and selection for surgery. In: Kulbertus HE, editor. Reentrant arrhythmias. Lancaster (UK): MTP; 1977. p. 334–50.
33. Fontaine G, Frank R, Gallais-Hamonno F, et al. Electrocardiographie des potentials tardifs du syndrome de post-excitation. Arch Mal Coeur Vaiss 1978;71:854–9 [in French].
34. Marcus FI. Introduction: past, present and future. In: Nava A, Rossi L, Thiene G, editors. Arrhythmogenic right ventricular cardiomyopathy/dysplasia. Amsterdam: Elsevier; 1997. p. 1–6.
35. Marcus FI, Fontaine G, Guiraudon G, et al. Right ventricular dysplasia. A report of 24 adult cases. Circulation 1982;65:384–98.
36. Guiraudon GM, Klein G, Gulamhusein SS, et al. Total disconnection of the right ventricle free wall: surgical treatment of right ventricular tachycardia associated with right ventricular dysplasia. Circulation 1983;67:463–70.
37. Nava A, Scognamiglio R, Thiene G, et al. A polymorphic form of familial arrhythmogenic right ventricular dyplasia. Am J Cardiol 1987;59:1405–9.
38. Nava A, Thiene G, Canciani B, et al. Familial occurrence of right ventricular dysplasia: a study involving nine families. J Am Coll Cardiol 1988;12:1222–8.
39. Buja G, Nava A, Daliento L, et al. Right ventricular cardiomyopathy in identical and non identical young twins. Am Heart J 1993;126:1187–93.
40. Rossi L, Thiene G. Recent advances in clinicohistopathologic correlates of sudden cardiac death. Am Heart J 1981;102:478–84.
41. Thiene G, Nava A, Corrado D, et al. Right ventricular cardiomyopathy and sudden death in young people. N Engl J Med 1988;318:129–33.
42. Maron BJ. Right ventricular cardiomyopathy. Another cause of sudden death in the young [editorial]. N Engl J Med 1988;318:178–9.
43. Protonotarios N, Tsatsopoulou A, Scampardonis G. Familial arrhythmogenic right ventricular dysplasia associated with palmoplantar keratosis [letter]. N Engl J Med 1988;319:174–6.
44. Protonotarios N, Tsatsopoulou A, Patsourakos P, et al. Cardiac abnormalities in familial palmoplantar keratosis. Br Heart J 1986;56:321–6.
45. Corrado D, Thiene G, Nava A, et al. Sudden death in young competitive athletes: clinicopathologic correlation in 22 cases. Am J Med 1990;89:588–96.
46. Wilson RM. The beloved physicians: Sir James Mackenzie. New York: Macmillan; 1926. p. 177.
47. Nava A, Canciani B, Buja G, et al. Electrovectorcardiographic study of negative T waves on precordial leads in arrhythmogenic right ventricular dysplasia. Relationship with right ventricular volumes. J Electrocardiol 1988;21:239–45.
48. Scognamiglio R, Fasoli G, Nava A, et al. Relevance of subtle echocardiographic findings in early diagnosis of the concealed form of right ventricular dysplasia. Eur Heart J 1989;10:27–8.
49. Daliento L, Rizzoli G, Thiene G, et al. Diagnostic accuracy of right ventriculography in arrhythmogenic right ventricular cardiomyopathy. Am J Cardiol 1990;66:741–5.
50. Wichter T, Hindricks G, Lerch H, et al. Regional myocardial sympathetic dysinnervation in arrhythmogenic right ventricular cardiomyopathy. An analysis using ^{123}I-meta-iodobenzylguanidine scintigraphy. Circulation 1994;89:667–83.
51. Oselladore L, Nava A, Buja G, et al. Signal-averaged electrocardiography in familial form of arrhythmogenic right ventricular cardiomyopathy. Am J Cardiol 1995;75:1038–41.
52. Angelini A, Thiene G, Boffa GM, et al. Endomyocardial biopsy in right ventricular cardiomyopathy. Int J Cardiol 1993;40:273–2826.
53. Menghetti L, Basso C, Nava A, et al. Spin-echo nuclear magnetic resonance for tissue characterisation in arrhythmogenic right ventricular cardiomyopathy. Heart 1996;76:467–70.
54. Turrini P, Corrado D, Basso C, et al. Dispersion of ventricular depolarisation-repolarization. A noninvasive marker for risk stratification in arrhythmogenic right ventricular cardiomyopathy. Circulation 2001;103:3075–80.
55. Folino AF, Buja G, Bauce B, et al. Heart rate variability in arrhythmogenic right ventricular cardiomyopathy correlation with clinical and prognostic features. Pacing Clin Electrophysiol 2002;25:1285–92.
56. Tandri H, Saranathan M, Rodriguez ER, et al. Noninvasive detection of myocardial fibrosis in arrhythmogenic right ventricular cardiomyopathy using delayed-enhancement magnetic resonance imaging. J Am Coll Cardiol 2005;45:98–103.
57. Corrado D, Basso C, Leoni L, et al. Three-dimensional electroanatomic voltage mapping increases accuracy of diagnosing arrhythmogenic right ventricular cardiomyopathy/dysplasia. Circulation 2005;111:3042–50.
58. McKenna WJ, Thiene G, Nava A, et al. Diagnosis of arrhythmogenic right ventricular dysplasia/cardiomyopathy. Br Heart J 1994;71:215–8.
59. Marcus FI, McKenna WJ, Sherrill D, et al. Diagnosis of arrhythmogenic right ventricular cardiomyopathy/dysplasia. Proposed modification of the Task Force criteria. Circulation 2010;121:1533–41; and Eur Heart J 2010;31:806–14.
60. Corrado D, Basso C, Pavei A, et al. Trends in sudden cardiovascular death in young competitive athletes after implementation of a preparticipation screening program. JAMA 2006;296:1593–601.
61. Wichter T, Borggrefe M, Haverkamp W, et al. Efficacy of antiarrhythmic drugs in patients with

arrhythmogenic right ventricular disease. Results in patients with inducible and noninducible ventricular tachycardia. Circulation 1992;86:29–37.
62. Dalal D, Jain R, Tandri H, et al. Long-term efficacy of catheter ablation of ventricular tachycardia in patients with arrhythmogenic right ventricular dysplasia/cardiomyopathy. J Am Coll Cardiol 2007;50:432–40.
63. Garcia FC, Bazan V, Zado ES, et al. Epicardial substrate and outcome with epicardial ablation of ventricular tachycardia in arrhythmogenic right ventricular cardiomyopathy/dysplasia. Circulation 2009;120:366–75.
64. Corrado D, Leoni L, Link MS, et al. Implantable cardioverter-defibrillator therapy for prevention of sudden death in patients with arrhythmogenic right ventricular cardiomyopathy/dysplasia. Circulation 2003;108:3084–91.
65. Corrado D, Calkins H, Link MS, et al. Prophylactic implantable defibrillator in patients with arrhythmogenic right ventricular cardiomyopathy/dysplasia and no prior ventricular fibrillation or sustained ventricular tachycardia. Circulation 2010;122:1144–52.
66. Basso C, Thiene G, Valente M, et al. Arrhythmogenic right ventricular cardiomyopathy: dysplasia, dystrophy or myocarditis? Circulation 1996;94: 983–91.
67. Valente M, Calabrese F, Angelini A, et al. In vivo evidence of apoptosis in arrhythmogenic right ventricular cardiomyopathy. Am J Pathol 1998; 152:479–84.
68. Calabrese F, Angelini A, Thiene G, et al. No detection of enteroviral genome in the myocardium of patients with arrhythmogenic right ventricular cardiomyopathy. J Clin Pathol 2000;53:382–7.
69. Richardson P, McKenna WJ, Bristow M, et al. Report of the 1995 WHO/ISFC Task Force on the definition and classification of cardiomyopathies. Circulation 1996;93:841–2.
70. Fox PR, Maron BJ, Basso C, et al. Spontaneously occurring arrhythmogenic right ventricular cardiomyopathy in the domestic cat: a new animal model similar to the human disease. Circulation 2000;102: 1863–70.
71. Basso C, Fox PR, Meurs KM, et al. Arrhythmogenic right ventricular cardiomyopathy causing sudden cardiac death in boxer dogs: a new animal model of human disease. Circulation 2004;109:1180–5.
72. Rampazzo A, Nava A, Danieli GA, et al. The gene for arrhythmogenic right ventricular cardiomyopathy maps to chromosome 14q23-q24. Hum Mol Genet 1994;3:959–62.
73. Rampazzo A, Danieli GA. Advances in genetics: dominant forms. In: Marcus FI, Nava A, Thiene G, editors. Arrhythmogenic right ventricular cardiomyopathy/dysplasia—recent advances. Milano (Italy): Springer; 2007. p. 7–14.
74. Ruiz P, Brinkmann V, Ledermann B, et al. Targeted mutation of plakoglobin in mice reveals essential functions of desmosomes in the embryonic heart. J Cell Biol 1996;135:215–25.
75. Coonar AS, Protonotarios N, Tsatsopoulou A, et al. Gene for arrhythmogenic right ventricular cardiomyopathy with diffuse nonepidermolytic palmoplantar keratoderma and woolly hair (Naxos disease) maps to 17q21. Circulation 1998;97: 2049–58.
76. McKoy G, Protonotarios N, Crosby A, et al. Identification of a deletion in plakoglobin in arrhythmogenic right ventricular cardiomyopathy with palmoplantar keratoderma and wolly hair (Naxos disease). Lancet 2000;355:2119–24.
77. Carvajal-Huerta L. Epidermolytic palmoplantar keratoderma with woolly hair and dilated cardiomyopathy. J Am Acad Dermatol 1998;39:418–21.
78. Norgett EE, Hatsell SJ, Carvajal-Huerta L, et al. Recessive mutation in desmoplakin disrupts desmoplakin-intermediate filament interactions and causes dilated cardiomyopathy, woolly hair and keratoderma. Hum Mol Genet 2000;9:2761–6.
79. Kaplan SR, Gard JJ, Carvajal-Huerta L, et al. Structural and molecular pathology of the heart in Carvajal syndrome. Cardiovasc Pathol 2004; 13:26–32.
80. Rampazzo A, Nava A, Malacrida S, et al. Mutation in human desmoplakin domain binding to plakoglobin causes a dominant form of arrhythmogenic right ventricular cardiomyopathy. Am J Hum Genet 2002;71:1200–6.
81. Bauce B, Basso C, Rampazzo A, et al. Clinical profile of four families with arrhythmogenic right ventricular cardiomyopathy caused by dominant desmoplakin mutations. Eur Heart J 2005;26: 1666–75.
82. Sen-Chowdhry S, Syrris P, Ward D, et al. Clinical and genetic characterization of families with arrhythmogenic right ventricular dysplasia/cardiomyopathy provides novel insights into patterns of disease expression. Circulation 2007;115:1710–20.
83. Tiso N, Stephan DA, Nava A, et al. Identification of mutations in the cardiac ryanodine receptor gene in families affected with arrhythmogenic right ventricular cardiomyopathy type 2 (ARVD2). Hum Mol Genet 2001;10:189–94.
84. Priori SG, Napolitano C, Tiso N, et al. Mutations in the cardiac ryanodine receptor gene (hRyR2) underlie catecholaminergic polymorphic ventricular tachycardia. Circulation 2001;103:196–200.
85. Coumel P, Fidelle J, Lucet V. Catecholamine-induced severe ventricular arrhythmias with Adams-Stokes syndrome in children: report of four cases. Br Heart J 1978;40(Suppl):28–37.
86. Gerull B, Heuser A, Wichter T, et al. Mutations in the desmosomal protein plakophilin-2 are common in

arrhythmogenic right ventricular cardiomyopathy. Nat Genet 2004;36:1162–4.

87. Pilichou K, Nava A, Basso C, et al. Mutations in desmoglein-2 gene are associated with arrhythmogenic right ventricular cardiomyopathy. Circulation 2006;113:1171–9.
88. Syrris P, Ward D, Evans A, et al. Arrhythmogenic right ventricular dysplasia/cardiomyopathy associated with mutations in the desmosomal gene desmocollin-2. Am J Hum Genet 2006;79:978–84.
89. Beffagna G, De Bortoli M, Nava A, et al. Missense mutations in desmocollin-2 N-terminus, associated with arrhythmogenic right ventricular cardiomyopathy, affect intracellular localization of desmocollin-2 in vitro. BMC Med Genet 2007;8:65.
90. Thiene G, Corrado D, Basso C. Cardiomyopathies: is it time for a molecular classification? Eur Heart J 2004;25:1772–5.
91. Maron BJ, Towbin JA, Thiene G, et al. Contemporary definitions and classification of the cardiomyopathies: an American Heart Association Scientific Statement from the Council on Clinical Cardiology, Heart Failure and Transplantation Committee; Quality of Care and Outcomes Research and Functional Genomics and Translational Biology Interdisciplinary Working Groups; and Council on Epidemiology and Prevention. Circulation 2006;113:1807–16.
92. Basso C, Czarnowska E, Della Barbera M, et al. Ultrastructural evidence of intercalated disc remodelling in arrhythmogenic right ventricular cardiomyopathy: an electron microscopy investigation on endomyocardial biopsies. Eur Heart J 2006; 27:1847–54.
93. Sen-Chowdry S, Syrris P, McKenna WJ. Role of genetic analysis in the management of patients with arrhythmogenic right ventricular dysplasia/cardiomyopathy. J Am Coll Cardiol 2007;50: 1813–21.
94. Kirchhof P, Fabritz L, Zwiener M, et al. Age and training dependent development of arrhythmogenic right ventricular cardiomyopathy in heterozygous plakoglobin deficient mice. Circulation 2006;114: 1799–806.
95. Garcia-Gras E, Lombardi R, Giocondo MJ, et al. Suppression of canonical Wnt/beta-catenin signaling by nuclear plakoglobin recapitulates phenotype of arrhythmogenic right ventricular cardiomyopathy. J Clin Invest 2006;116:1825–8.
96. Yang Z, Bowles NE, Scherer SE, et al. Desmosomal dysfunction due to mutations in desmoplakin causes arrhythmogenic right ventricular dysplasia/cardiomyopathy. Circ Res 2006;99:646–55.
97. Pilichou K, Remme CA, Basso C, et al. Myocyte necrosis underlies progressive myocardial dystrophy in mouse dsg2-related arrhythmogenic right ventricular cardiomyopathy. J Exp Med 2009;206:1787–802.
98. Basso C, Corrado D, Thiene G. Arrhythmogenic right ventricular cardiomyopathy: what's in a name? From a congenital defect (dysplasia) to a genetically determined cardiomyopathy (dystrophy). Am J Cardiol 2010;106:275–7.
99. Asimaki A, Tandri H, Huang H, et al. A new diagnostic test for arrhythmogenic right ventricular cardiomyopathy. N Engl J Med 2009;360:1075–84.
100. Corrado D, Fontaine G, Marcus FI, et al. Arrhythmogenic right ventricular dysplasia/cardiomyopathy: need for an International Registry. Circulation 2000;101:e101–6.
101. Basso C, Wichter T, Danieli GA, et al. Arrhythmogenic right ventricular cardiomyopathy: clinical registry and database, evaluation of therapies, pathology registry, DNA banking. Eur Heart J 2004;25:531–4.
102. Marcus F, Towbin JA, Zareba W, et al, ARVD/C Investigators. Arrhythmogenic right ventricular dysplasia/cardiomyopathy (ARVD/C): a multidisciplinary study: design and protocol. Circulation 2003;107:2975–8.
103. Marcus FI, Nava A, Thiene G. Arrhythmogenic right ventricular cardiomyopathy/dysplasia—recent advances. Milano (Italy): Springer; 2007.
104. Rossi L. History of the disease. In: Nava A, Rossi L, Thiene G, editors. Arrhythmogenic right ventricular cardiomyopathy/dysplasia. Amsterdam (Netherlands): Elsevier; 1997. p. 7–14.

Pathobiology of Arrhythmogenic Cardiomyopathy

Cristina Basso, MD, PhD[a,*], Kalliopi Pilichou, PhD[a], Elisa Carturan, PhD[a], Stefania Rizzo, MD[a], Barbara Bauce, MD, PhD[b], Gaetano Thiene, MD[a]

KEYWORDS

- Animal models
- Arrhythmogenic right ventricular cardiomyopathy/dysplasia
- Pathobiology • Pathology

This article discusses recent advances in the pathology and pathogenesis of arrhythmogenic cardiomyopathy (AC) that have led to the current perspective of a genetically determined cardiomyopathy.[1–6]

AC was initially believed to be a developmental defect of the right ventricular (RV) myocardium, thus justifying the original designation of dysplasia. Only in the 1980s was AC recognized to be a heredofamilial heart disease, usually transmitted as an autosomal dominant trait with variable penetrance.[7] Nowadays, up to 50% of probands affected with AC carry 1 or more mutations in genes encoding desmosomal proteins.[2,5]

PATHOLOGY

The original systematic description of morphologic abnormalities of AC dates back to 1988, when Thiene and colleagues[8] investigated a series of juvenile sudden deaths that occurred in the northeast of Italy, thus recognizing that the disease is a major cause of cardiac arrest in the young. Since then, the pathologic diagnosis of AC has been traditionally based on gross and histologic evidence of transmural myocardial loss with fibrofatty replacement of the RV free wall, extending from the epicardium toward the endocardium.

RV aneurysms, whether single or multiple, located in the so-called triangle of dysplasia (ie, inflow, apex, and outflow tract)[9] are considered a pathognomonic feature of AC, although not necessarily present in all cases.[10] Hearts with end-stage disease and congestive heart failure consistently showed a higher prevalence of biventricular involvement, usually with multiple aneurysms and a parchment-like appearance of the free wall.[10,11]

However, all the morphologic features mentioned earlier refer to the classic AC picture. Recently, it has been shown that the disease can have a phenotypic spectrum much wider than previously believed, with grossly normal hearts at one end, in whom only a careful histopathology investigation can reveal AC features in one or both ventricles, and hearts with massive RV involvement, with or without left ventricular (LV) involvement, at the opposite end (**Figs. 1** and **2**).

The wide variability in reported pathologic features mostly depends on the selection bias (ie, whether the cases come from referral centers for arrhythmias/sudden death or for heart failure/cardiac transplantation).

Transmural fibrofatty myocardial replacement of the RV free wall has always been considered the "conditio sine qua non" for pathologic diagnosis

[a] Cardiovascular Pathology, Department of Medical-diagnostic Sciences and Special Therapies, University of Padua Medical School, Via A. Gabelli, 35121 Padua, Italy
[b] Division of Cardiology, Department of Cardiac, Thoracic and Vascular Sciences, University of Padua Medical School, Via Giustiniani, 2-35121 Padua, Italy
* Corresponding author.
E-mail address: cristina.basso@unipd.it

Card Electrophysiol Clin 3 (2011) 193–204
doi:10.1016/j.ccep.2011.02.001
1877-9182/11/$ – see front matter

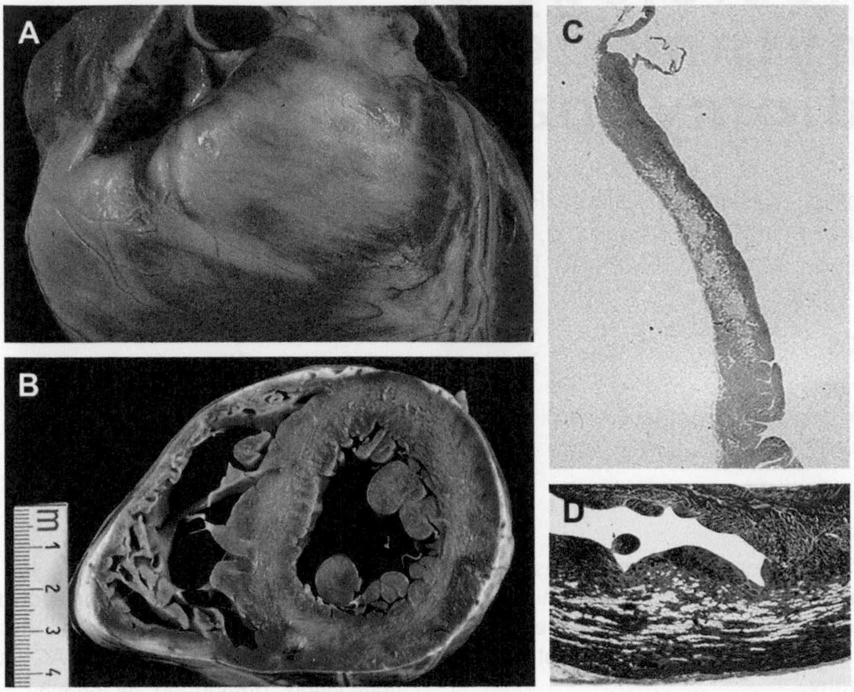

Fig. 1. AC (segmental form) in a 26-year-old athlete who died suddenly. (*A*) Anterior view of the RV outflow tract, which appears mildly dilated. (*B*) Cross section of the heart showing the absence of RV free wall aneurysms: note the spotty involvement of the posterior right ventricular free wall. (*C*) Histology of the RV outflow tract; note the regional loss of myocardium with fibrofatty replacement. (*D*) Histology of the posterior RV free wall; note the fibrofatty replacement of the myocardium in the absence of wall thinning. (*Modified from* Basso C, Thiene G, Corrado D, et al. Arrhythmogenic right ventricular cardiomyopathy: dysplasia, dystrophy or myocarditis? Circulation 1996;94:986; with permission.)

of AC, which might explain why several cases with early segmental RV involvement (ie, not yet full thickness deepening from epicardium to endocardium) or those with predominant or isolated LV disease, usually without wall thinning and aneurysm formation, escape the diagnosis.[1–3] The existence of cases with biventricular involvement or predominantly either LV or RV should suggest the use of the more comprehensive term AC.

Histologic examination reveals islands of surviving myocytes interspersed within fibrous and fatty tissue.[8,10,11] Clusters of myocytes may be seen dying at histology, providing evidence of the acquired nature of myocardial atrophy, and are frequently associated with inflammatory infiltrates, which probably plays a major role in triggering life-threatening arrhythmias (**Fig. 3**).[10,12]

Rather than being a continuous process, disease progression may occur during periodic bursts of an otherwise stable disease that can be clinically silent in most patients but sometimes may be characterized by life-threatening arrhythmic exacerbation. Environmental factors, such as exercise or inflammation, may facilitate disease onset and progression.

Fatty infiltration of the RV per se is not a sufficient morphologic hallmark of AC.[13] A certain amount of intramyocardial fat is present in the RV anterolateral and apical region even in the normal heart, and increases with age and body size. Moreover, AC is distinct from adipositas cordis.[14] Presence of replacement-type fibrosis and myocyte degenerative changes are essential to provide a clear-cut diagnosis, besides remarkable fatty replacement.

Transvenous endomyocardial biopsy may be of help in the diagnostic work-up for an in vivo tissue characterization through histologic evidence of fibrofatty myocardial replacement.[15–17] Samples should be retrieved from the RV free wall, because the fibrofatty replacement is herein usually transmural and thus detectable from the endocardial approach, whereas the ventricular septum is usually spared. A residual amount of myocardium (<60%), caused by fibrous or fibrofatty replacement, has been proved to have a high diagnostic accuracy and is now considered a major criterion for AC diagnosis (**Fig. 4**).[17,18] To improve the diagnostic sensitivity for AC, an endomyocardial biopsy procedure guided either by voltage mapping or by magnetic resonance imaging has been

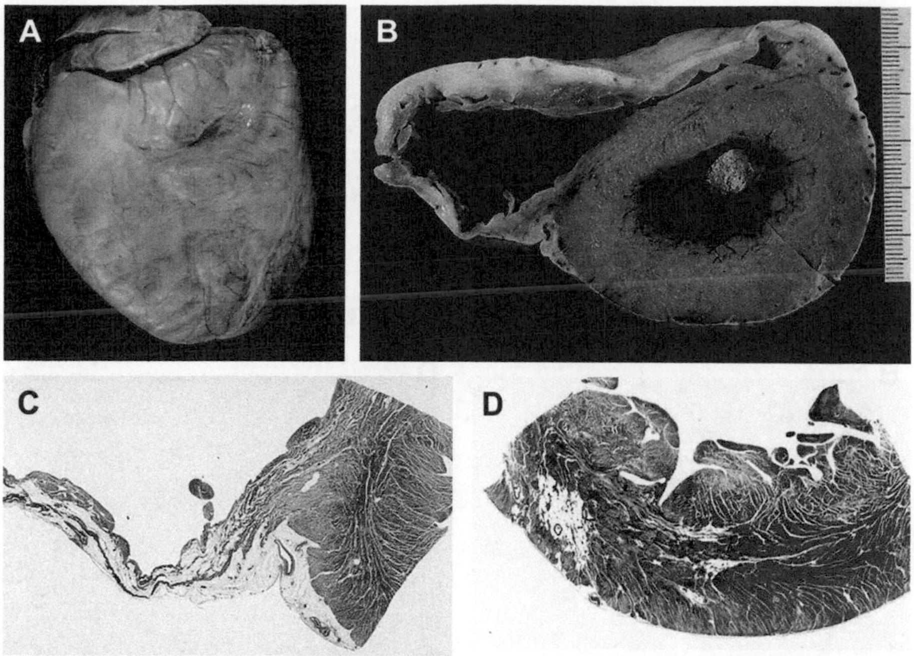

Fig. 2. AC (diffuse form) in a 14-year-old boy who died suddenly during a soccer game. (*A*) Anterior view of the heart; note the yellow appearance and the RV outflow tract aneurysm. (*B*) Cross section of the heart showing the presence of anterior and posterior aneurysms as well as patchy involvement of the LV free wall, posterolateral region. (*C*) Histology of the aneurysmal posteroinferior wall of the RV; note the loss of myocardium with fibrofatty replacement. (*D*) Histology of the LV free wall in the areas of fibrofatty replacement. (*Modified from* Basso C, Thiene G, Corrado D, et al. Arrhythmogenic right ventricular cardiomyopathy: dysplasia, dystrophy or myocarditis? Circulation 1996;94:985; with permission.)

suggested.[19] Moreover, endomyocardial biopsy is essential to rule out the so-called AC phenocopies, such as myocarditis, sarcoidosis, or idiopathic RV outflow tract tachycardia, particularly when dealing with probands with a sporadic AC form.[20–24]

DISCOVERY OF THE GENETIC BACKGROUND AND INTERCELLULAR JUNCTION INVESTIGATION

Despite the early recognition in the 1980s of the heredofamilial character of the disease in at least 50% of cases,[7,25] the first AC-causing gene (plakoglobin) was identified only in 2000,[26] in the recessive cardiocutaneous syndrome called Naxos disease. Soon after, a recessive mutation of desmoplakin was found to cause another cardiocutaneous syndrome (Carvajal disease), characterized by biventricular involvement.[27,28] Desmoplakin was the first defective gene to be associated with autosomal dominant AC by Rampazzo and colleagues[29] in 2002. Subsequently, a variety of mutations in plakophilin-2, desmoglein-2, and desmocollin-2 genes have been found,[30–32] and plakoglobin has been reported even in dominant forms.[33] More recently, desmin has been identified as a novel AC gene,[34] and should be included in the molecular genetic screening of patients with AC. Thus, with the exception of a few other genes unrelated to cell adhesion complex, such as ryanodine 2 receptor, the transforming growth factor β3, and the transmembrane protein 43 encoding genes,[35–37] the most common disease genes encode for desmosomal proteins, and double or compound heterozygosity is commonly reported.[38–40] This consistent type of protein alteration supports the concept of a final common pathway of genetically determined cardiomyopathies, AC being deemed to be a desmosomal disease, hypertrophic cardiomyopathy a sarcomeric disease, and dilated cardiomyopathy a cytoskeletal disease (**Fig. 5**).[6,41]

For these reasons, morphologic and molecular studies of intercellular junctions became a major issue both in humans and experimental pathology.

Ultrastructural investigation of endomyocardial biopsies in gene-positive patients with AC revealed intercalated disc remodeling with desmosomal abnormalities.[42] In particular, the number of desmosomes was significantly lower, the desmosomal gap widened, and desmosomal

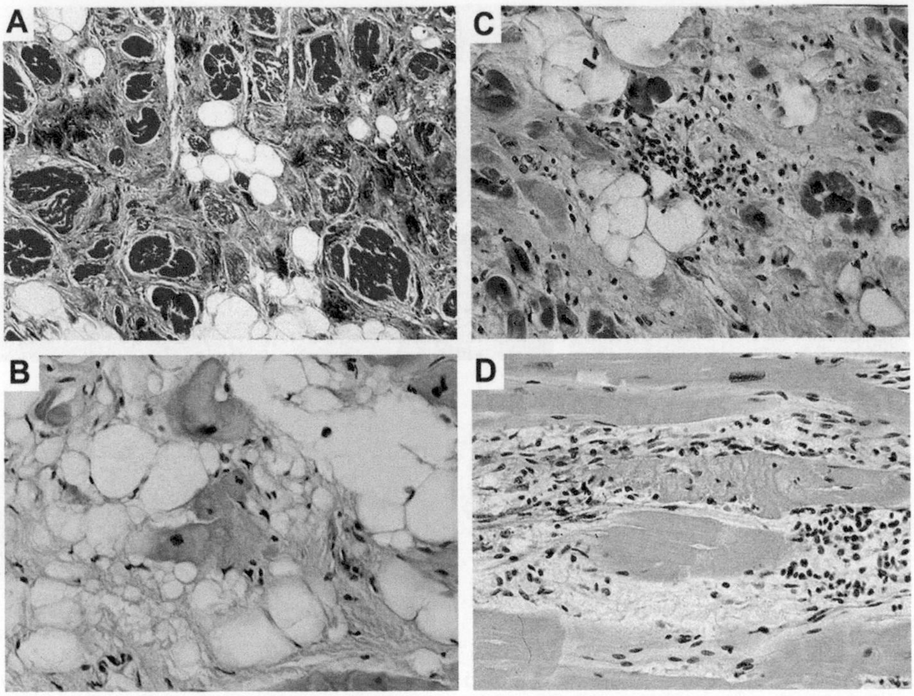

Fig. 3. Histologic features of AC. (*A*) Residual myocytes entrapped within fibrous and fatty tissue. (*B*) Adipogenesis in areas of myocyte injury. (*C*) Inflammatory infiltrates within fibrofatty areas. (*D*) Myocyte contraction band necrosis.

length higher in AC than in controls. Moreover, abnormally located desmosomes were identified in most cases, often with pale internal plaques.

Later, immunohistochemical and molecular studies of intercellular junction proteins showed plakoglobin redistribution from intercellular junctions to other locations within the cell in Naxos disease and Carvajal syndrome.[43,44] These data provided the first evidence that a mutation in a single desmosomal protein may disrupt the subcellular distribution of another intercellular junction protein that is not genetically altered.

More recently, Asimaki and colleagues[45] found that, in nearly every case of AC, the signal for the intracellular linker protein, plakoglobin, is diminished at intercalated disks and seems to be specific for AC (**Fig. 6**). From these findings, the investigators suggested that the evaluation of abnormal localization of desmosomal proteins by immunohistochemistry analysis on endomyocardial biopsy samples represents a promising test for AC diagnosis. Redistribution of plakoglobin from junctions to intracellular pools could be part of a final common pathway in disease

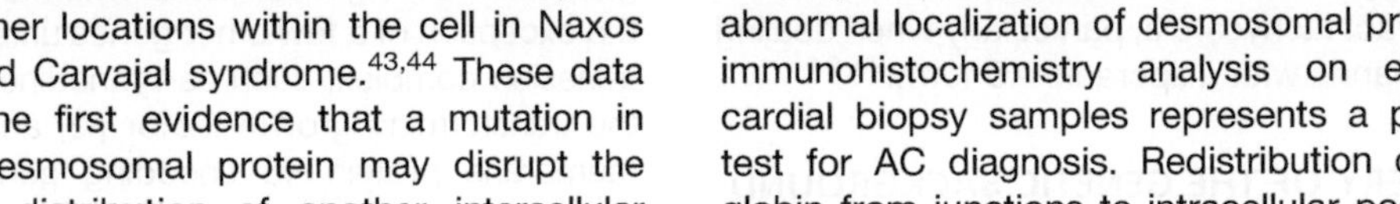

Fig. 4. Diagnostic endomyocardial biopsy in AC (major criterion); each of the 3 biopsy samples shows a significant amount of myocardial atrophy (less than 60% of the surface area) with fibrous and fibrofatty replacement. (*From* Marcus FI, McKenna WJ, Sherrill D, et al. Diagnosis of arrhythmogenic right ventricular cardiomyopathy/dysplasia: proposed modification of the task force criteria. Circulation 2010;121:1538; with permission.)

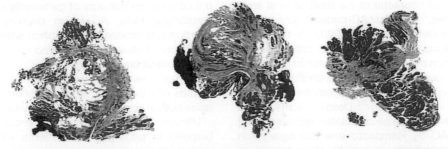

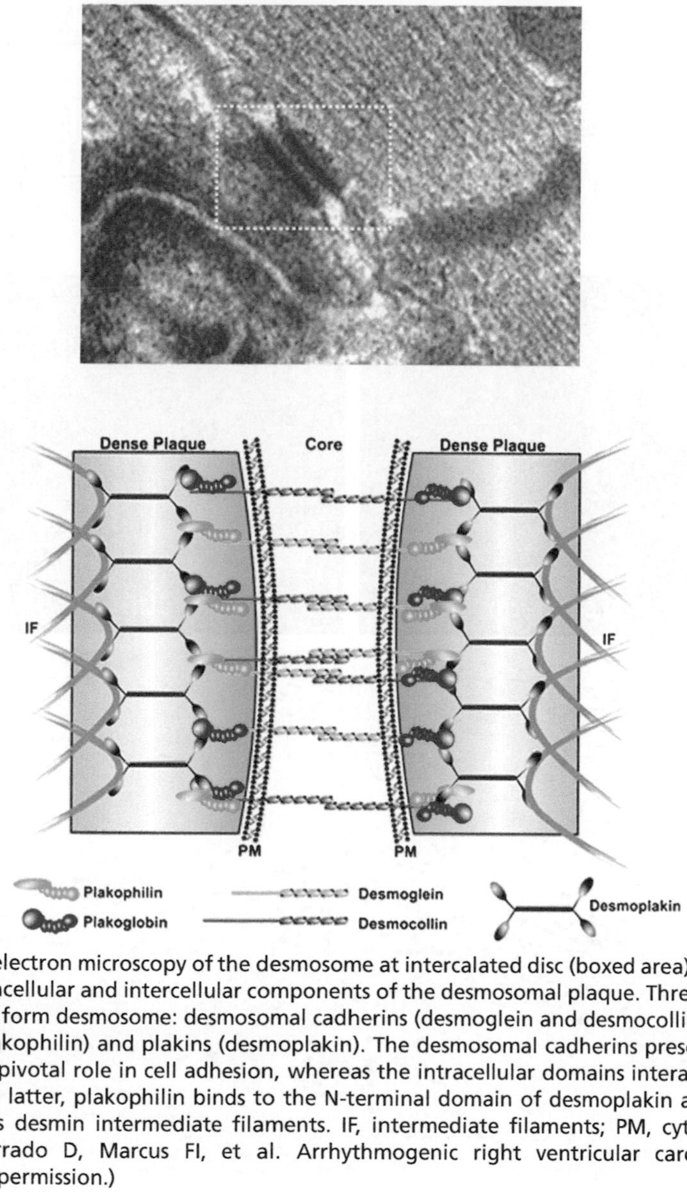

Fig. 5. Transmission electron microscopy of the desmosome at intercalated disc (boxed area) and schematic representation of the intracellular and intercellular components of the desmosomal plaque. Three separate families of proteins assemble to form desmosome: desmosomal cadherins (desmoglein and desmocollin), armadillo proteins (plakoglobin and plakophilin) and plakins (desmoplakin). The desmosomal cadherins present with extracellular domains that play a pivotal role in cell adhesion, whereas the intracellular domains interact with the armadillo proteins. Among the latter, plakophilin binds to the N-terminal domain of desmoplakin and the C terminal of desmoplakin anchors desmin intermediate filaments. IF, intermediate filaments; PM, cytoplasmic membrane. (*From* Basso C, Corrado D, Marcus FI, et al. Arrhythmogenic right ventricular cardiomyopathy. Lancet 2009;373:1290; with permission.)

pathogenesis and impaired mechanical coupling might account for abnormal electrical coupling by gap junction remodeling. Immunohistochemical and electron microscopy studies in Naxos disease revealed reduced localization of mutant plakoglobin to cell-cell junctions, diminished expression of the gap junction protein connexin-43 (Cx43), and a decreased number and size of gap junctions.[43] In Carvajal syndrome, immunoreactive signals for both desmoplakin and plakoglobin were markedly diminished at intercalated disks, as were signals for desmin and connexin-43.[44] More recently, similar changes in the various intercalated disk proteins were observed in the classic form of AC without cardiocutaneous manifestations caused by plakophilin-2 mutations.[46] These preliminary findings suggest that gap junction remodeling might provide an alternative mechanism for conduction delay and RV electrical instability, which may result in potentially fatal arrhythmias before fibrofatty myocardial replacement occurs at histology. However, large-scale clinicopathologic series, including patients without AC, are needed before using this test in the routine diagnostic work-up.

ETIOPATHOGENETIC THEORIES

To explain the loss of the ventricular myocardium being substituted by fibrous and fatty tissue,

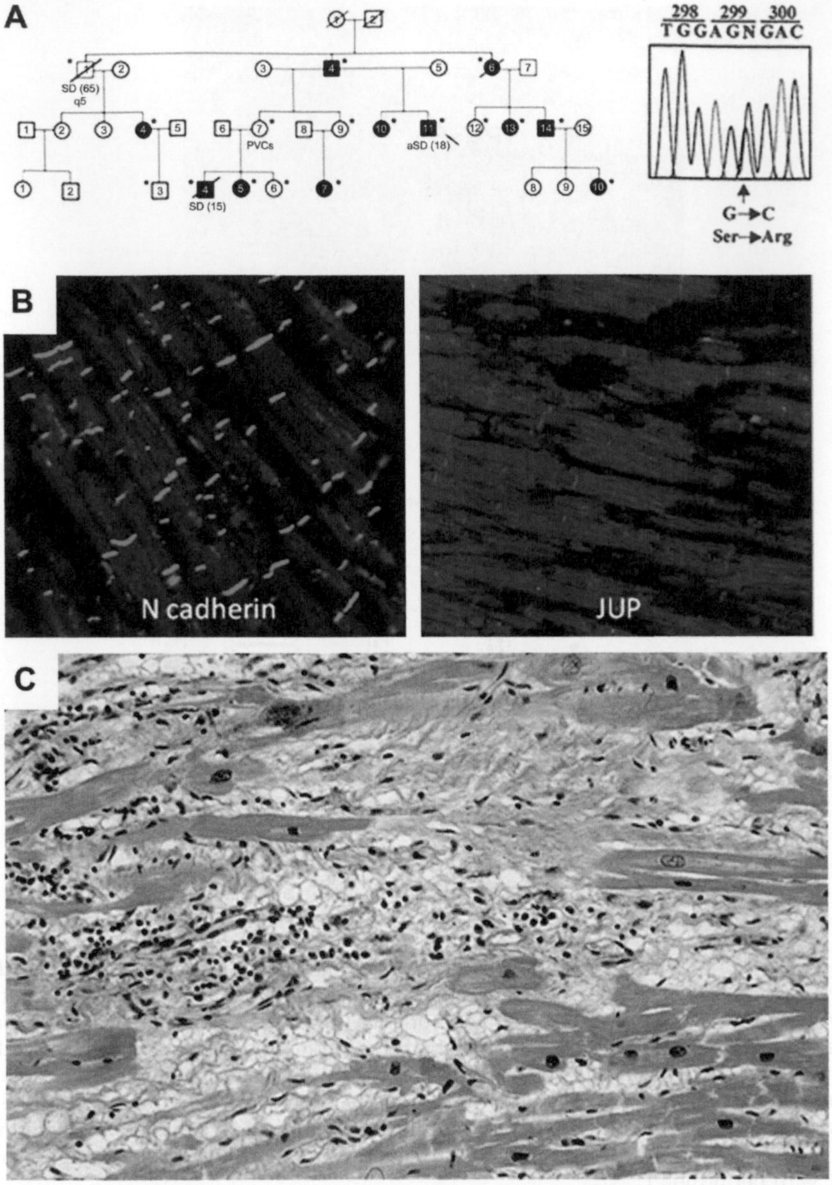

Fig. 6. Immunoreactive plakoglobin signal and histologic features in a sudden death victim from familial AC caused by a mutant desmoplakin gene. (*A*) Family pedigree of the AC family and identified mutation (S299R) in exon 7 of desmoplakin gene. (*B*) Immunohistochemical analysis of human myocardial samples of the proband from patients who died suddenly at the age of 15 years shows a marked reduction in immunoreactive signal levels for plakoglobin but normal signal levels for the nondesmosomal adhesion molecule N-cadherin. (*C*) Histology of the ventricular myocardium showing ongoing cardiomyocyte death with early fibrofatty replacement. (*From* Corrado D, Basso C, Pilichou K, et al. Molecular biology and the clinical management of arrhythmogenic right ventricular cardiomyopathy/dysplasia. Heart 2011;97:530–9; with permission.)

several etiopathogenetic theories have been put forward.[3,10]

The original concept was that of a congenital abnormality (dysplasia, aplasia, or hypoplasia) characterized by maldevelopment of the RV myocardium. Confusion in the literature about AC has been created by the misuse of the term Uhl's anomaly, which was described as an almost total absence of the myocardium of the RV in a 7-month-old infant, with the epicardium applied directly to endocardium in the absence of intervening fat.[47] In contrast, in AC there is always fat and fibrous tissue with residual myocytes between the epicardial and endocardial layers. Additional features in differential diagnosis with Uhl's anomaly include the lack of family history, heart failure as clinical picture, infrequency of arrhythmias, and a significantly earlier age of presentation, usually in childhood. In AC, myocardial atrophy is the consequence of cell death occurring after birth, usually during childhood, and is progressive with time, as distinct from Uhl's disease, a congenital heart defect in which the RV myocardium fails to develop at the embryonic stage.[10]

As for the inflammatory theory, it has been a matter of debate whether the inflammatory cells are a reaction to cell death or the consequence of infective or immune mechanisms.[10,12] Cardiotropic viruses, such as adenovirus, hepatitis C virus, and parvovirus B19, have been reported in the myocardium of some patients with AC, and they have been proposed as possible causal agents, thus supporting an infective pathogenesis.[48,49] However, the viral agent might be just an innocent bystander or play a secondary, but still important, role. According to the latter hypothesis, the genetically dystrophic myocardium could favor viral settlement (superimposed myocarditis), leading to progression or the precipitation of the disease phenotype. Similar pathologic features of inflammation have been described in spontaneous animal models of AC, with a clinical picture dominated by right heart failure and ventricular arrhythmias at risk of sudden death.[50] Moreover, recent evidence of massive inflammatory cell infiltrates following acute myocyte necrosis in the early stages of the disease onset in AC transgenic mice supports the reactive nature of myocarditis.[51]

To explain the fibrofatty phenomenon, even a transdifferentiation theory has been put forward, according to which cardiomyocytes transform into fibrocytes and/or adipocytes.[52] However, this theory is questionable because of the limited dedifferentiation capabilities of adult cardiomyocytes.

The most likely etiopathogenetic theory remains the dystrophic one (myocardial dystrophy), which was postulated before the discovery of the disease-causing genes.[10] The idea came from the observation of the similarities of histopathologic features of AC and of skeletal muscle dystrophies (such as Duchenne or Becker), that is, a progressive and acquired muscular atrophy with replacement by exuberant fatty and fibrous tissue.[10] Thus, in AC cardiomyocyte death, either by apoptosis or necrosis, could account for a genetically determined progressive loss of the ventricular myocardium.[53,54] The discovery of the first disease gene (plakoglobin) made it possible to identify additional genes in the autosomal dominant variants of AC (ie, desmoplakin, plakophilin-2, desmoglein-2, and desmocollin-2).[26–33]

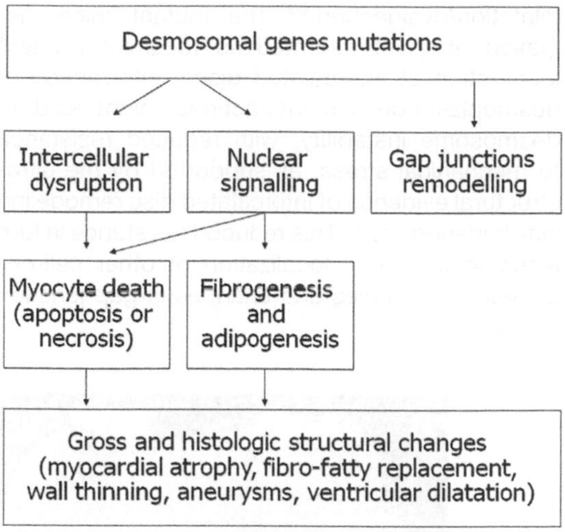

Fig. 7. The current hypotheses on AC pathogenesis: cascade of events leading from desmosomal gene mutations to structural changes.

According to the widely accepted defective desmosome hypothesis, genetically determined disruption of desmosomal integrity is the key factor leading to the development of AC. Although desmosomes are traditionally considered specialized structures that provide mechanical attachment between cells, they are emerging as mediators of intracellular and intercellular signal transduction pathways.[55–57] Some desmosomal proteins fulfill roles both as structural proteins in cell-cell adhesion junctions and as signaling molecules in pathways mediated by Wnt ligands. Evidence is increasing that mutations in desmosomal proteins can perturb the normal balance of critical proteins in junctions and the cytosol, which, in turn, could alter gene expression by circumventing normal Wnt signaling pathways. Moreover, there is increasing evidence that components of the desmosome are essential for the proper function and distribution of the gap junction protein Cx43, supporting the notion of a molecular crosstalk between desmosomal and gap junction proteins (**Fig. 7**).[43,58,59]

RECENT ADVANCES IN DISEASE PATHOBIOLOGY: THE LESSON OF TRANSGENIC ANIMAL MODELS

Transgenic animal models recapitulating the AC phenotype have recently been developed.

A transgenic mouse with cardiac-restricted overexpression of the C-terminal mutant (R2834H) desmoplakin has been shown to develop increased cardiomyocyte apoptosis, myocardial fibrosis, and lipid accumulation as well as biventricular dilatation/dysfunction.[60] The mutant mice displayed aberrant intermediate (desmin) filament localization at intercalated discs. Interruption of desmoplakin-desmin interactions might lead to desmosome instability, with reduced resistance to mechanical stress, as supported by the ultrastructural evidence of intercalated disc remodeling with widened gaps. This reduced resistance in turn leads to abnormal localization of other cell-cell adhesion molecules and changes in gap junction components.

Data from Garcia-Gras and colleagues[61] on cardiac desmoplakin-deficient mice suggest an alternative molecular mechanism of disease that implicates inhibition of the canonical Wnt/β-catenin signaling through Tcf/Lef transcription factors in the pathogenesis of AC. In this study, cardiac-specific loss of the desmosomal protein desmoplakin was sufficient to cause nuclear translocation of plakoglobin, increased expression of adipogenic and fibrogenic genes, and the development of an AC-like phenotype consisting of

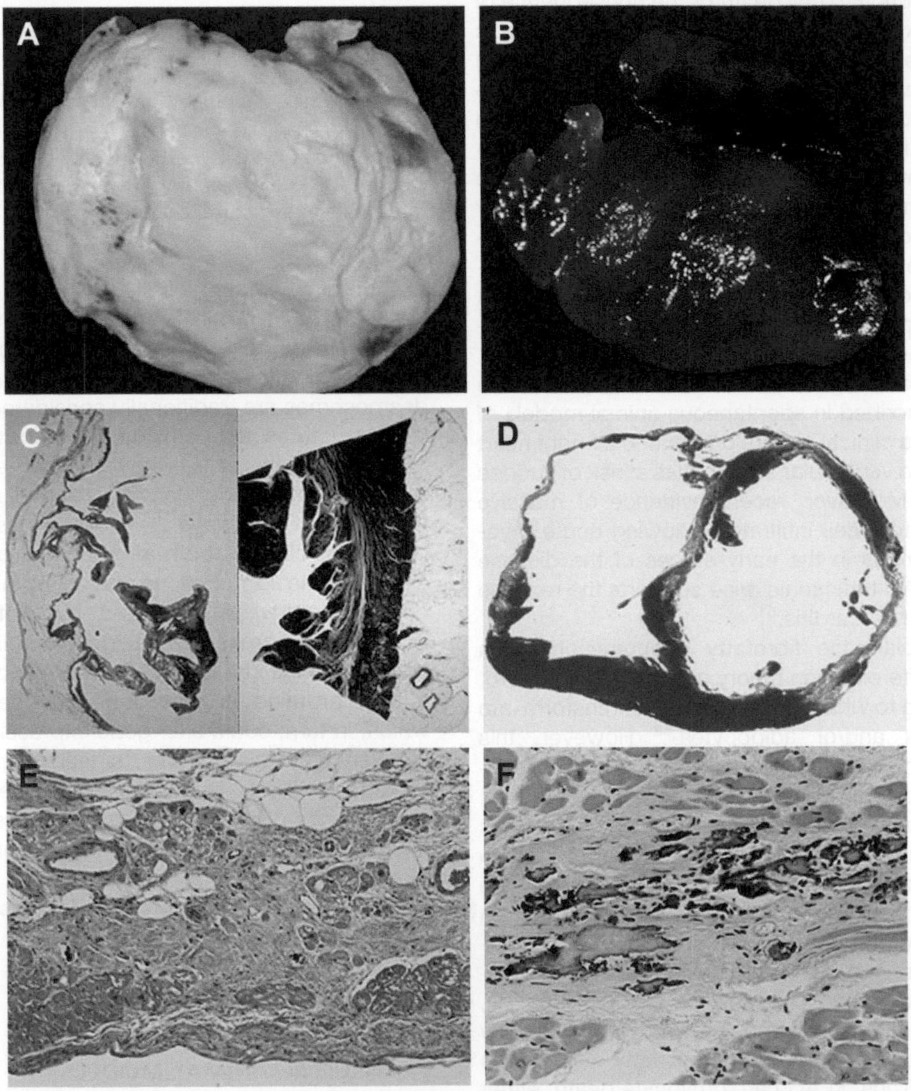

Fig. 8. AC in a human patient with Dsg2 mutation (*A, C, E*) and in the experimental transgenic mouse with Dsg2 mutation overexpression (*B, D, F*). (*A, B*) Gross anterior view of the fatty heart showing ventricular chamber dilatation and aneurysms. (*C, D*) Trichrome staining on full-thickness RV and LV free walls (*C*, human heart) and on transverse section of the heart (*D*, mouse heart) showing biventricular myocardial atrophy with fibrofatty and fibrous tissue repair, respectively, and with wall thinning and aneurysm formation. (*E, F*) Hematoxylin-eosin staining at higher magnification with abnormal residual cardiomyocytes and spotty calcification. (*From* Pilichou K, Remme CA, Basso C, et al. Myocyte necrosis underlies progressive myocardial dystrophy in mouse dsg2-related arrhythmogenic right ventricular cardiomyopathy. J Exp Med 2009;206:1789; with permission.)

myocardial fibrofatty infiltration, cavity enlargement, and ventricular arrhythmias. This evidence for potential Wnt/β-catenin signaling defects implicates a role of cell adhesion proteins not only as passive players in providing mechanical attachment between cells, but as regulators in cardiac development, in myocyte differentiation, and in the maintenance of the myocardial architecture.[62]

Another study on heterozygous plakoglobin-deficient mice showed that mutant animals had increased RV volume, reduced RV function, and more frequent and severe ventricular tachycardia of RV origin.[63] In this animal model, endurance training accelerated the development of RV dysfunction and arrhythmias. However, the clinical phenotype of this heterozygous plakoglobin-deficient mutant mouse showed only limited similarity to the human forms of AC, because none of the mutant mice were found to have myocardial fibrofatty replacement, and only inconsistent RV dilation was noted. The same group recently demonstrated that load-reducing therapy (furosemide and nitrates) prevents training-induced (daily swimming) development of AC in plako(+/-) mice.[64]

Further insights into the pathobiologic mechanisms involved in AC (onset and progression) are provided by the study of a transgenic mouse model (Tg-NS) with cardiac overexpression of desmoglein-2 gene mutation N271S.[51] Transgenic mice reproduced the clinical features of AC, including spontaneous ventricular arrhythmias, cardiac dysfunction, biventricular dilatation with aneurysms, and sudden death at young age. Investigation of transgenic lines with different levels of transgene expression attested to a dose-dependent dominant-negative effect of the mutation. The study showed for the first time that myocyte necrosis is the key initiator of myocardial injury. Myocyte necrosis was the first manifestation of disease in all Tg-NS hearts studied. Electron microscopic evaluation in Tg-NS/H mice between 2 and 3 weeks old showed disruption of the sarcolemma, disgregation of myofilaments and other cytoplasmic elements, and mitochondrial swelling, all ultrastructural features consistent with cardiomyocyte necrosis. Myocardial cell death subsequently triggers an inflammatory response and massive calcification within the myocardium, followed later by injury repair with fibrous tissue replacement and aneurysm formation (**Fig. 8**). More recently, an inducible cardiorestricted knockout of the plakoglobin gene was generated in mice.[65] Plakoglobin knockout mice exhibited a phenotype similar to that of AC patients. Desmosomal proteins from the intercalated disc were decreased, consistent with altered desmosome ultrastructure. Ablation of plakoglobin caused increase β-catenin stabilization associated with activated AKT and inhibition of glycogen synthase kinase 3β.

SUMMARY

Functional analysis of cellular and transgenic animal models with mutant desmosomal genes may help to elucidate the cascade of cellular and molecular events involved in the AC phenotype development and the clinical relevance of different desmosomal gene variants, either isolated or together. Knowledge of the mechanisms leading from the mutant protein to the clinical phenotype, and the search for genetic or environmental factors that influence the expression of these defective proteins, will allow to identify potential molecular targets for therapeutic intervention to stop disease onset and progression.

REFERENCES

1. Marcus FI, Nava A, Thiene G. Arrhythmogenic right ventricular cardiomyopathy/dysplasia: recent advances. Milan: Springer-Verlag; 2007.
2. Thiene G, Corrado D, Basso C. Arrhythmogenic right ventricular cardiomyopathy/dysplasia. Orphanet J Rare Dis 2007;2:45.
3. Basso C, Corrado D, Marcus FI, et al. Arrhythmogenic right ventricular cardiomyopathy. Lancet 2009;373:1289–300.
4. Basso C, Corrado D, Thiene G. Arrhythmogenic right ventricular cardiomyopathy: what's in a name? From a congenital defect (dysplasia) to a genetically determined cardiomyopathy (dystrophy). Am J Cardiol 2010;106:275–7.
5. Corrado D, Basso C, Pilichou K, et al. Molecular biology and the clinical management of arrhythmogenic right ventricular cardiomyopathy/dysplasia. Heart 2011;97:530–9.
6. Maron BJ, Towbin JA, Thiene G, et al. Contemporary definitions and classification of the cardiomyopathies: an American Heart Association Scientific Statement from the Council on Clinical Cardiology, Heart Failure and Transplantation Committee; Quality of Care and Outcomes Research and Functional Genomics and Translational Biology Interdisciplinary Working Groups; and Council on Epidemiology and Prevention. Circulation 2006;113:1807–16.
7. Nava A, Thiene G, Canciani B, et al. Familial occurrence of right ventricular dysplasia: a study involving nine families. J Am Coll Cardiol 1989;12:1222–8.
8. Thiene G, Nava A, Corrado D, et al. Right ventricular cardiomyopathy and sudden death in young people. N Engl J Med 1988;318:129–33.

9. Marcus F, Fontaine G, Guiraudon G, et al. Right ventricular dysplasia: a report of 24 adult cases. Circulation 1982;65:384–98.
10. Basso C, Thiene G, Corrado D, et al. Arrhythmogenic right ventricular cardiomyopathy: dysplasia, dystrophy or myocarditis? Circulation 1996;94:983–91.
11. Corrado D, Basso C, Thiene G, et al. Spectrum of clinicopathologic manifestations of arrhythmogenic right ventricular cardiomyopathy/dysplasia: a multicenter study. J Am Coll Cardiol 1997;30:1512–20.
12. Thiene G, Corrado D, Nava A, et al. Right ventricular cardiomyopathy: is there evidence of an inflammatory aetiology? Eur Heart J 1991;12:22–5.
13. Basso C, Thiene G. Adipositas cordis, fatty infiltration of the right ventricle, and arrhythmogenic right ventricular cardiomyopathy. Just a matter of fat? Cardiovasc Pathol 2005;14:37–41.
14. Marcus F, Basso C, Gear K, et al. Pitfalls in the diagnosis of arrhythmogenic right ventricular cardiomyopathy/dysplasia. Am J Cardiol 2010;105:1036–9.
15. Angelini A, Basso C, Nava A, et al. Endomyocardial biopsy in arrhythmogenic right ventricular cardiomyopathy. Am Heart J 1996;132:203–6.
16. McKenna WJ, Thiene G, Nava A, et al. Diagnosis of arrhythmogenic right ventricular dysplasia/cardiomyopathy. Task Force of the Working Group Myocardial and Pericardial Disease of the European Society of Cardiology and of the Scientific Council on Cardiomyopathies of the International Society and Federation of Cardiology. Br Heart J 1994;71:215–8.
17. Basso C, Ronco F, Marcus F, et al. Quantitative assessment of endomyocardial biopsy in arrhythmogenic right ventricular cardiomyopathy/dysplasia: an in vitro validation of diagnostic criteria. Eur Heart J 2008;29:2760–71.
18. Marcus FI, McKenna WJ, Sherrill D, et al. Diagnosis of arrhythmogenic right ventricular cardiomyopathy/dysplasia: proposed modification of the task force criteria. Circulation 2010;121:1533–41; and Eur Heart J 2010;31:806–14.
19. Avella A, d'Amati G, Pappalardo A, et al. Diagnostic value of endomyocardial biopsy guided by electroanatomic voltage mapping in arrhythmogenic right ventricular cardiomyopathy/dysplasia. J Cardiovasc Electrophysiol 2008;19:1127–34.
20. Corrado D, Basso C, Leoni L, et al. Three-dimensional electroanatomical voltage mapping and histologic evaluation of myocardial substrate in right ventricular outflow tract tachycardia. J Am Coll Cardiol 2008;51:731–9.
21. Corrado D, Basso C, Leoni L, et al. Three-dimensional electroanatomic voltage mapping increases accuracy of diagnosing arrhythmogenic right ventricular cardiomyopathy/dysplasia. Circulation 2005;111:3042–50.
22. Ladyjanskaia GA, Basso C, Hobbelink MG, et al. Sarcoid myocarditis with ventricular tachycardia mimicking ARVD/C. J Cardiovasc Electrophysiol 2010;21:94–8.
23. Vasaiwala SC, Finn C, Delpriore J, et al. Prospective study of cardiac sarcoid mimicking arrhythmogenic right ventricular dysplasia. J Cardiovasc Electrophysiol 2009;20:473–6.
24. Corrado D, Thiene G. Cardiac sarcoidosis mimicking arrhythmogenic right ventricular cardiomyopathy/dysplasia: the renaissance of endomyocardial biopsy? J Cardiovasc Electrophysiol 2009;20:477–9.
25. Nava A, Bauce B, Basso C, et al. Clinical profile and long-term follow-up of 37 families with arrhythmogenic right ventricular cardiomyopathy. J Am Coll Cardiol 2000;36:2226–33.
26. McKoy G, Protonotarios N, Crosby A, et al. Identification of a deletion in plakoglobin in arrhythmogenic right ventricular cardiomyopathy with palmoplantar keratoderma and woolly hair (Naxos disease). Lancet 2000;355:2119–24.
27. Norgett EE, Hatsell SJ, Carvajal-Huerta L, et al. Recessive mutation in desmoplakin disrupts desmoplakin-intermediate filament interactions and causes dilated cardiomyopathy, woolly hair and keratoderma. Hum Mol Genet 2000;9:2761–6.
28. Alcalai R, Metzger S, Rosenheck S, et al. A recessive mutation in desmoplakin causes arrhythmogenic right ventricular dysplasia, skin disorder, and woolly hair. J Am Coll Cardiol 2003;42:319–27.
29. Rampazzo A, Nava A, Malacrida S, et al. Mutation in human desmoplakin domain binding to plakoglobin causes a dominant form of arrhythmogenic right ventricular cardiomyopathy. Am J Hum Genet 2002;71:1200–6.
30. Gerull B, Heuser A, Wichter T, et al. Mutations in the desmosomal protein plakophilin-2 are common in arrhythmogenic right ventricular cardiomyopathy. Nat Genet 2004;36:1162–4.
31. Pilichou K, Nava A, Basso C, et al. Mutations in desmoglein-2 gene are associated with arrhythmogenic right ventricular cardiomyopathy. Circulation 2006;113:1171–9.
32. Syrris P, Ward D, Evans A, et al. Arrhythmogenic right ventricular dysplasia/cardiomyopathy associated with mutations in the desmosomal gene desmocollin-2. Am J Hum Genet 2006;79:978–84.
33. Asimaki A, Syrris P, Wichter T, et al. A novel dominant mutation in plakoglobin causes arrhythmogenic right ventricular cardiomyopathy. Am J Hum Genet 2007;81:964–73.
34. Klauke B, Kossmann S, Gaertner A, et al. De novo desmin-mutation N116S is associated with arrhythmogenic right ventricular cardiomyopathy. Hum Mol Genet 2010;19:4595–607.
35. Tiso N, Stephan DA, Nava A, et al. Identification of mutations in the cardiac ryanodine receptor gene

in families affected with arrhythmogenic right ventricular cardiomyopathy type 2 (ARVD2). Hum Mol Genet 2001;10:189–94.
36. Beffagna G, Occhi G, Nava A, et al. Regulatory mutations in transforming growth factor-beta3 gene cause arrhythmogenic right ventricular cardiomyopathy type 1. Cardiovasc Res 2005;65:366–73.
37. Merner ND, Hodgkinson KA, Haywood AF, et al. Arrhythmogenic right ventricular cardiomyopathy type 5 is a fully penetrant, lethal arrhythmic disorder caused by a missense mutation in the TMEM43 gene. Am J Hum Genet 2008;82:809–21.
38. Corrado D, Thiene G. Arrhythmogenic right ventricular cardiomyopathy/dysplasia: clinical impact of molecular genetic studies. Circulation 2006;113: 1634–7.
39. Bauce B, Nava A, Beffagna G, et al. Multiple mutations in desmosomal proteins encoding genes in arrhythmogenic right ventricular cardiomyopathy/ dysplasia. Heart Rhythm 2010;7:22–9.
40. Xu T, Yang Z, Vatta M, et al. Multidisciplinary Study of Right Ventricular Dysplasia Investigators. Compound and digenic heterozygosity contributes to arrhythmogenic right ventricular cardiomyopathy. J Am Coll Cardiol 2010;55:587–97.
41. Thiene G, Corrado D, Basso C. Cardiomyopathies: is it time for a molecular classification? Eur Heart J 2004;25:1772–5.
42. Basso C, Czarnowska E, Della Barbera M, et al. Ultrastructural evidence of intercalated disc remodelling in arrhythmogenic right ventricular cardiomyopathy: an electron microscopy investigation on endomyocardial biopsies. Eur Heart J 2006;27: 1847–54.
43. Kaplan SR, Gard JJ, Protonotarios N, et al. Remodeling of myocyte gap junctions in arrhythmogenic right ventricular cardiomyopathy due to a deletion in plakoglobin (Naxos disease). Heart Rhythm 2004;1:3–11.
44. Kaplan SR, Gard JJ, Carvajal-Huerta L, et al. Structural and molecular pathology of the heart in Carvajal syndrome. Cardiovasc Pathol 2004;13:26–32.
45. Asimaki A, Tandri H, Huang H, et al. A new diagnostic test for arrhythmogenic right ventricular cardiomyopathy. N Engl J Med 2009;360:1075–84.
46. Fidler LM, Wilson GJ, Liu F, et al. Abnormal connexin43 in arrhythmogenic right ventricular cardiomyopathy caused by plakophilin-2 mutations. J Cell Mol Med 2009;13:4219–28.
47. Uhl HS. A previously undescribed congenital malformation of the heart: almost total absence of the myocardium of the right ventricle. Bull Johns Hopkins Hosp 1952;91:197–209.
48. Bowles NE, Ni J, Marcus F, et al. The detection of cardiotropic viruses in the myocardium of patients with arrhythmogenic right ventricular dysplasia/ cardiomyopathy. J Am Coll Cardiol 2002;39:892–5.
49. Calabrese F, Basso C, Carturan E, et al. Arrhythmogenic right ventricular cardiomyopathy/dysplasia: is there a role for viruses? Cardiovasc Pathol 2006; 15:11–7.
50. Fox PR, Maron BJ, Basso C, et al. Spontaneously occurring arrhythmogenic right ventricular cardiomyopathy in the domestic cat: A new animal model similar to the human disease. Circulation 2000;102: 1863–70.
51. Pilichou K, Remme CA, Basso C, et al. Myocyte necrosis underlies progressive myocardial dystrophy in mouse dsg2-related arrhythmogenic right ventricular cardiomyopathy. J Exp Med 2009;206:1787–802.
52. d'Amati G, di Gioia CR, Giordano C, et al. Myocyte transdifferentiation: a possible pathogenetic mechanism for arrhythmogenic right ventricular cardiomyopathy. Arch Pathol Lab Med 2000;124: 287–90.
53. Mallat Z, Tedgui A, Fontaliran F, et al. Evidence of apoptosis in arrhythmogenic right ventricular dysplasia. N Engl J Med 1996;335:1190–6.
54. Valente M, Calabrese F, Thiene G, et al. In vivo evidence of apoptosis in arrhythmogenic right ventricular cardiomyopathy. Am J Pathol 1998;152: 479–84.
55. Huber O. Structure and function of desmosomal proteins and their role in development and disease. Cell Mol Life Sci 2003;60:1872–90.
56. Desai BV, Harmon RM, Green KJ. Desmosomes at a glance. J Cell Sci 2009;122:4401–7.
57. Green KJ, Getsios S, Troyanovsky S, et al. Intercellular junction assembly, dynamics, and homeostasis. Cold Spring Harb Perspect Biol 2010;2: a000125.
58. Sato PY, Musa H, Coombs W, et al. Loss of plakophilin-2 expression leads to decreased sodium current and slower conduction velocity in cultured cardiac myocytes. Circ Res 2009;105:523–6.
59. Delmar M, McKenna WJ. The cardiac desmosome and arrhythmogenic cardiomyopathies: from gene to disease. Circ Res 2010;107:700–14.
60. Yang Z, Bowles NE, Scherer SE, et al. Desmosomal dysfunction due to mutations in desmoplakin causes arrhythmogenic right ventricular dysplasia/cardiomyopathy. Circ Res 2006;99:646–55.
61. Garcia-Gras E, Lombardi R, Giocondo MJ, et al. Suppression of canonical Wnt/beta-catenin signaling by nuclear plakoglobin recapitulates phenotype of arrhythmogenic right ventricular cardiomyopathy. J Clin Invest 2006;116:2012–21.
62. Lombardi R, Dong J, Rodriguez G, et al. Genetic fate mapping identifies second heart field progenitor cells as a source of adipocytes in arrhythmogenic right ventricular cardiomyopathy. Circ Res 2009; 104:1076–84.
63. Kirchhof P, Fabritz L, Zwiener M, et al. Age- and training-dependent development of arrhythmogenic

right ventricular cardiomyopathy in heterozygous plakoglobin-deficient mice. Circulation 2006;114: 1799–806.

64. Fabritz L, Hoogendijk MG, Scicluna BP, et al. Load-reducing therapy prevents development of arrhythmogenic right ventricular cardiomyopathy in plakoglobin-deficient mice. J Am Coll Cardiol 2011; 57:740–50.

65. Li J, Swope D, Raess N, et al. Cardiac tissue-restricted deletion of plakoglobin results in progressive cardiomyopathy and activation of {beta}-catenin signaling. Mol Cell Biol 2011;31:1134–44.

Clinical Impact of Genetics in Arrhythmogenic Cardiomyopathy

Srijita Sen-Chowdhry, MBBS, MD[a,b], Petros Syrris, PhD[a], Giovanni Quarta, MD[c,d], William J. McKenna, MD, DSc[a,c,*]

KEYWORDS

- Arrhythmogenic right ventricular cardiomyopathy/dysplasia
- Diagnosis • Gene testing • Genetics • Sudden death

Electrophysiologists commonly consider the possibility of arrhythmogenic cardiomyopathy (AC) when investigating arrhythmia of right ventricular origin. The patient may present with palpitation or symptoms of impaired consciousness; ventricular arrhythmia of left bundle branch block is apparent on surface electrocardiography (ECG). A monomorphic configuration, with inferior axis and transition at V3/4, is further suggestive of a right ventricular outflow tract (RVOT) focus. By conventional dictum, the benign diagnosis here is idiopathic RVOT arrhythmia.[1] In spite of its infrequent association with malignant ventricular fibrillation, prognosis is generally good and radiofrequency ablation may be curative.[1–3] The main differential diagnosis is AC, widely perceived to be a rare disease of youth, associated with sudden cardiac death (SCD) and heart failure.

This traditional view of AC has proved tenacious, although 2 decades of research have overturned many of its central tenets. With a prevalence of 1 in 1,000 and likely clinical under-recognition, AC is not rare.[4] Nor does it present exclusively in youth and middle age. On the contrary, there is accumulating evidence of age-related expression, implying that late-onset disease may simply be underdiagnosed.[5–8] AC is most commonly inherited as an autosomal-dominant trait, but the impetus to evaluate relatives lags behind that in hypertrophic cardiomyopathy, in which familial evaluation is standard practice. Prospective follow-up of familial cohorts with AC has revealed favorable outcomes in most, contrasting with an annual appropriate discharge rate of 5% to 8% among index cases with implantable cardioverter defibrillators (ICDs).[9–11]

CHANGING PERSPECTIVES ON AC

In the classic natural history of AC, regional right ventricular disease progresses to isolated right

Disclosures: The authors have no conflicts of interest to declare.
SSC and PS are supported by the British Heart Foundation. GQ is supported by a PhD Fellowship from the University "La Sapienza" of Rome and by a European Society of Cardiology Research Training Fellowship. WJM is supported by EU 5th Framework Program Research & Technology Development – QLG1-CT-2000-01091 and by British Heart Foundation Program Grant RG/04/010. University College London receives a proportion of funding from the Department of Health's NIHR Biomedical Research Centers funding scheme.
[a] Department of Cardiovascular Medicine, University College London, London WC1E 6JF, UK
[b] Department of Epidemiology, Imperial College, St Mary's Campus, Norfolk Place, London W2 1NY, UK
[c] The Heart Hospital, University College London Hospitals NHS Trust, 16-18 Westmoreland Street, London W1G 8PH, UK
[d] Department of Cardiology, S. Andrea Hospital, University "La Sapienza", Rome, Italy
* Corresponding author. The Heart Hospital, University College London Hospitals NHS Trust, 16-18 Westmoreland Street, London W1G 8PH, UK.
E-mail address: william.mckenna@uclh.nhs.uk

Card Electrophysiol Clin 3 (2011) 205–215
doi:10.1016/j.ccep.2011.02.011
1877-9182/11/$ – see front matter

heart failure before the onset of left ventricular involvement. It is now recognized that AC represents one extreme of a broader disease spectrum. There are biventricular and left-dominant variants characterized by early left-sided disease.[12,13] Clinical markers of left ventricular involvement include inverted T-waves in the left ventricular leads, ventricular arrhythmia of right bundle branch block configuration, and regional or global left ventricular dilation or dysfunction, which mirror the classic right-sided changes.[12,13] Late gadolinium enhancement on cardiovascular magnetic resonance (CMR) is a marker for the presence of fibrous or fibrofatty substrate on histology.[14,15] Nonclassic disease subtypes are distinguished from dilated cardiomyopathy primarily on clinical grounds, by recognizing a propensity toward arrhythmia that exceeds the degree of morphologic abnormality and systolic impairment.[7,13] The proposed designation of AC underscores not only the breadth of disease expression but the myriad possible presentations, which exceed arrhythmia of right ventricular origin.[7,12]

This contemporary perspective on AC has its foundations in the investigation of families. The disease may present with SCD, providing a clinical mandate for presymptomatic screening of relatives, despite certain practical limitations. Reduced penetrance, coupled with evaluation of small nuclear families in clinical practice, may lead to underestimation of heritable disease. The other major impediment is variable expressivity, with family members commonly showing milder phenotypes. Incomplete disease expression in relatives is the primary reason that family history alone, even a detailed multigeneration pedigree, is no substitute for prospective evaluation in establishing inheritance. The challenge lies in differentiating mild or atypical manifestations in relatives from phenocopies (nonhereditary states that mimic the genetically determined disease) without definite knowledge of gene-carrier status.

In the past decade, elucidation of the genetic etiology of AC has shed light on the cellular and molecular mechanisms underlying the disease. In addition to its diagnostic utility, genetic testing has provided a more stringent benchmark for analysis of heterogeneous disease expression. Genotype-phenotype correlation has built on earlier familial studies to redefine the natural history of the disease and its pleiomorphic manifestations.[8,16–18] This review provides an up-to-date summary of the genetics of AC as a prelude to discussion of its effect on clinical diagnosis, prognostication, and therapy.

GENETICS OF AC

The clinical features of AC are diverse and nonspecific, complicating diagnosis and determination of severity. For example, an individual might have nonsustained ventricular tachycardia (VT), inverted T-waves in the right precordial leads, late potentials on signal-averaged ECG, and a family history of SCD, but minimal structural abnormalities. In contrast, other patients might have prominent ventricular dysfunction and aneurysms, but lack ECG changes or documented ventricular arrhythmia. The Task Force diagnostic guidelines incorporate multiple aspects of the disease, subdivided into major and minor criteria according to their specificity. The criteria have been valuable in standardizing clinical diagnosis of AC, but in their original 1994 incarnation lacked sensitivity for early and familial disease.[19] At least 2 major familial studies reported borderline status in 10% to 11% of relatives, who had characteristic clinical abnormalities that were insufficient, in isolation, for Task Force diagnosis.[7,8,16] Revisions have since been made, although the 2010 version is still under evaluation in varied clinical settings.[20]

A DISEASE OF THE DESMOSOME

From the standpoint of mutation analysis, uncertainty as to whether family members are genetically affected complicates both linkage mapping and candidate gene sequencing. Consequently, more than a decade elapsed from observation of familial clustering in AC[21] to isolation of the first disease-causing gene in 2000.[22] In the interim, multiple disease loci were mapped, but the causal genes remained elusive. The successful strategy involved genetic studies in a highly penetrant form with a readily discernible phenotype: Naxos syndrome. The characteristic triad of AC, palmoplantar keratoderma, and woolly hair was first described in families from the Greek island of Naxos, where its name originates. Its prevalence there exceeds 1 in 1000 in spite of autosomal-recessive inheritance, raising suspicion of a founder effect.[23,24] The skin and hair phenotype is expressed from infancy, facilitating recognition of affected individuals, whereas cardiac symptoms typically develop during adolescence. Linkage analysis mapped the disease locus to 17q21,[24] where a homozygous 2-base-pair deletion in the plakoglobin gene was subsequently detected.[22]

The junctional plakoglobin gene (*JUP*) encodes a component of desmosomes: the specialized adhesive junctions that enable cardiac and epithelial tissue to withstand mechanical stress.[25] Shortly thereafter, a homozygous mutation in another desmosomal gene (desmoplakin, DSP) was implicated in Carvajal syndrome. The cutaneous features of Carvajal syndrome are similar to Naxos disease, but the cardiac phenotype most closely resembles the left-dominant and biventricular subtypes of AC.[26,27] Desmoplakin also became the first gene implicated in autosomal-dominant AC in 2002, paving the way for screening of related desmosomal components using a candidate gene approach. Rare sequence variants in plakophilin-2 (PKP2), desmoglein-2 (DSG2), and desmocollin-2 (DSC2) have since been isolated in index cases and families with AC (**Table 1**).[18,28–36]

EXTRADESMOSOMAL GENES

Three of the genes hitherto linked to AC do not encode desmosomal proteins. Mutations in the cardiac ryanodine receptor gene *RyR2* cause a distinct clinical entity, ARVD2, characterized by juvenile SCD and effort-induced polymorphic VT. Affected individuals do not develop the typical electrocardiographic features of AC, and structural abnormalities are limited to mild regional wall motion abnormalities of the right ventricle, with maintained global systolic function. The ARVD2 phenotype bears closer resemblance to familial catecholaminergic polymorphic VT, which is also associated with mutations in RyR2.[37,38]

Mutations in the untranslated regions of transforming growth factor (*TGF-β3*), predicted to result in overexpression, have been identified in one large family and a single, unrelated proband with ARVD1 linkage (locus 14q24.3). The protein product stimulates production of components of the extracellular matrix and, in vitro, modulates expression of desmosomal genes. Two ARVD1

Table 1
Genetic causes of AC

Gene	Encoded Protein	Chromosomal Location	OMIM[a]	Mode of Inheritance	Comment
Desmosomal					
JUP	Plakoglobin	17q21	#173325	Autosomal dominant Autosomal recessive	 Naxos disease (nonepidermolytic palmoplantar keratoderma, woolly hair; OMIM #601214)
DSP	Desmoplakin	6p24	#125647	Autosomal dominant Autosomal recessive	 Carvajal syndrome (dilated cardiomyopathy, keratoderma, woolly hair; OMIM #605676)
PKP2	Plakophilin-2	12p11	#602861	Autosomal dominant Autosomal recessive	—
DSG2	Desmoglein-2	18q12	#125671	Autosomal dominant	—
DSC2	Desmocollin-2	18q12	#125645	Autosomal dominant Autosomal recessive	 Mild palmoplantar keratoderma, woolly hair
Nondesmosomal					
RYR2	Cardiac ryanodine receptor	1q42–q43	#180902	Autosomal dominant	Catecholaminergic polymorphic VT
TGF-β3	Transforming growth factor β3	14q23–q24	#190230	Autosomal dominant	—
TMEM43	Transmembrane protein 43	3p25	#612048	Autosomal dominant	—

[a] OMIM, Online Mendelian Inheritance in Man, http://www.ncbi.nlm.nih.gov/omim/.

kindreds lacked mutations in TGF-β3, precluding definitive inferences concerning its overall contribution to AC.[25,39,40]

A missense mutation in the gene encoding transmembrane protein 43 (*TMEM43*) has been identified in the Newfoundland founder population.[6] The associated phenotype, termed ARVD5, is characterized by ventricular extrasystoles, right precordial R-wave reduction on the 12-lead ECG, early and prominent left ventricular involvement, and relatively high incidence of SCD and heart failure in survivors. Little is presently known regarding the function of the TMEM43 protein product, although the gene contains a response element for peroxisome proliferator-activated receptor-γ (PPARγ), an adipogenic transcription factor, which has the potential to promote the characteristic myocardial fatty replacement of AC.[6] PPARγ is also involved in epithelial cell differentiation, consistent with the premise that impaired desmosomal function may be the final common pathway in AC.

DIAGNOSTIC USEFULNESS OF GENOTYPING

Prospective evaluation of the relatives of index cases with AC remains the remit of referral centers for several reasons. Optimal imaging requires operators and readers who specialize in the disease, handling large numbers of cases on a regular basis.[14,41] Both echocardiography and CMR are best performed with dedicated protocols that are more intensive than routine examinations. Interpretation of wall motion abnormalities in the thin-walled, trabeculated, pyramidal right ventricle is not straight forward.[41] Both CMR and CT offer tissue characterization, but normal penetration of epicardial fat into the myocardium may be difficult to distinguish from the pathologic fatty replacement of AC. Although these challenges are also inherent to the investigation of index cases, they are further complicated in family screening programs by limited and atypical phenotypic expression and the current lack of consensus diagnostic criteria for nonclassic subtypes. Consequently, both general cardiologists and electrophysiologists may prefer to recommend family screening at specialist units and focus their own efforts on establishing the diagnosis in putative index cases. A pivotal issue, therefore, is whether genetic analysis might facilitate diagnosis when other investigations are borderline.[38]

CONFIRMATORY CLINICAL DIAGNOSIS IN INDEX CASES

Confirmatory testing has been defined as the use of genotyping to corroborate clinical suspicion of disease in an index case. As such, it should be distinguished from genetic screening of relatives. The primary clinical precedent comes from Huntington disease; in a patient with the characteristic cognitive, motor, or psychiatric symptoms, the presence of an expanded trinucleotide repeat on the short arm of chromosome 4 is diagnostic.[38] The use of genotyping to clinch a clinical diagnosis is less well established in inherited cardiovascular disease, although its appeal is wide. In the present context, the most topical question might be: does genetic analysis facilitate the differentiation of AC from idiopathic RVOT arrhythmia?

The answer is more complicated than immediately apparent. Between 30% and 60% of cases of AC harbor rare sequence variants in 1 of the 5 desmosomal genes (*JUP*, *DSP*, *PKP2*, *DSG2*, and *DSC2*).[38,42] *PKP2, DSP,* and *DSG2* account for most isolated variants.[38] The contribution of mutations in *TMEM43* to disease outside the Newfoundland population is unresolved. Nevertheless, both the estimated success rate of genotyping and the genetic profile vary according to the cohort. Founder effects contribute to the 70% reported prevalence of PKP2 mutations among AC families in the Netherlands.[42] Early data also suggest that *PKP2* disease is more likely to follow the classic, right-dominant course.[30] Cohorts recruited predominantly from index cases with arrhythmia of right ventricular origin may therefore show a preponderance of *PKP2* variants (~40%–50%).[29] In contrast, the London and Padua cohorts include nonclassic subtypes in their case mix and have a higher prevalence of *DSP* mutations.[38]

Because ~50% of cases of AC do not harbor a defect in a known causal gene, genotyping can never exclude the disease. In a patient with features compatible with AC (such as arrhythmia of right ventricular origin) the presence of a rare variant in 1 of the known causal genes raises the index of suspicion. It may not, however, be diagnostic per se. This lack of a certainty is down to the marked allelic heterogeneity shown by the main desmosomal genes and the high prevalence of private mutations.[38] If the variant identified has been previously reported and causally linked to AC, then the diagnosis is confirmed. Mutation screening may, however, yield a novel variant. In the latter scenario, causality must first be demonstrated by some combination of in vitro functional studies, in silico molecular modeling (to determine predicted effect on the gene product), and clinical correlation within families.

The importance of this process has been highlighted by accumulating evidence that many published mutations in *PKP2* may not be causal in isolation. Three missense changes originally believed to be causal were subsequently identified in 0.5% to 1.4% of healthy controls.[43] Of these variants, 2 (PKP2-D26N and PKP2-V587I) do not alter the polarity of the affected amino acid, whereas the third (PKP2-S140F) is not highly conserved across species. Nevertheless, all 3 were selectively enriched in AC cases compared with controls, suggesting a contributory rather than a causal role. Awareness has also been growing that PKP2 mutations, including nonsense and frameshift changes, are frequently nonpenetrant in family members.[5] Among a series of 38 index cases with AC harboring PKP2 defects, 9 were compound heterozygotes, whereas 16 (42%) were double heterozygotes, with an additional rare variant in another desmosomal gene.[44] Early data suggest, as might be expected, that disease severity is greater in digenic patients.[45] These findings further emphasize the need to screen every coding region of all known disease-causing genes, even after identification of a putative pathogenic mutation.

As the most prevalent genetic change observed in AC, *PKP2* variants require guarded interpretation. Doubts have also surfaced regarding the pathogenicity of certain variants in *DSG2*. The E713K, V56M, V158G, and V920G alleles in *DSG2*, initially presumed causal, have since been identified in healthy control individuals at frequencies of 13.9%, 0.5%, 2.2%, and 0.8%, respectively.[46] Nevertheless, among a series of 538 patients with dilated cardiomyopathy, 13 (2.4%) were carriers of DSG2-V56M, a significant overrepresentation compared with controls. Immunostaining and electron microscopy of explanted left ventricular myocardium from these patients revealed irregularly shaped intercalated disks and, in a homozygous carrier, shortening of the desmosome. *DSG2*-V56M therefore seems to be a susceptibility allele for dilated cardiomyopathy, and potentially for AC.[47] The same may be true of many desmosomal gene variants: instead of being necessary and sufficient for AC in any particular carrier, they may influence the risk of disease development.

What, then, is the role of genetic analysis in the diagnosis of index cases? A positive result from mutation screening is supportive but not always confirmatory, whereas a negative result is noncontributory. Even in tertiary referral centers, genotyping is not a routine component of the initial evaluation for AC. In years to come, however, genotyping may become indispensible in this setting, because of its capacity to detect the disease in its earliest stages. Timely diagnosis is of particular importance in AC because of the characteristic concealed phase, when clinical abnormalities are subtle or absent, but individuals may nonetheless be at risk of SCD.

A remarkable example of concealed AC has been reported in a child homozygous for the Naxos mutation. The cutaneous phenotype was fully expressed from infancy; by the age of 5 years, a cardiovascular evaluation had revealed more than 14,000 ventricular extrasystoles/24 hours, mainly of right ventricular origin, and epsilon waves. After her death from leukemia 2 years later, her heart appeared grossly normal on postmortem. Extensive histologic assessment failed to identify any fibrofatty atrophy of the myocardium, leukemic infiltrates, or chemotherapy-related injury. Electron microscopy and immunofluorescence revealed reduced localization of mutant plakoglobin to intercellular junctions, diminished expression of the gap junction protein connexin-43, and a decrease in the number and size of gap junctions.[48]

Gap junction remodeling has since been observed in Carvajal syndrome and autosomal-dominant AC, but always in the setting of histologically overt disease.[49,50] Reduction in the immunoreactive signal for plakoglobin at intercalated disks is a recurrent feature in myocardium from patients with AC, a molecular signature that has potential as a diagnostic test. In a recent series of 11 patients with AC and an equal number of control individuals, immunohistochemical analysis had a sensitivity of 91% and a specificity of 82% for the disease.[51] Yet the Naxos case remains unique in that a significant burden of ventricular arrhythmia and typical ECG changes were documented in the absence of morphologic and histologic disease. Because imaging abnormalities are lacking in such a scenario, genotyping is the sole noninvasive test that might establish a diagnosis of AC. Nevertheless, the genetic complexity of AC must be better understood before genetic analysis can assume a primary diagnostic role.

POSTMORTEM DIAGNOSIS IN INDEX CASES

Molecular genetic analysis and genotype-phenotype correlation studies have wrought a sea change in our perception of AC. Fibrofatty atrophy of the myocardium, once considered the defining feature of the disease, seems now to arise relatively late in its evolution, preceded and perhaps instigated by characteristic molecular changes. Yet many questions remain unanswered. For instance: if genetically affected individuals can develop frequent ventricular extrasystoles without underlying histologic substrate, might they also suffer SCD? Should SCD occur in the prehistology stage, a standard postmortem examination, no matter how rigorous, would be negative, yielding a default diagnosis of sudden arrhythmic death syndrome (SADS).

Evaluation of the surviving relatives of individuals with SADS elicits a diagnosis of AC in 7% to 9% of cases.[52,53] The missed diagnosis in the index cases is generally attributed to incomplete or nonexpert postmortem examination, or mild histopathologic abnormalities that were either insufficient to fulfill diagnostic criteria or beneath the notice even of an expert.[52] A proportion of these cases may, however, represent prehistologic SCD. Establishing this requires extensive examination of both the whole heart and its sections, followed by a molecular autopsy.[54] For AC, this second-line assessment might include electron microscopy and immunohistochemistry, seeking evidence of diminished plakoglobin signal at the intercalated disk and, perhaps, gap junction remodeling. Although the latter occurs in a variety of settings, including ischemic heart disease and dilated cardiomyopathy, its presence in a histologically normal heart would be noteworthy and perhaps supportive of AC.[51]

The usefulness of diminished plakoglobin signal for the detection of early AC is unresolved. Diminished plakoglobin signal at the intercalated disk was present in the original case of the Naxos child, but the subsequent work was performed on myocardial samples from patients with a definitive clinical or pathologic diagnosis.[48,51] Data from animal models are too limited to be conclusive. At the age of 10 months, heterozygous plakoglobin-deficient mice had right ventricular dilation, systolic dysfunction, and spontaneous ventricular extrasystoles.[55] Histology, however, remained unremarkable, as did the appearance of the desmosomal junction on microscopy. Immunohistochemistry failed to show any alteration in the distribution or density of connexin-43 compared with wild-type littermates.[55] The observed ventricular arrhythmia cannot therefore be ascribed to gap junction remodeling; there has been speculation about mechanoelectric feedback as a possible mechanism.[38] Nevertheless, the study of $JUP^{+/-}$ mice preceded development of the new immunohistochemistry protocol, so specific data regarding the plakoglobin signal at intercalated disks are lacking. More recently, transgenic mice overexpressing DSG2-N271S were shown to have ultrastructurally normal desmosomes, even in the presence of sarcolemmal disruption and myocyte necrosis. The distribution of plakoglobin at the intercalated disks was apparently normal.[56]

If even the molecular signature of AC lacks sensitivity for early disease, but arrhythmogenicity is sufficient to cause SCD on occasion, then genotyping might prove the only recourse for diagnosis. Screening of archived tissue from sudden unexplained death syndrome (SUDS) cases for ion channel genes is described, but the desmosomal genes have been less obvious targets.[54] Genetic analysis in a postmortem setting would be attended the same limitations as its use in confirmatory clinical diagnosis and awaits resolution of the complex genetics of AC. Its applications might ultimately include pathologically overt cases, to facilitate subsequent family assessment; idiopathic myocardial fibrosis, which may be part of the same spectrum as AC; SUDS; and isolated myocarditis, which occurred early in the disease course of DSG2-N271S mice and was the predominant pathologic feature in a 15-year-old boy with a *DSP* mutation who suffered SCD.[13,17,56]

PREDICTIVE TESTING IN RELATIVES

In some families with AC, notably those with nonsense/frameshift mutations in *DSP*, penetrance approaches 100% from late adolescence or adulthood.[13,17,18] In contrast, the low pathogenicity of PKP2 variants, coupled with the presence of unidentified contributory alleles, may obscure Mendelian inheritance patterns in other pedigrees. Predictive testing of relatives is the main indication for genetic analysis in AC, but its implementation suffers from most of the caveats that apply to confirmatory testing.

Before any novel variant is used for predictive testing in a family, it is imperative to determine whether it is necessary and sufficient for clinical disease. Demonstrating cosegregation with clinical status may be challenging because phenotypic expression is highly variable and atypical disease forms are difficult to distinguish from phenocopies. As such, it should not be the sole means of determining pathogenicity unless the results are unequivocal. Conversely, performing functional studies for every private allele may impose on resources to the point of being impractical.

Without definite proof of pathogenicity, a relative with a benign variant may be subjected to protracted clinical follow-up. This scenario is, however, less troubling than the alternative. Complex trait genetics have underscored the contribution of sequence variants with modest effects; some of these patients may show formes frustes of the disease. Furthermore, lifelong periodic rescreening is recommended in families without identifiable mutations, and the recommended workup for asymptomatic individuals is noninvasive. Relatives followed up for noncausal variants therefore experience little change in their management. Where there is no obligation to disclose the results of genetic testing to insurance companies, the main personal repercussion for misdiagnosed carriers may be the false belief that they have a 50% chance of transmitting the allele to their children. The genetic counseling process should emphasize that it is the allele, rather than the disease, that is transmitted, particularly in families with apparently low penetrance. Proscriptive reproductive counseling is generally not justified in AC when treatment options are available.[38]

The more concerning possibility is that relatives are falsely reassured that they do not harbor the family mutation, when the allele being tested is merely a modifier, and the culprit primary mutation has yet to be identified. For this reason, symptoms or borderline clinical abnormalities in a family member should not be dismissed as unrelated to AC unless the genetic diagnosis is incontestable.

A definitive genetic diagnosis allows cascade screening of the family. In the setting of monogenic autosomal-dominant inheritance, ~50% of those tested are negative for the primary mutation, affording them a lifetime of reassurance and obviating the need to offer genetic analysis to their children.[38] Resources may be targeted toward evaluation and follow-up of proven gene carriers. So appealing is this prospect that there is a strong argument for more widespread integration of genotyping into clinical practice despite the difficulties. Until recently, the major technical obstacle has been the prohibitive costs of screening a genomic region exceeding 40 kb by conventional direct sequencing.[38] With increased availability of cost-effective, high-throughput genomics, genotyping may rapidly become routine at any center that performs family evaluation for AC.

ROLE OF GENOTYPING IN PROGNOSTICATION

The main impact of genotyping in prognostication has been to draw attention to the limitations of our present knowledge base. Proposed predictors of arrhythmic events in AC include syncope, VT with hemodynamic compromise, severe right ventricular dilation, left ventricular dysfunction, and male sex.[9–11,57] Nevertheless, most of the patients in existing studies underwent ICD placement for previous ventricular fibrillation arrest, sustained VT, or syncope. Units specializing in family evaluation have long been aware of the growing cohort of affected relatives with incomplete phenotypes, for whom risk stratification protocols derived from index cases with advanced disease are not applicable. Although outcomes in familial disease are generally favorable, some affected relatives experience events in the absence of conventional risk factors.[8,17] The advent of genetic testing has led to increased identification of individuals about whom still less is currently known: gene carriers with minimal disease expression.

The optimal timing of predictive genetic testing for AC remains unresolved. Although there is no convincing justification for prenatal genotyping, many parents choose to have their children tested in infancy. Age-dependent expression is well documented for carriers of PKP2 variants and in the Newfoundland founder population, who harbor a missense variant in TMEM43; clinical observation suggests that it is a phenomenon common to all known disease-causing genes.[5,6] Childhood onset of clinical disease is therefore rare but not unheard of. It is more common for the disease to manifest during the pubertal growth spurt or in adulthood. As reported in the Newfoundland cohort, the disease may become penetrant in the seventh and eighth decades of life.[6] Delayed onset is not an assurance of benign disease; there have been reports of patients experiencing a first arrhythmic event after middle age.[13,17] Lifelong follow-up is therefore indicated for all gene carriers, but risk stratification remains largely unresolved.

Part of the challenge is that index cases and relatives offer different windows on the same disease. For example, subtype discordance has been reported in 67% of families.[12] The relatives of index cases with classic right-dominant disease often show a biventricular subtype. But whereas nonclassic disease in family member might be dismissed as phenocopy, genotype-phenotype correlation studies are free from this limitation. Cases of left-dominant AC had been reported for at least a decade before its relation to AC became accepted, as a direct corollary of its recognition in a family with a *DSP* mutation.[13,16,58,59] Prognostication in the nonclassic subtypes is, however, still to be addressed. Compounding this challenge is the observation that relatives frequently have early disease, which behaves differently from the overt form, perhaps because the mechanisms underlying arrhythmia are distinct.

The traditional conception of stable macroreentrant circuits arising around islands of fibrofatty tissue remains valid. This mechanism is liable to dominate late in the disease course, and underlies sustained, monomorphic VT, which is inducible on programmed ventricular stimulation and shows entrainment. In contrast, gap junction remodeling and mechanoelectric feedback must be invoked to account for the propensity toward ventricular arrhythmia in prehistologic disease. A third putative mechanism is extension of the disease process to previously unaffected regions of the myocardium. At a cellular level, the key feature is probably acute or subacute myocyte necrosis, which may be accompanied by an inflammatory response.[17] This transient myocarditis may be clinically silent or instigate mild symptomatic flare-ups that punctuate an otherwise stable disease course. Occasionally, however, the result may be an unheralded arrhythmic event. Besides encouraging symptomatic vigilance and periodic reassessment, there is currently no means to ascertain or predict so-called hot phases.[38]

A family history of premature SCD does not seem to be a key indicator of adverse prognosis in AC; on the contrary, index cases and relatives harboring the same causal mutation tend to have different disease courses and outcomes.[8,10,16] Thus, the contribution of primary mutation analysis to prognostication is also likely to be limited.[38] Chain-termination mutations are associated with a higher prevalence of ventricular arrhythmia, non-sustained VT, and left ventricular involvement; there is also some evidence that certain risk factors have reduced predictive capacity in *PKP2* disease.[12,36] Both these findings have advanced our understanding of genotype-phenotype associations, while making little difference to the clinical risk stratification process. In the Newfoundland founder population, the high incidence of arrhythmic events may justify ICD placement based on genotype; but even here, the role of genetic analysis is to facilitate timely diagnosis rather than prognostication.[60] As the complex genetics of AC are gradually unraveled, a comprehensive genomic profile incorporating both primary mutation and modifiers may ultimately prove of greater value in risk prediction.

ROLE OF GENOTYPING IN CLINICAL MANAGEMENT

It has long been accepted that adrenergic stimulation during extreme exertion may trigger ventricular tachyarrhythmia in individuals with underlying cardiovascular disease.[61] For this reason foremost, a diagnosis of any inherited cardiovascular disease results in permanent disqualification from competitive sports. In AC, however, the effects of strenuous activity may be more complex. In heterozygous plakoglobin-deficient mice, endurance exercise accelerated phenotypic maturation, including right ventricular systolic dysfunction.[55] In a cohort of 200 patients with AC, indices of structural severity were increased among the 11 who had been long-term endurance athletes before diagnosis.[12] The genetic cause of AC provides a possible explanation for this observation.

Most of the known disease-causing genes are components of the desmosome, the specialized intercellular junctions that anchor intermediate filaments to the cytoplasmic membrane in adjoining cells, thereby forming a supportive network. Desmosomes are commonly found in tissues exposed to frictional and shear stress, such as the myocardium and epithelium, where they play a key role in imparting mechanical strength, both via intercellular adhesion and through transmission of force between the junctional complex and the intermediate filaments in the cytoskeleton. Hence, a desmosomal gene mutation may compromise either cell-cell adhesion, or intermediate filament function, or both, depending on its precise location and effect on protein structure and function.[25,38] The right ventricle may be particularly vulnerable to impaired cell adhesion, because of its thin walls and high distensibility, an adaptation to wide physiologic variations in preload. In contrast, defects causing truncation of the C-terminus of desmosomal proteins may result in dominant and/or severe left ventricular involvement through disruption of intermediate filament binding, a mechanism that may take on particular importance in desmoplakin mutants because of its direct interaction with desmin.[12,62]

This model successfully accounts for many aspects of the clinical phenotype of AC, including age-related penetrance, which may be a consequence of accumulated wear and tear, and the finding of structurally severe disease in long-term endurance athletes.[25] It also presents a challenge to the cardiologist who, in the absence of additional confirmatory data, must weigh the merits of more stringent exercise restrictions against the benefits of an active lifestyle in the prevention of coronary artery disease. The purported role of mechanical stress in disease progression also suggests that β-blocker therapy might have benefits beyond arrhythmia suppression. Long-term follow-up and intervention studies in large cohorts are needed to address many of these questions.

SUMMARY

Between 30% and 60% of individuals with AC harbor a rare sequence variant in a desmosomal gene. The genetics of AC are, however, more complex than previously appreciated. Some of the alleles identified are of low pathogenicity and emerging evidence suggests that more than 1 hit may be required for clinical disease expression in many cases. These considerations complicate mutation screening in AC, although both confirmatory and predictive testing are feasible when the genetic diagnosis is definitive. Genotype-phenotype correlation analysis has built on family studies to expand the recognized disease spectrum and redefine its natural history. Early exploration of the mechanisms underlying ventricular arrhythmia has shed light on the differences between concealed and overt disease. The desmosomal model of AC points to lifestyle measures and therapies that reduce mechanical stress on the heart.

REFERENCES

1. Arya A, Piorkowski C, Sommer P, et al. Idiopathic outflow tract tachycardias: current perspectives. Herz 2007;32:218–25.
2. Noda T, Shimizu W, Taguchi A, et al. Malignant entity of idiopathic ventricular fibrillation and polymorphic ventricular tachycardia initiated by premature extrasystoles originating from the right ventricular outflow tract. J Am Coll Cardiol 2005; 46:1288–94.
3. Viskin S, Antzelevitch C. The cardiologists' worst nightmare sudden death from "benign" ventricular arrhythmias. J Am Coll Cardiol 2005;46:1295–7.
4. Peters S, Trummel M, Meyners W. Prevalence of right ventricular dysplasia-cardiomyopathy in a non-referral hospital. Int J Cardiol 2004;97:499–501.
5. Dalal D, James C, Devanagondi R, et al. Penetrance of mutations in plakophilin-2 among families with arrhythmogenic right ventricular dysplasia/cardiomyopathy. J Am Coll Cardiol 2006;48: 1416–24.
6. Merner ND, Hodgkinson KA, Haywood AF, et al. Arrhythmogenic right ventricular cardiomyopathy type 5 is a fully penetrant, lethal arrhythmic disorder caused by a missense mutation in the TMEM43 gene. Am J Hum Genet 2008;82:809–21.
7. Sen-Chowdhry S, Morgan RD, Chambers JC, et al. Arrhythmogenic cardiomyopathy: etiology, diagnosis, and treatment. Annu Rev Med 2010;61: 233–53.
8. Nava A, Bauce B, Basso C, et al. Clinical profile and long-term follow-up of 37 families with arrhythmogenic right ventricular cardiomyopathy. J Am Coll Cardiol 2000;36:2226–33.
9. Wichter T, Paul M, Wollmann C, et al. Implantable cardioverter/defibrillator therapy in arrhythmogenic right ventricular cardiomyopathy: single-center experience of long-term follow-up and complications in 60 patients. Circulation 2004;109:1503–8.
10. Corrado D, Leoni L, Link MS, et al. Implantable cardioverter-defibrillator therapy for prevention of sudden death in patients with arrhythmogenic right ventricular cardiomyopathy/dysplasia. Circulation 2003;108:3084–91.
11. Roguin A, Bomma CS, Nasir K, et al. Implantable cardioverter-defibrillators in patients with arrhythmogenic right ventricular dysplasia/cardiomyopathy. J Am Coll Cardiol 2004;43:1843–52.
12. Sen-Chowdhry S, Syrris P, Ward D, et al. Clinical and genetic characterization of families with arrhythmogenic right ventricular dysplasia/cardiomyopathy provides novel insights into patterns of disease expression. Circulation 2007;115:1710–20.
13. Sen-Chowdhry S, Syrris P, Prasad SK, et al. Left-dominant arrhythmogenic cardiomyopathy: an under-recognized clinical entity. J Am Coll Cardiol 2008;52:2175–87.
14. Sen-Chowdhry S, Prasad SK, Syrris P, et al. Cardiovascular magnetic resonance in arrhythmogenic right ventricular cardiomyopathy revisited: comparison with task force criteria and genotype. J Am Coll Cardiol 2006;48:2132–40.
15. Tandri H, Saranathan M, Rodriguez ER, et al. Noninvasive detection of myocardial fibrosis in arrhythmogenic right ventricular cardiomyopathy using delayed-enhancement magnetic resonance imaging. J Am Coll Cardiol 2005;45:98–103.
16. Hamid MS, Norman M, Quraishi A, et al. Prospective evaluation of relatives for familial arrhythmogenic right ventricular cardiomyopathy/dysplasia reveals a need to broaden diagnostic criteria. J Am Coll Cardiol 2002;40:1445–50.
17. Bauce B, Basso C, Rampazzo A, et al. Clinical profile of four families with arrhythmogenic right ventricular cardiomyopathy caused by dominant desmoplakin mutations. Eur Heart J 2005;26:1666–75.
18. Norman M, Simpson M, Mogensen J, et al. Novel mutation in desmoplakin causes arrhythmogenic left ventricular cardiomyopathy. Circulation 2005; 112:636–42.
19. McKenna WJ, Thiene G, Nava A, et al. Diagnosis of arrhythmogenic right ventricular dysplasia/cardiomyopathy. Task Force of the Working Group Myocardial and Pericardial Disease of the European Society of Cardiology and of the Scientific Council on Cardiomyopathies of the International Society and Federation of Cardiology. Br Heart J 1994;71: 215–8.
20. Marcus FI, McKenna WJ, Sherrill D, et al. Diagnosis of arrhythmogenic right ventricular cardiomyopathy/ dysplasia. Proposed modification of the task force criteria. Circulation 2010;121:1533–41; and Eur Heart J 2010;31:806–14.
21. Nava A, Thiene G, Canciani B, et al. Familial occurrence of right ventricular dysplasia: a study involving nine families. J Am Coll Cardiol 1988;12:1222–8.
22. McKoy G, Protonotarios N, Crosby A, et al. Identification of a deletion in plakoglobin in arrhythmogenic right ventricular cardiomyopathy with palmoplantar keratoderma and woolly hair (Naxos disease). Lancet 2000;355:2119–24.
23. Protonotarios NI, Tsatsopoulou AA, Gatzoulis KA. Arrhythmogenic right ventricular cardiomyopathy caused by a deletion in plakoglobin (Naxos disease). Card Electrophysiol Rev 2002;6:72–80.

24. Coonar AS, Protonotarios N, Tsatsopoulou A, et al. Gene for arrhythmogenic right ventricular cardiomyopathy with diffuse nonepidermolytic palmoplantar keratoderma and woolly hair (Naxos disease) maps to 17q21. Circulation 1998;97:2049–58.
25. Sen-Chowdhry S, Syrris P, McKenna WJ. Genetics of right ventricular cardiomyopathy. J Cardiovasc Electrophysiol 2005;16:927–35.
26. Norgett EE, Hatsell SJ, Carvajal-Huerta L, et al. Recessive mutation in desmoplakin disrupts desmoplakin-intermediate filament interactions and causes dilated cardiomyopathy, woolly hair and keratoderma. Hum Mol Genet 2000;9:2761–6.
27. Protonotarios N, Tsatsopoulou A. Naxos disease and Carvajal syndrome: cardiocutaneous disorders that highlight the pathogenesis and broaden the spectrum of arrhythmogenic right ventricular cardiomyopathy. Cardiovasc Pathol 2004;13:185–94.
28. Rampazzo A, Nava A, Malacrida S, et al. Mutation in human desmoplakin domain binding to plakoglobin causes a dominant form of arrhythmogenic right ventricular cardiomyopathy. Am J Hum Genet 2002;71:1200–6.
29. Gerull B, Heuser A, Wichter T, et al. Mutations in the desmosomal protein plakophilin-2 are common in arrhythmogenic right ventricular cardiomyopathy. Nat Genet 2004;36:1162–4.
30. Syrris P, Ward D, Asimaki A, et al. Clinical expression of plakophilin-2 mutations in familial arrhythmogenic right ventricular cardiomyopathy. Circulation 2006; 113:356–64.
31. Gandjbakhch E, Fressart V, Bertaux G, et al. Sporadic arrhythmogenic right ventricular cardiomyopathy/dysplasia due to a de novo mutation. Europace 2009;11:379–81.
32. Awad MM, Dalal D, Tichnell C, et al. Recessive arrhythmogenic right ventricular dysplasia due to novel cryptic splice mutation in PKP2. Hum Mutat 2006;27:1157.
33. Pilichou K, Nava A, Basso C, et al. Mutations in desmoglein-2 gene are associated with arrhythmogenic right ventricular cardiomyopathy. Circulation 2006;113:1171–9.
34. Syrris P, Ward D, Asimaki A, et al. Desmoglein-2 mutations in arrhythmogenic right ventricular cardiomyopathy: a genotype-phenotype characterization of familial disease. Eur Heart J 2007;28:581–8.
35. Syrris P, Ward D, Evans A, et al. Arrhythmogenic right ventricular dysplasia/cardiomyopathy associated with mutations in the desmosomal gene desmocollin-2. Am J Hum Genet 2006;79:978–84.
36. Dalal D, Molin LH, Piccini J, et al. Clinical features of arrhythmogenic right ventricular dysplasia/cardiomyopathy associated with mutations in plakophilin-2. Circulation 2006;113:1641–9.
37. Tiso N, Stephan DA, Nava A, et al. Identification of mutations in the cardiac ryanodine receptor gene in families affected with arrhythmogenic right ventricular cardiomyopathy type 2 (ARVD2). Hum Mol Genet 2001;10:189–94.
38. Sen-Chowdhry S, Syrris P, McKenna WJ. Role of genetic analysis in the management of patients with arrhythmogenic right ventricular dysplasia/cardiomyopathy. J Am Coll Cardiol 2007;50: 1813–21.
39. Beffagna G, Occhi G, Nava A, et al. Regulatory mutations in transforming growth factor-beta3 gene cause arrhythmogenic right ventricular cardiomyopathy type 1. Cardiovasc Res 2005;65:366–73.
40. Nattel S, Schott JJ. Arrhythmogenic right ventricular dysplasia type 1 and mutations in transforming growth factor beta3 gene regulatory regions: a breakthrough? Cardiovasc Res 2005;65:302–4.
41. Sen-Chowdhry S, McKenna WJ. The utility of magnetic resonance imaging in the evaluation of arrhythmogenic right ventricular cardiomyopathy. Curr Opin Cardiol 2008;23:38–45.
42. van Tintelen JP, Entius MM, Bhuiyan ZA, et al. Plakophilin-2 mutations are the major determinant of familial arrhythmogenic right ventricular dysplasia/ cardiomyopathy. Circulation 2006;113:1650–8.
43. Christensen AH, Benn M, Tybjaerg-Hansen A, et al. Missense variants in plakophilin-2 in arrhythmogenic right ventricular cardiomyopathy patients: disease-causing or innocent bystanders? Cardiology 2010; 115:148–54.
44. Xu T, Yang Z, Vatta M, et al. Compound and digenic heterozygosity contributes to arrhythmogenic right ventricular cardiomyopathy. J Am Coll Cardiol 2010;55:587–9.
45. Bauce B, Nava A, Beffagna G, et al. Multiple mutations in desmosomal proteins encoding genes in arrhythmogenic right ventricular cardiomyopathy/ dysplasia. Heart Rhythm 2010;7:22–9.
46. Posch MG, Posch MJ, Perrot A, et al. Variations in DSG2: V56M, V158G and V920G are not pathogenic for arrhythmogenic right ventricular dysplasia/ cardiomyopathy. Nat Clin Pract Cardiovasc Med 2008;5:E1.
47. Posch MG, Posch MJ, Geier C, et al. A missense variant in desmoglein-2 predisposes to dilated cardiomyopathy. Mol Genet Metab 2008;95:74–80.
48. Kaplan SR, Gard JJ, Protonotarios N, et al. Remodeling of myocyte gap junctions in arrhythmogenic right ventricular cardiomyopathy due to a deletion in plakoglobin (Naxos disease). Heart Rhythm 2004;1:3–11.
49. Kaplan SR, Gard JJ, Carvajal-Huerta L, et al. Structural and molecular pathology of the heart in Carvajal syndrome. Cardiovasc Pathol 2004;13:26–32.
50. Fidler LM, Wilson GJ, Liu F, et al. Abnormal connexin43 in arrhythmogenic right ventricular cardiomyopathy caused by plakophilin-2 mutations. J Cell Mol Med 2008;13:4219–28.

51. Asimaki A, Tandri H, Huang H, et al. A new diagnostic test for arrhythmogenic right ventricular cardiomyopathy. N Engl J Med 2009;360:1075–84.
52. Behr ER, Dalageorgou C, Christiansen M, et al. Sudden arrhythmic death syndrome: familial evaluation identifies inheritable heart disease in the majority of families. Eur Heart J 2008;29:1670–80.
53. Tan HL, Hofman N, van Langen IM, et al. Sudden unexplained death: heritability and diagnostic yield of cardiological and genetic examination in surviving relatives. Circulation 2005;112:207–13.
54. Chugh SS, Senashova O, Watts A, et al. Postmortem molecular screening in unexplained sudden death. J Am Coll Cardiol 2004;43:1625–9.
55. Kirchhof P, Fabritz L, Zwiener M, et al. Age- and training-dependent development of arrhythmogenic right ventricular cardiomyopathy in heterozygous plakoglobin-deficient mice. Circulation 2006;114: 1799–806.
56. Pilichou K, Remme CA, Basso C, et al. Myocyte necrosis underlies progressive myocardial dystrophy in mouse dsg2-related arrhythmogenic right ventricular cardiomyopathy. J Exp Med 2009;206: 1787–802.
57. Piccini JP, Dalal D, Roguin A, et al. Predictors of appropriate implantable defibrillator therapies in patients with arrhythmogenic right ventricular dysplasia. Heart Rhythm 2005;2:1188–94.
58. Collett BA, Davis GJ, Rohr WB. Extensive fibrofatty infiltration of the left ventricle in two cases of sudden cardiac death. J Forensic Sci 1994;39:1182–7.
59. Gallo P, d'Amati G, Pelliccia F. Pathologic evidence of extensive left ventricular involvement in arrhythmogenic right ventricular cardiomyopathy. Hum Pathol 1992;23:948–52.
60. Hodgkinson KA, Parfrey PS, Bassett AS, et al. The impact of implantable cardioverter-defibrillator therapy on survival in autosomal-dominant arrhythmogenic right ventricular cardiomyopathy (ARVD5). J Am Coll Cardiol 2005;45:400–8.
61. Corrado D, Basso C, Rizzoli G, et al. Does sports activity enhance the risk of sudden death in adolescents and young adults? J Am Coll Cardiol 2003;42: 1959–63.
62. Sen-Chowdhry S, Syrris P, McKenna WJ. Desmoplakin disease in arrhythmogenic right ventricular cardiomyopathy: early genotype-phenotype studies. Eur Heart J 2005;26:1582–4.

Arrhythmogenic Cardiomyopathy Diagnostic Criteria: An Update

Frank I. Marcus, MD

KEYWORDS

- Arrhythmogenic right ventricular cardiomyopathy/dysplasia
- Diagnostic criteria • Genetics

Multiple criteria are needed to diagnose arrhythmogenic cardiomyopathy (AC) because there is no single criterion that is sufficiently specific to reliably establish the diagnosis. Thus, there is no "gold standard."[1] In about 50% of patients, a desmosomal genetic abnormality can be identified. However, even if a desmosomal abnormality is present, it does not indicate that the individual is or will be affected because the penetrance is so variable.[2]

In the early stages the disease may be difficult to differentiate from normal, and in the advanced stage the diagnosis may be obvious. Even so, several diseases such as cardiac sarcoidosis can mimic the clinical presentation of AC.[3]

Usually the patient will come to medical attention for evaluation of palpitations, due to premature ventricular beats (PVBs) or nonsustained ventricular tachycardia.[4] Other clinical presentations are sustained ventricular tachycardia, syncope, or resuscitated sudden death. Evaluation may be requested because of AC in a family member. Uncommonly, the patient can present with right heart failure with or without ventricular arrhythmias.[5] Then the differential diagnosis includes congenital or acquired heart disease that primarily affects the right heart such as atrial septal defect, Ebstein anomaly and congenital or acquired tricuspid regurgitation, primary pulmonary hypertension, or pulmonary hypertension secondary to pulmonary emboli. Rarely, chest trauma with injury to the right heart may cause an aneurysm of the right ventricular (RV) outflow tract that may lead to suspicion of AC. Recognition of the disease has now been extended to patients with desmosomal abnormalities who present with primarily left or biventricular involvement associated with ventricular arrhythmias. This possibility raises the question of whether the disease should be called "arrhythmogenic cardiomyopathy" rather than "arrhythmogenic RV cardiomyopathy."

The original description of the clinical profile of 24 patients with this disease was based on experience with patients in the more advanced stage of the disease, generally unresponsive to antiarrhythmic drugs, who were referred to a tertiary care electrophysiology center for treatment of recurrent ventricular tachycardia.[6] Twenty-one of the 24 patients had electrocardiograms (ECGs) with T-wave inversion in V_1 to V_4. Nine patients had incomplete right bundle branch block (RBBB) and one patient had complete RBBB. Postexcitation or epsilon waves were present in 7 patients. By echocardiogram, the RV/left ventricle (LV) ratio was increased in all patients. The LV size and contractility was normal in all but one patient.

As is common with many newly diagnosed diseases, the index cases with severe disease are followed by those with lesser severity of the disease as well as variations from the original description. In a recent study of 108 newly diagnosed patients with AC, only 30 of 95 (32%) patients had T-wave inversion beyond V_3. Epsilon

Division of Internal Medicine, University of Arizona and Sarver Heart Center, 1501 North Campbell, Room 5153, Tucson, AZ 85724–5037, USA
E-mail address: Fmarcus@shc.arizona.edu

Card Electrophysiol Clin 3 (2011) 217–226
doi:10.1016/j.ccep.2011.02.007
1877-9182/11/$ – see front matter

waves were present in 1 of 95 ECGs, severe wall motion abnormalities by 2-dimensional (2-D) echocardiogram in 44 of 93 (47%), and markedly reduced global RV function in 24 of 85 (28%).[7]

The observation that there were patients with AC who had fewer and less severe clinical features of the disease was soon recognized after the first clinical profile was published in 1982. It became evident that the disease can be exceedingly difficult to diagnose, particularly in those with minimal structural and/or functional alterations of the RV.

This corollary led to the formation of a Task Force that in 1994 proposed major and minor criteria to aid in the diagnosis.[8] This report achieved the goal of standardizing diagnostic criteria. With time and experience, it became evident that these criteria lack diagnostic sensitivity.[9] Therefore, a second Task Force was assembled in 2007 to modify these criteria, and the revised criteria have recently been published (**Table 1**).[10]

Several modifications, particularly those relating to the ECG, deserve emphasis because the 12-lead ECG can alert the physician to strongly suspect this diagnosis. For example, in the 1994 guidelines, ventricular tachycardia with left bundle branch block (LBBB) configuration was considered a minor criterion. It has become evident that patients who have ventricular arrhythmias arising from the right ventricle can be further categorized as those who have LBBB with an inferior axis versus LBBB with a superior axis. In those with LBBB and inferior axis (QRS positive in leads 2, 3, and aVF, and negative in lead aVL), the differential diagnosis is that of RV outflow tract tachycardia (RVOT), a relatively benign condition, and AC, which may have a serious prognosis. Patients with this configuration of ventricular arrhythmia who have T-wave inversion in leads V_1 to V_3 on the standard 12-lead ECG are more likely to have AC than benign idiopathic RVOT. Morin and colleagues[11] recently reported that in patients with ventricular tachycardia of LBBB and inferior QRS axis, there were 35 of 94 (37%) patients with AC who had T-wave inversion in V_1 to V_3, but only 5 of 121 (4%) patients with idiopathic RVOT tachycardia had this ECG finding. Patients who have ventricular ectopy not originating from the RVOT, characterized by LBBB configuration with a superior QRS axis (negative QRS in leads 2, 3, and aVF, and positive in lead aVL) are more likely to have AC. This information is reflected in the revised criteria that categorize ventricular arrhythmias of LBBB configuration with an inferior QRS as a minor criterion while grading those with superior QRS axis as a major criterion. Also, T-wave inversion in leads V_1, V_2, V_3 or beyond is now listed as a major ECG criterion rather than minor. In addition, T-wave inversion beyond V_3 in the presence of RBBB is listed as a new minor criterion, because this finding is uncommon in patients with RBBB who do not have AC.[12]

A new ECG finding considered to be a minor criterion is slurring and delay of the upslope of the QRS complex in V_1, V_2, or V_3 caused by prolonged depolarization in the RV. This criterion is defined as "terminal activation duration of QRS $\geq$55 msecs measured from the nadir of the S wave to the end of the QRS, including R prime in V_1, V_2, or V_3 in the absence of complete RBBB."[13]

The definition of an abnormal signal-averaged ECG has been changed in the modified criteria. In the previous criteria, the standard interpretation of an abnormal signal-averaged ECG was 2 of the 3 abnormal measurements of late potentials. It has been found that there is similar sensitivity and specificity with any one of the three measurements; the filtered QRS duration (fQRS $\geq$114 milliseconds), duration of terminal QRS less than 40 μV (low-amplitude signal $\geq$38 milliseconds), or the root mean squared voltage of the terminal 40 milliseconds (root mean square $\leq$20 μV). The presence of only one abnormal parameter in the absence of QRS duration of 110 milliseconds or more on the standard ECG is now a minor criterion for late potentials in the modified Task Force criteria.

There were no criteria for the diagnosis of AC by magnetic resonance imaging (MRI) in the 1994 guidelines because there was little diagnostic experience with this imaging modality at that time. MRI is now an important diagnostic tool, and specific quantitative measures for the RV have been established by comparing AC probands with a large series of normal individuals.[14,15] Quantitative parameters are also provided for abnormal criteria by echocardiography, and methods to analyze RV angiograms for volume and wall motion abnormalities are now available.[16,17]

In the 1994 Task Force criteria patients with moderate to severe decrease in LV function were excluded. This restriction has been eliminated in the modified criteria because it is clear that patients with desmosomal abnormalities can present with predominant left or biventricular involvement.[18]

Documentation of familial involvement has been clarified. There is also recognition of the relatively newly discovered genetic abnormalities. The presence of a pathogenic mutation probably associated with AC in the proband or family members under evaluation is now recognized as a major criterion.[19]

The new criteria include modified diagnostic terminology. Patients formerly were classified as

Table 1
Comparison of original and revised task force criteria[a]

Original Task Force Criteria	Revised Task Force Criteria	
Global and/or Regional Dysfunction and Structural Alterations	Global and/or Regional Dysfunction and Structural Alterations[a]	
Major	Major (by 2-D echo)	
Severe dilatation and reduction of RV ejection fraction with no (or only mild) LV impairment	Regional RV akinesia, dyskinesia, or aneurysm	
Localized RV aneurysms (akinetic or dyskinetic areas with diastolic bulging)	and one of the following (end diastole):	
Severe segmental dilatation of the RV	Parasternal long-axis view RVOT (PLAX)	$\geq$32 mm
	Corrected for body size (PLAX/BSA)	$\geq$19 mm/m^2
	Parasternal short-axis view RVOT (PSAX)	$\geq$36 mm
	Corrected for body size (PSAX/BSA)	$\geq$21 mm/m^2
	or	
	Fractional area change (FAC)	$\leq$33%
—	Major (by MRI)	
	Regional RV akinesia or dyskinesia or dyssynchronous RV contraction	
	and one of the following:	
	RVEDV/BSA	$\geq$110 ml/m^2 male $\geq$100 ml/m^2 female
	or	
	RVEF	$\leq$40%
—	Major (by RV angiography)	
	Regional RV akinesis, dyskinesis, or aneurysm	
Minor	Minor (by 2D echo)	
Mild global RV dilatation and/or ejection fraction reduction with normal LV	Regional RV akinesia or dyskinesia	
Mild segmental dilatation of the RV	and one of the following (end diastole):	
Regional RV hypokinesia	Parasternal long-axis view RVOT (PLAX)	$\geq$29 to <32 mm
	Corrected for body size (PLAX/BSA)	$\geq$16 to <19 mm/m^{2i}
	Parasternal short-axis view RVOT (PSAX)	$\geq$32 to <36 mm
	Corrected for body size (PSAX/BSA)	$\geq$18 to <21 mm/m^2
	or	
	FAC	>33% to $\leq$40%

(*continued on next page*)

Table 1
(continued)

Original Task Force Criteria	Revised Task Force Criteria
—	Minor (by MRI) Regional RV akinesia or dyskinesia or dyssynchronous RV contraction And one of the following: RVEDV/BSA $\geq$100 to <110 ml/m^2 male; $\geq$90 to <100 ml/m^2 female or RVEF >40% to $\leq$45%
Tissue Characterization of Wall Major Fibrofatty replacement of myocardium on endomyocardial biopsy	Tissue Characterization of Wall Major Residual myocytes <60% by morphometric analysis, (or <50% if estimated), with fibrous replacement of the RV free wall myocardium in at least 1 sample, with or without fatty replacement of tissue
—	Minor Residual myocytes 60%–75% by morphometric analysis, (or 50%–65% if estimated), with fibrous replacement of the RV free wall myocardium in at least 1 sample, with or without fatty replacement of tissue
Repolarization Abnormalities Minor Inverted T waves in right precordial leads (V_2 and V_3) (people aged >12 years, in absence of RBBB)	Repolarization Abnormalities Major Inverted T waves in right precordial leads (V_1, V_2, V_3) or beyond in individuals >14 years old (in the absence of complete RBBB QRS $\geq$120 ms) Minor Inverted T waves in leads V_1 and V_2 in individuals >14 years of age (in the absence of complete RBBB), or in V_4, V_5, or V_6 Inverted T waves in leads V_1, V_2, V_3, and V_4 in individuals >14 years old in the presence of complete RBBB
Depolarization/Conduction Abnormalities Major Epsilon waves or localized prolongation (>110 ms) of the QRS complex in right precordial leads (V_1–V_3)	Depolarization/Conduction Abnormalities Major Epsilon wave (reproducible low amplitude signals between end of QRS complex to onset of the T wave) in the right precordial leads (V_1–V_3)

Minor Late potentials (signal-averaged ECG)	Minor Late potentials by signal-averaged ECG in at least 1 of 3 parameters in the absence of a QRS duration of $\geq$110 ms on the standard ECG Filtered QRS duration (fQRS) $\geq$114 ms Duration of terminal QRS <40 μV (LAS) $\geq$38 ms RMS voltage of terminal 40 ms $\leq$20 μV Terminal activation duration of QRS $\geq$55 ms measured to the end of the QRS, including R prime, in V_1 or V_2 or V_3, in the absence of complete RBBB
Arrhythmias Minor LBBB type ventricular tachycardia (sustained and nonsustained) (ECG, Holter, exercise testing) Frequent ventricular extrasystoles (>1000/24 h) (Holter)	Arrhythmias Major Nonsustained or sustained VT of LBBB morphology with superior axis (negative or indeterminate QRS in II, III, aVF, and positive in aVL) Minor Nonsustained or sustained VT of RV outflow configuration, LBBB morphology with inferior axis (positive QRS in II, III, aVF, and negative in aVL) or of unknown axis Greater than 500 ventricular extrasystoles/24 h by Holter
Family History Major Familial disease confirmed at necropsy or surgery	Family History Major AC confirmed in a first-degree relative who meets current Task Force criteria AC confirmed pathologically at autopsy or surgery in a first-degree relative Identification of a pathogenic mutation[b] categorized as associated or probably associated with AC in the patient under evaluation
Minor Family history of premature sudden death (<35 y) due to suspected AC Family history (clinical diagnosis based on present criteria)	Minor History of AC in a first-degree relative in whom it is not possible or practical to determine if the family member meets current Task Force Criteria Premature sudden death (<35 y) due to suspected AC in a first-degree relative
Diagnostic terminology for original criteria This diagnosis is fulfilled by the presence of 2 major criteria, or 1 major plus 2 minor criteria, or 4 minor criteria from different groups	Diagnostic terminology for revised criteria Definite diagnosis: 2 major criteria, or 1 major and 2 minor criteria, or 4 minor criteria from different categories Borderline: 1 major and 1 minor, or 3 minor criteria from different categories Possible: 1 major, or 2 minor criteria from different categories

Abbreviations: BSA, body surface area; 2-D, 2-dimensional; ECG, electrocardiogram; FAC, fractional area change; LAS, low-amplitude signal; LBBB, left bundle branch block; LV, left ventricle; MRI, magnetic resonance imaging; PLAX, parasternal long axis; PSAX, parasternal short axis; RBBB, right bundle branch block; RMS, root mean square; RV, right ventricle; RVEDV, RV end-diastolic volume; RVEF, RV ejection fraction; RVOT, RV outflow tract tachycardia; VT, ventricular tachycardia.

[a] Hypokinesis is not included in this or subsequent definitions of RV regional wall motion abnormalities for the proposed modified criteria.

[b] A pathogenic mutation is a DNA alteration associated with AC that alters or is expected to alter the encoded protein, is unobserved or rare in a large non-AC control population, and either alters or is predicted to alter the structure or function of the protein or has demonstrated linkage to the disease phenotype in a conclusive pedigree.

Data From Marcus FI, McKenna WJ, Sherrill D, et al. Diagnosis of arrhythmogenic RV cardiomyopathy/dysplasia; proposed modification of the Task Force criteria. Circulation 2010;121:1533–41; Eur Heart J 2010;31:806–14.

affected or not affected, based on meeting Task Force criteria. It is now realized that this sharp division should be changed because there are patients who almost meet the criteria and are thought to be affected. Some of these patients have a desmosomal abnormality. The new terminology for diagnosis consists of definite: 2 major criteria, or 1 major and 2 minor criteria, or 4 minor criteria from different categories; borderline: 1 major and 1 minor, or 3 minor criteria from different categories; possible: 1 major or 2 minor criteria from different categories.

The revised criteria were applied post hoc to 108 newly diagnosed probands enrolled in the Multidisciplinary Study of Right Ventricular Dysplasia, a study supported by the National Institutes of Health.[10] Not including genetic results, of the 28 probands classified as borderline (met some but not all of the original Task Force criteria—ie, 1 major and 1 minor or 3 minor), 16 were reclassified by the new criteria as affected, 5 remained borderline, and 7 were classified as possible AC. Of 7 probands previously classified as unaffected, 4 became possible, 1 became affected, and 2 became borderline. Therefore, the major effect of the revised criteria is to increase the sensitivity of the classification, primarily in probands previously classified as borderline. The sensitivity of the revised criteria is not perfect. For example, 9 of 28 probands classified as borderline by original criteria have gene variants consistent with AC. When genetic abnormalities were not included, the proposed criteria classified 4 as affected, 3 as borderline, and 2 as possible. Including the proposed genetic criteria resulted in all 9 being classified as affected.

It has been observed that family members of probands may have the disease but with reduced penetrance. Family members may have some clinical manifestations of AC and/or the genetic abnormality, but do not meet the new Task Force criteria for probands. Therefore, guidelines have been proposed for family members and have been adopted as part of the modified Task Force criteria.[19] According to these recommendations, in the context of proven AC in a first-degree relative, the diagnosis of familial AC is based on the documentation of one of the following in a family member:

1. T-wave inversion in right precordial leads, V_1, V_2, and V_3 in individuals older than 14 years
2. Late potentials by signal-averaged ECG
3. Ventricular tachycardia of LBBB morphology on ECG, Holter monitor, or during exercise testing, or >200 premature ventricular contractions (PVCs) in 24 hours
4. Mild global dilatation and/or reduction in RV ejection fraction with normal left ventricle or mild segmental dilatation of the right ventricle
5. Regional RV hypokinesis.

A typical AC case and 2 other cases are presented to illustrate that the disease can be difficult to diagnose with certainty. A recent publication provides illustration of the misdiagnosis of AC with resultant inappropriate insertion of an implantable cardioverter defibrillator (ICD).[20]

CASE PRESENTATIONS

Case 1: Typical Case of AC

A 45-year-old woman, previously well, had the sudden onset on rapid heartbeat, lightheadedness, and dizziness. She went to the emergency department where she was diagnosed as having supraventricular tachycardia at a rate of 240 beats/min. This condition was unresponsive to chemical cardioversion, and sinus rhythm was restored with a DC shock. Thereafter she was treated with amiodarone and discharged.

Three months later she had recurrent tachycardia for 12 to 13 hours. In the emergency room an ECG showed wide complex tachycardia of LBBB morphology with superior axis; the rate was 160 beats/min (**Fig. 1**). After cardioversion her ECG showed sinus rhythm. T waves were inverted in the inferior leads as well as in the precordial leads V_1 to V_6 (see **Fig. 1**). A 2-D echocardiogram showed that her LV was normal in size and function; the LV ejection fraction was 65%. However, the RV was moderately dilated with markedly depressed RV function, a fractional area change of 16%. An RV angiogram showed an akinetic area in the subtricuspid region. An ICD was inserted.

Comment

This patient has all the classic features of AC including the ECG, the QRS morphology during ventricular tachycardia, 2-D echocardiographic changes, and RV angiographic abnormalities. She meets the modified Task Force criteria for AC: ECG, T-wave inversion beyond V_3 is a major criterion (Category III, repolarization abnormalities). Ventricular tachycardia of the specific morphology described is also a major criterion (Category V, arrhythmias). Imaging studies showed RV fractional area change of 16% and an akinetic area in the subtricuspid region, which is a major criterion (Category I, imaging). The epsilon wave is also a major criterion (Category IV, repolarization). Therefore the diagnosis is well established according to the modified Task Force criteria.

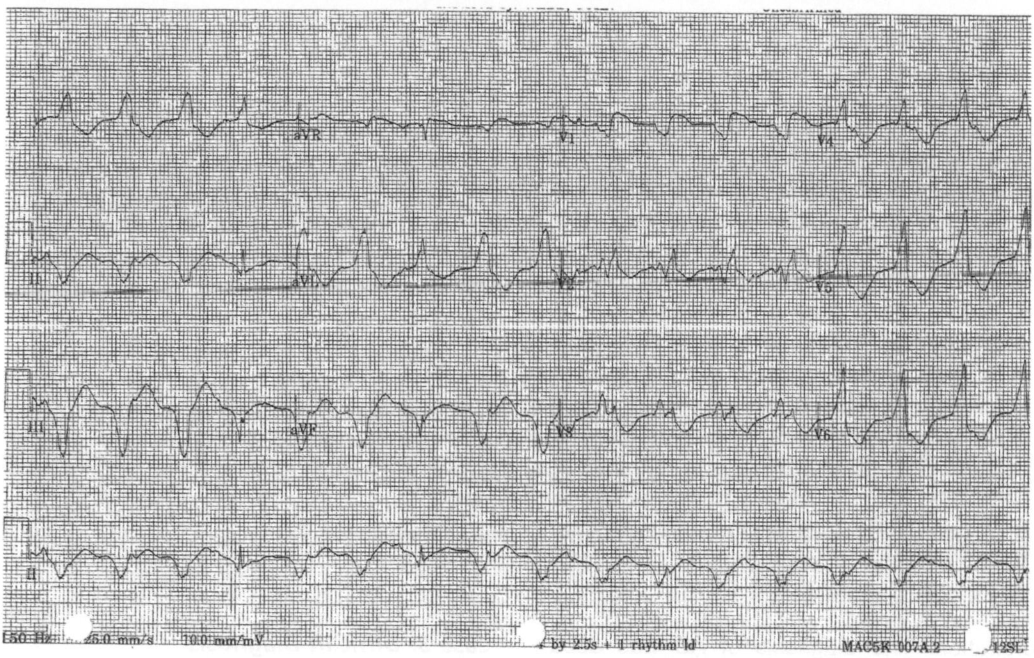

Fig. 1. Patient #1. Ventricular tachycardia has a QRS morphology of LBBB with superior QRS axis negative in leads 2, 3, and aVF and positive in aVL, indicating its origin from the body of the RV and not from the RV outflow tract.

Case 2: Unusual Presentation of AC

This 36-year-old woman was asymptomatic but had cardiac evaluation in 2001 because of family history of heart disease. Although the patient was asymptomatic, the ECG showed sinus rhythm with generalized low QRS voltage (**Fig. 2**). There was poor R-wave progression in the precordial leads and the T waves were inverted in leads V_1 to V_4. In addition, she had PVCs of LBBB morphology with an inferior QRS axis. The QRS axis of the PVCs was isoelectric in aVL. A 2-D echocardiogram showed an enlarged RV. An electrophysiological study was done, but ventricular tachycardia could not be induced with a pacing cycle length of 400 milliseconds with 1, 2, and 3 extra stimuli. Even though the patient was asymptomatic, an ICD was implanted because of the findings suggestive of AC including the ECG and imaging studies. She has not had ventricular tachycardia and her only ICD therapy was inappropriate shocks, due to lead fractures requiring replacement twice over 9 years. In 2006 she had the onset of symptoms of right heart failure that have increased over the subsequent 4 years. Repeated 2-D echocardiograms have shown massive enlargement of the RV and right atrium, with severe tricuspid regurgitation. The tricuspid valve appeared to be tethered, suggestive of primary tricuspid abnormality possibly related to Ebstein malformation. There were no RV wall motion abnormalities observed by serial echoes and MRI studies. RV function was depressed, and the LV size and function appeared to be normal. Cardiac catheterization performed in 2009 documented massive tricuspid regurgitation; the pulmonary pressure was 29/16 mm Hg and the wedge pressure was 8 mm.

Exploratory surgery was performed in 2009 because it was considered she might have an unusual malformation of the tricuspid valve that could be repaired. However, at surgery the RV was thin and was found to have massive scar tissue and only isolated areas of muscle. Biopsy was not performed, and tricuspid repair was not attempted because of the severity of the RV dysfunction. The patient is being considered for cardiac transplantation.

Further details of the cardiac disease in the family history were as follows. One brother died at the age of 33 years after being in a vegetative state for 11 years. He had mitral valve replacement for mitral stenosis at the age of 17. At the age of 23 he had ventricular tachycardia followed by cardiac arrest. He was resuscitated but had irreversible anoxic encephalopathy, and died 11 years later. His echocardiogram showed decreased LV function, pulmonary hypertension, massive RV enlargement, and moderate to severe tricuspid

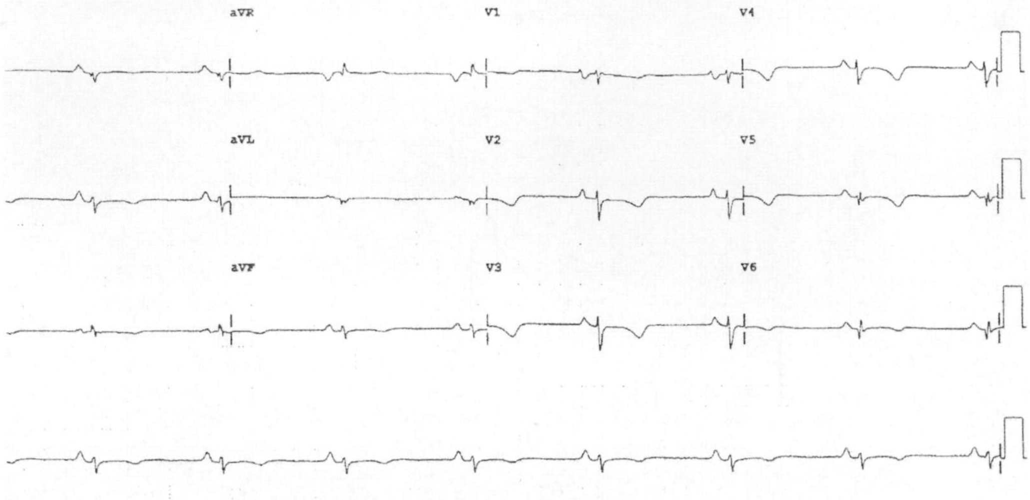

Fig. 2. Patient #2. Twelve-lead ECG showing the typical T-wave inversion in V_1 to V_6.

regurgitation. The diagnosis of AC was documented at autopsy. The patient's other brother was an athlete who at the age of 19 years had ventricular tachycardia, and was diagnosed as having AC. An MRI showed a dilated hypokinetic RV particularly of the anterior wall. There was no LV enlargement. He had an ICD implanted, and had several episodes of ventricular tachycardia terminated by ICD shock. His 12-lead ECG showed T-wave inversion in V_1, V_2, and V_3, and PVCs of LBBB morphology with a superior axis. The diagnosis of AC was substantiated based on his ECG, ventricular tachycardia morphology, and imaging studies.

Comment

This patient was asymptomatic when AC was diagnosed. Clinical findings were dominated by diffuse RV enlargement, but she did not have ventricular tachycardia over a 9-year follow up. She has generalized, severe, RV involvement causing right heart failure and has severe tricuspid regurgitation undoubtedly due to the markedly enlarged and hypokinetic RV. If the family history were unknown or were not well documented, she would not fit the diagnostic criteria for AC because she had only one major criterion, specifically the ECG changes. Although the RV was markedly involved there was no akinesia, dyskinesia, or aneurysm. The imaging criteria would not be met because of the absence of wall motion abnormalities, as noted above. Therefore she would be classified as "possible." With the addition of the strong family history of AC, she would have 2 major criteria and therefore would be classified as "affected."

Case 3: Difficult Diagnosis

This 26-year-old man was first seen at age 17 years. At that time he was a competitive long-distance runner. He had true syncope on 3 occasions, twice after completing a race. One syncopal episode occurred toward the end of the race. He was noted to be cyanotic and lost bladder control. He was not taking any medication. There was no family history of sudden cardiac death. His ECG was normal; the T waves were upright in leads V_1 to V_6. The signal-averaged ECG was unremarkable. An echocardiogram was interpreted as normal. The RV end-diastolic diameter was 2.5 cm (normal 0.8–2 cm). This slight enlargement of the RV was interpreted as consistent with an athletic heart. Cardiac MRI was also interpreted as normal. There was a comment that there was a slight decrease in LV contractility, but overall LV and RV function were normal. On a stress test he exercised for 17 minutes, achieving a heart rate of greater than 200 beats/min. There were no arrhythmias and no symptoms of near syncope. A Holter monitor did not show any arrhythmias. An MRI of the brain was negative. Because of the severity of his symptoms that were unexplained by these tests, an electrophysiologic study was performed. No ventricular arrhythmias were induced before and during isoproterenol infusion with 1, 2, and 3 extra stimuli. Immediately after the electrophysiologic study and while there was venous access, an RV angiogram was done. There was normal RV volume, and global contractility and function. However, in the lateral view there was an unexplained akinetic area in the inferior (diaphragmatic) portion of the RV (**Fig. 3**).

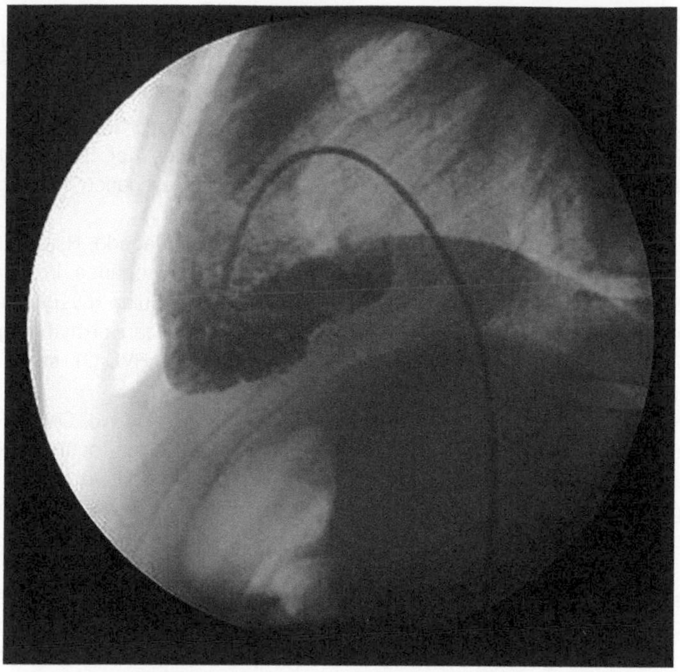

Fig. 3. Patient #3. Lateral view of the RV angiogram. Note the apparent outpouching of the inferior wall.

In summary, this 17-year-old competitive athlete had 3 episodes of syncope. He had a complete cardiac evaluation that was normal except for a localized hypokinetic region in the inferior RV that was seen only in the RV angiogram.

Does this patient have AC? Should he have an ICD? Because the reason for suspecting this diagnosis was a hypokinetic area seen only in the RV angiogram, he was told that there was a suspicion of ventricular structural abnormality. He was advised not to continue with competitive sports. He has been evaluated at intervals for 8 years, with no further syncopal episodes. There has been no change in his ECG, signal-averaged ECG, 2-D echocardiogram, stress test, or cardiac MRI. By the modified Task Force criteria, he would have only one major criterion (category I, regional RV akinesis by angiography). Therefore he would be classified as "possible AC."

This case illustrates the difficulty in diagnosing AC. Of note, the patient did not meet previous Task Force criteria or the modified Task Force criteria for this diagnosis. The cause of his syncopal episodes remains unexplained.

SUMMARY

Multiple criteria are needed to diagnose AC because there is no single criterion ("gold standard") that is sufficiently specific to reliably establish the diagnosis. For these reasons, in 1994 a Task Force proposed major and minor criteria to aid in the diagnosis. This report achieved the goal of standardizing diagnostic criteria. However, with time and experience, it became evident that these criteria lack diagnostic sensitivity. Therefore, a second Task Force was assembled in 2007 to increase sensitivity, but with the important requisite of maintaining specificity.

The 3 cases reported here illustrate the spectrum of patients who are suspected of having AC and the utility of the modified Task Force criteria in the assessment of the disease. The modification of the original Task Force criteria represents a working framework to improve the diagnosis and management of AC.

REFERENCES

1. Corrado D, Thiene G. Diagnosis of right ventricular cardiomyopathy/dysplasia: is there a single gold standard test? J Cardiovasc Electrophysiol 2004; 15:307–9.
2. Xu T, Yang Z, Vatta M, et al. Compound and digenic heterozygosity contributes to arrhythmogenic right ventricular cardiomyopathy. J Am Coll Cardiol 2010;55:587–97.
3. Vasaiwala SC, Finn C, Delpriore J, et al. Prospective study of cardiac sarcoid mimicking arrhythmogenic right ventricular dysplasia. J Cardiovasc Electrophysiol 2009;20:473–6.

4. Basso C, Corrado D, Marcus FI, et al. Arrhythmogenic right ventricular cardiomyopathy. Lancet 2009;373: 1289–300.
5. Sen-Chowdhry S, Syrris P, Ward D, et al. Clinical and genetic characterization of families with arrhythmogenic right ventricular dysplasia/cardiomyopathy provides novel insights into patterns of disease expression. Circulation 2007;115:1710–20.
6. Marcus FI, Fontaine GH, Guiraudon G, et al. Right ventricular dysplasia: a report of 24 adult cases. Circulation 1982;65:384–98.
7. Marcus FI, Zareba W, Calkins H, et al. Arrhythmogenic right ventricular cardiomyopathy/dysplasia clinical presentation and diagnostic evaluation: results from the North American Multidisciplinary Study. Heart Rhythm 2009;6:984–92.
8. McKenna WJ, Thiene G, Nava A, et al. Diagnosis of arrhythmogenic right ventricular dysplasia/cardiomyopathy. Br Heart J 1994;71:215–8.
9. Marcus FI, Sherrill D. Strengths and weaknesses of the task force criteria—proposed modifications. In: Marcus FI, Nava A, Thiene G, editors. Arrhythmogenic right ventricular cardiomyopathy/dysplasia. Milan (Italy): Springer-Verlag; 2007. p. 97–104.
10. Marcus FI, McKenna WJ, Sherrill D, et al. Diagnosis of arrhythmogenic right ventricular cardiomyopathy/dysplasia; proposed modification of the Task Force Criteria. Circulation 2010;121:1533–41; and Eur Heart J 2010;31;806–14.
11. Morin DP, Mauer AC, Gear K, et al. Usefulness of precordial T-wave inversion to distinguish arrhythmogenic right ventricular cardiomyopathy from idiopathic ventricular tachycardia arising from the right ventricular outflow tract. Am J Cardiol 2010;105:1821–4.
12. Jain R, Dalal D, Daly A, et al. Electrocardiographic features of arrhythmogenic right ventricular dysplasia. Circulation 2009;120:477–87.
13. Cox MG, van der Smagt JJ, Wilde AA, et al. New ECG criteria in arrhythmogenic right ventricular dysplasia/cardiomyopathy. Circ Arrhythm Electrophysiol 2009;2:524–30.
14. Tandri H, Daya SK, Khurran N, et al. Normal reference values for the adult right ventricle by magnetic resonance imaging. Am J Cardiol 2006; 98:1660–4.
15. Tandri H, Macedo R, Calkins H, et al. Role of magnetic resonance imaging in arrhythmogenic right ventricular dysplasia: insights from the North American arrhythmogenic right ventricular dysplasia (ARVD/C) study. Am Heart J 2008; 155:147–53.
16. Indik JH, Dallas WJ, Ovitt T, et al. Do patients with right ventricular outflow ventricular arrhythmias have normal right ventricular wall motion? A quantitative analysis compared to normal subjects. Cardiology 2005;104:10–5.
17. Indik JH, Wichter T, Gear K, et al. Quantitative assessment of angiographic right ventricular wall motion in arrhythmogenic right ventricular dysplasia/cardiomyopathy (ARVD/C). J Cardiovasc Electrophysiol 2008;19:39–45.
18. Sen-Chowdhry S, Syrris P, Prasad SK, et al. Left-dominant arrhythmogenic cardiomyopathy an under-recognized clinical entity. J Am Coll Cardiol 2008;52:2175–87.
19. Hamid MS, Norman M, Quraishi A, et al. Prospective evaluation of relatives for familial arrhythmogenic right ventricular cardiomyopathy/dysplasia reveals a need to broaden diagnostic criteria. J Am Coll Cardiol 2002;40:1445–50.
20. Marcus F, Basso C, Gear K, et al. Pitfalls in the diagnosis of arrhythmogenic right ventricular cardiomyopathy/dysplasia (ARVC/D). Am J Cardiol 2010; 105:1036–9.

Arrhythmogenic Cardiomyopathy: Clinical Presentation

Nikos Protonotarios, MD*, Adalena Tsatsopoulou, MD

KEYWORDS

- Arrhythmogenic right ventricular cardiomyopathy/dysplasia
- Desmosome mutations • Heart failure • Naxos disease
- Sudden death

Arrhythmogenic cardiomyopathy (AC) is a heart muscle disorder characterized by progressive myocyte degeneration with fibrous or fibrofatty replacement, resulting in intraventricular conduction abnormalities and reentrant ventricular arrhythmias occasionally leading to sudden death.[1–3] The incidence of disease in the general population ranges from 1:5000 up to 1:2000.[1] AC has been characterized as a disease of cell-cell adhesion.[4,5] Mutations in genes encoding desmosomal proteins plakoglobin (JUP), desmoplakin (DSP), plakophilin-2 (PKP2), desmoglein-2 (DSG2), and desmokollin-2 (DSC2) have been identified as the causative molecular defects in more than 50% of probands.[5–15] These proteins secure structural and functional integrity of myocyte cell-cell adhesion.[4,16] The mode of inheritance is both dominant and recessive. The dominant form is the most common variant, with incomplete penetrance reaching 60%.[17–20] The recessive form presents full penetrance by adolescence, being associated with cutaneous abnormalities consisting of woolly hair and palmoplantar keratoderma.[21,22]

AC was reported at 1982 as a disease causing episodes of recurrent ventricular tachycardia of right ventricular origin, and soon after it was recognized as a major cause of sudden death in the young and the main cause of sudden death in competitive athletes in the Veneto Region, Italy.[23–25] Right ventricular structural/functional alterations usually predominate; however, left ventricular involvement has been increasingly recognized.[26] In the absence of a clinical gold standard for diagnosis, international Task Force criteria were established at 1994, aiming to diagnose overt and severe disease and differentiate it from other cardiomyopathies.[27] Subsequent studies on familial disease revealed a broad clinical spectrum including minor clinical forms misdiagnosed with the established criteria, although harboring the risk of sudden death.[28,29] These observations led to recent modifications of Task Force criteria in order to improve diagnostic sensitivity at early disease stages.[30]

In this article the authors aim to provide the clinical presentation at various stages of disease evolution with respect to symptoms, electrocardiographic abnormalities, and functional/structural alterations on conventional imaging.

PHASES OF CLINICAL DISEASE EXPRESSION

During disease evolution 3 phases of clinical expression have been observed: the early subclinical phase with concealed structural abnormalities ("concealed disease"), the clinical phase in which the established structural criteria are fulfilled ("overt disease"), and the advanced disease phase with severe structural progression ("end-stage disease").

Concealed Disease

Individuals with concealed disease are often asymptomatic but may nonetheless be at risk of sudden cardiac death. Functional/structural

Yannis Protonotarios Medical Centre, Hora Naxos, Naxos 84300, Greece
* Corresponding author.
E-mail address: nikos.protonotarios@otenet.gr

Card Electrophysiol Clin 3 (2011) 227–235
doi:10.1016/j.ccep.2011.02.013

alterations are subtle or absent on conventional imaging. However, 12-lead resting electrocardiography (ECG) and signal-averaged ECG may reveal minor abnormalities. Asymptomatic ventricular extrasystoles in excess of 200 may be recorded on 24-h ambulatory ECG. Delayed-enhancement imaging in cardiac magnetic resonance might be informative, particularly in early left ventricular involvement.[31] The clinician usually is confronted with the concealed type of disease while evaluating members of affected families.[32,33]

The disease onset and expression at early concealed phase have been studied in children homozygous for recessive JUP mutation (Naxos disease).[34–36] In these individuals, woolly hair and palmoplantar keratoderma appear from infancy, with the cardiomyopathy presenting full penetrance by adolescence.[22] These cutaneous manifestations enable identification of children who are going on to develop AC. It was observed that frequent ventricular extrasystoles and depolarization abnormalities preceded any structural alteration.[37] In a 7-year-old child with Naxos disease presenting this early electrical/arrhythmic phenotype, detailed postmortem evaluation by experts, following a noncardiac death, failed to reveal any macroscopic or histologic cardiac abnormality.[37] However, immunohistology of the heart revealed that mutant plakoglobin failed to localize at intercellular junctions. Connexin 43 was significantly reduced in both right and left ventricles with reduced number and size of gap junctions, leading to the hypothesis that abnormalities in the mechanical junctions may modify the function of electrical coupling and cause intraventricular conduction defects and reentrant ventricular arrhythmias before the development of pathologic myocardial changes.[37,38] In another 15-year-old boy from Italy, a carrier of dominant DSP mutation who died suddenly, resting ECG shortly before death showed minor nondiagnostic abnormalities.[17] Post mortem, a subepicardial band of acute-subacute myocyte necrosis with granulation tissue and fibrous and fatty tissue repair was revealed on the posterolateral wall of the left ventricle. It has been suggested that myocardial destruction with fibrofatty replacement may be episodic rather than gradual and continuous.[17] Delayed-enhancement imaging in cardiac magnetic resonance might be informative in this case.[31]

Therefore, it is of practical significance that individuals with signs suggesting concealed AC are followed up serially by 12-lead, signal-averaged, and 24-h ambulatory ECG and, potentially, cardiac magnetic resonance with late-enhancement imaging. This follow-up is most important for familial disease in which family members, particularly the carriers of pathogenic mutations, are at risk of disease development.[39] In the concealed phase of AC, differential diagnosis from benign ventricular extrasystoles and acute/subacute myocarditis is important and should be based on characteristics of arrhythmia, ECG abnormalities, cardiac magnetic resonance with late enhancement, family history, and molecular genetic results.

Overt Disease

Individuals with overt disease present with symptomatic arrhythmias, and right ventricular morphologic/functional abnormalities are readily discernible by conventional imaging.[40–42] The disease usually presents between the second and fifth decade of life.[17,19,43] The initial event is usually syncope or sustained palpitation, while sudden death may be the first manifestation of the disease.[17,19,43] Chest pain with elevated myocardial enzymes has been reported in some cases.[17,44] At the time of event, 12-lead ECG may reveal sustained ventricular tachycardia of left bundle branch block (LBBB) morphology.[44,45] All symptomatic patients exhibit diagnostic findings on 12-lead ECG and 2-dimensional echocardiography applying the established criteria.[43,45] Event-free survival is almost 60% at the beginning of the fifth decade of life.[17,19]

End-Stage Disease

Heart disease progresses over time, involving the right or mostly both ventricles. Structural progression detected by serial echocardiography is usually associated with severe potentially lethal ventricular arrhythmias.[22] Close follow-up of patients with recessive AC revealed that disease evolution follows a stepwise progression.[45] In each step an arrhythmic storm precedes morphologic/functional deterioration of the right and left ventricles.[45] In cases with grossly diffuse right ventricular involvement and right atrial dilatation, atrial fibrillation and paroxysmal atrial tachycardia have been observed.[45] Symptoms of heart failure, with fatigue, gastrointestinal disorders, hepatomegaly, and ascites, appear in the final stages when the right or both ventricles are severely affected.[45,46] AC is one of the rare heart disorders causing heart failure without pulmonary hypertension. Arrhythmic activity is almost totally suppressed at the end stages of evolution.[47]

Cardiac sarcoidosis mimics clinical presentation of AC with respect to arrhythmic, electrocardiographic, and structural findings. It should be considered in cases with biventricular involvement in the absence of family history, and differential diagnosis is based mainly on histologic findings.[48] When AC involves both ventricles severely or there is predominantly left ventricular involvement, it is difficult to differentiate clinically from dilated cardiomyopathy.[34,46,49] Arrhythmogenicity exceeding the degree of structural profile and family history of right-dominant disease support AC diagnosis. Endomyocardial biopsy and molecular genetic investigation further assist in establishing disease diagnosis.

EXPRESSION ON ELECTROCARDIOGRAPHY

Resting 12-lead ECG is abnormal in up to 95% of patients with overt disease,[19,50] revealing repolarization and/or depolarization abnormalities mainly detected in leads V_1 to V_3 (**Fig. 1**). T-wave inversion, QRS complex width greater than 110 milliseconds, parietal block (QRS width in V_1 to V_3 that exceeds the QRS width in lead V_6 by >25 milliseconds), terminal activation duration of QRS complex (from the nadir of the S wave to the end of the QRS, including R′) more than or equal to 55 milliseconds and epsilon waves are the most frequent ECG findings.[19,50,51] T-wave inversion in leads V_1 and V_2 in patients older than 14 years and in the absence of complete right bundle branch block (RBBB) is the most sensitive ECG finding with specificity more than 90%, and it was included in the revised Task Force criteria.[50,52] Epsilon waves are the most specific ECG finding observed in up to one-third of patients.[19,46,50] These waves are low-amplitude postexcitation waves appearing at the end of QRS complex or at the beginning of ST-segment (**Fig. 2**).[23,42] Epsilon waves are considered to be the result of delayed depolarization of surviving myocardial fibers interspersed with fibrous tissue within the residual right ventricular myocardium.[42] Signal-averaged ECG reveals low-amplitude late potentials at the end of the QRS complex, which correspond to epsilon waves on surface ECG.[53] Signal-averaged ECG should be performed using time-domain analysis with a bandpass filter of 40 Hz in individuals with QRS complex duration of less than 110 milliseconds on standard ECG. According to revised diagnostic criteria, it is considered positive for late potentials if at least 1 of the following 3 parameters is present: (1) filtered QRS duration 114 milliseconds or more; (2) low-amplitude signal duration (LAS) 38 milliseconds or more; or (3) root-mean-square voltage of terminal 40 milliseconds 20 μV or less.[30] Comparing ECG findings in affected carriers with PKP2 dominant mutations versus homozygous carriers of recessive JUP mutation, the prevalence of T-wave inversion was higher among PKP2 carriers whereas depolarization abnormalities

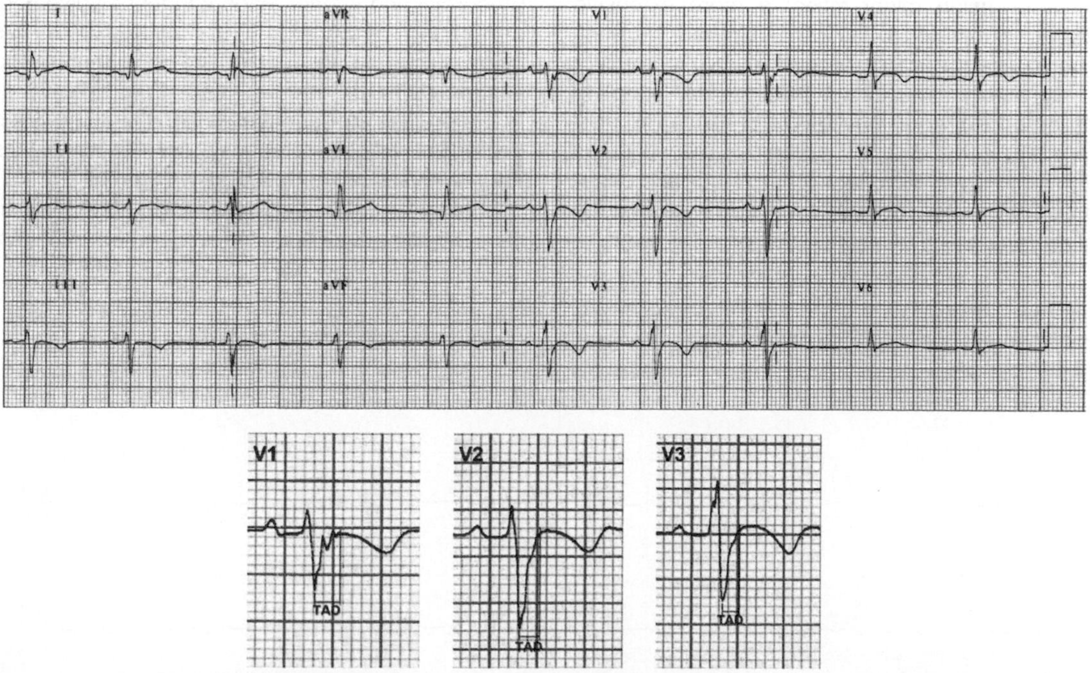

Fig. 1. (*Top*) Baseline 12-lead ECG recording (25 mm/s, 10 mm/mV) of a 16-year-old boy with AC. There is T-wave inversion in leads V_1 to V_4 and epsilon waves in lead V_1. (*Bottom*) Determination of terminal activation duration of QRS complex (TAD) is illustrated in V_1, V_2, and V_3 at 98, 76, and 62 milliseconds, respectively.

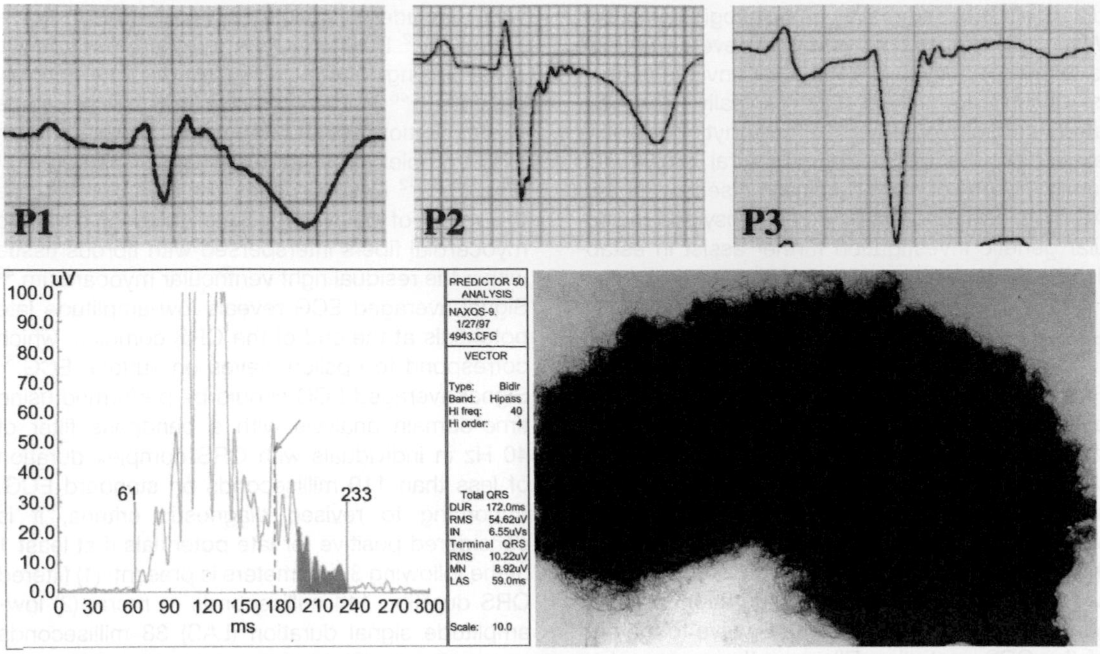

Fig. 2. "Woolly epsilon waves" in lead V_1 (50 mm/s, 20 mm/mV) in 3 patients (P1, P2, and P3) with Naxos disease (*top*) resembling the "woolly hair" phenotype (*bottom right*). There are multiple low/variable-amplitude signals between the end of QRS complex to the onset of T wave. Signal-averaged ECG (*bottom left*) reveals low-amplitude late potentials at the end of the QRS complex (filtered QRS duration = 172 milliseconds; LAS = 59 milliseconds; root mean square voltage = 10 μV).

(QRS complex prolongation and epsilon waves) were more prominent among JUP carriers.[19] T-wave inversion might reflect a more extensive fibrotic substitution in PKP2-affected carriers, whereas depolarization abnormalities might reflect a more extensive defect in electrical coupling attributed to gap junction remodeling in JUP homozygous carriers.[19] Other ECG findings consist of low QRS voltage in limp leads and occasionally in precordial leads, inverted T-waves in the inferior leads, and the presence of a QS wave or ST-segment elevation in leads V_1 to V_3.[54,55] T-wave inversion and/or abnormal Q waves in left precordial and inferior leads suggest involvement of the left ventricle.[17,26] Complete RBBB has been described in up to 10% of patients and incomplete RBBB in up to 25% of patients.[22,50,51] In the presence of complete RBBB, ECG findings consistent with AC diagnosis are epsilon waves and T-wave inversion beyond V_3 (**Fig. 3**).[30]

Ventricular extrasystoles of LBBB configuration have been recorded in the majority of patients.

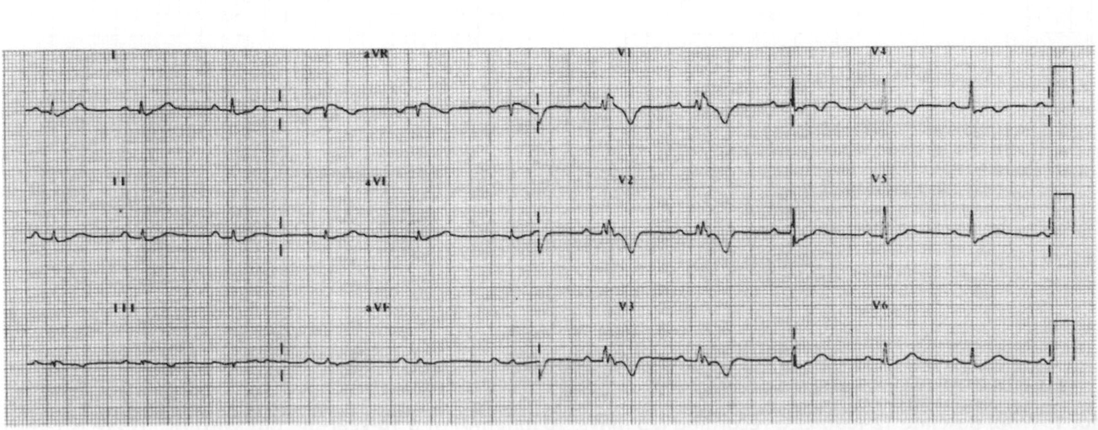

Fig. 3. Baseline 12-lead ECG recording (25 mm/s, 10 mm/mV) of a 58-year-old man with AC showing complete right bundle branch block. There is low voltage, T-wave inversion up to lead V_4 and epsilon waves in leads V_1 to V_3.

Ventricular extrasystoles of RBBB configuration are less common, suggesting left ventricular involvement.[26] Surface 12-lead ECG during ventricular tachycardia shows an LBBB pattern with inferior axis (positive QRS in leads II, III, and aVF, and negative in lead aVL) or superior axis (negative or indeterminate QRS in leads II, III, and aVF, and positive in lead aVL) (**Fig. 4**).

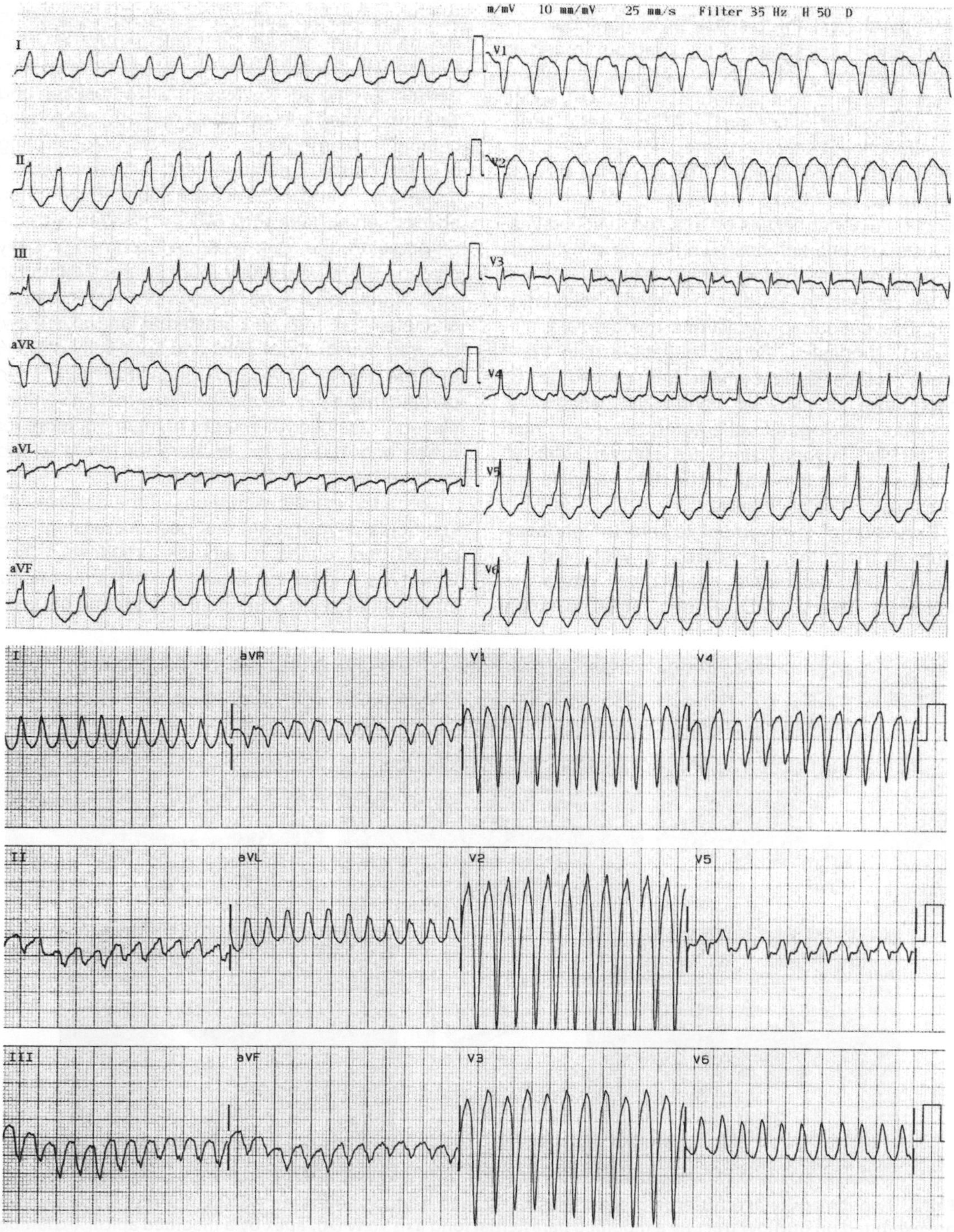

Fig. 4. Surface 12-lead ECG recordings (25 mm/s, 10 mm/mV) during sustained ventricular tachycardia in patients with AC. There is a left bundle branch block configuration with inferior axis (positive QRS in leads II, III, and aVF, and negative in lead aVL) (*top*) and superior axis (negative QRS in leads II, III, and aVF, and positive in lead aVL) (*bottom*).

Ventricular arrhythmias of LBBB morphology with superior axis are more specific for the disease.[30]

EXPRESSION ON IMAGING

At early stages, the disease involves subepicardial/mediomural layers of myocardium in certain regions of right ventricular free wall as the outflow tract, apex, and posterodiaphragmatic wall, called the "triangle of dysplasia."[23] At this stage structural/functional alterations may not be detectable by conventional imaging.[30] Therefore, the disease cannot be excluded in the absence of structural/functional abnormalities on imaging in young individuals with characteristics ventricular arrhythmias or positive family history for AC. Alternatively, late enhancement in cardiac magnetic resonance might reveal subepicardial/mid-myocardial distribution, suggesting fibrous substitution in these areas.[56] Late enhancement has proved to be informative for early left ventricular involvement, whereas analogous characterization of right ventricular myocardium has proved difficult because of the thin wall of the right ventricle and possible confusion with fat.[56,57]

Extension of involvement toward the endocardium in more than two-thirds of wall thickness results in detectable functional alterations (Gaetano Thiene, MD, Padua, Italy, personal communication) appearing as hypokinesia, akinesia, dyskinesia, or aneurysm (akinetic or dyskinetic area with diastolic bulging). All patients with overt disease present these regional wall motion abnormalities at the "triangle of dysplasia" on 2-dimensional echocardiography (see **Fig. 5**A–C), cardiac magnetic resonance, or angiography.[23,32,58–60] Regional hypokinesia may be prone to overinterpretation, leading to false-positive results, and was excluded from the revised diagnostic criteria.[30] Morphologic abnormalities consisting of trabecular derangement, hyperreflective moderator band, and sacculations have been also observed (see **Fig. 5**D).[32,34,59] With disease progression, the right ventricle becomes globally dilated. Right ventricular outflow tract dilatation on 2-dimensional echocardiography (end-diastolic diameter ≥32 mm on parasternal long-axis view) showed sensitivity of 75% and specificity of 95% in large series of AC probands (**Fig. 5**E).[30] On cardiac magnetic resonance it shows right ventricular end-diastolic volume of 110 mL/m^2 or more for males and 100 mL/m^2 or more for females, and ejection fraction of 40% or less.[30]

Since the initial descriptions of the disease, left ventricular involvement has been increasingly reported and related to adverse prognosis.[34,42,61] Genotype-phenotype evaluation with conventional imaging has related the degree and time of onset

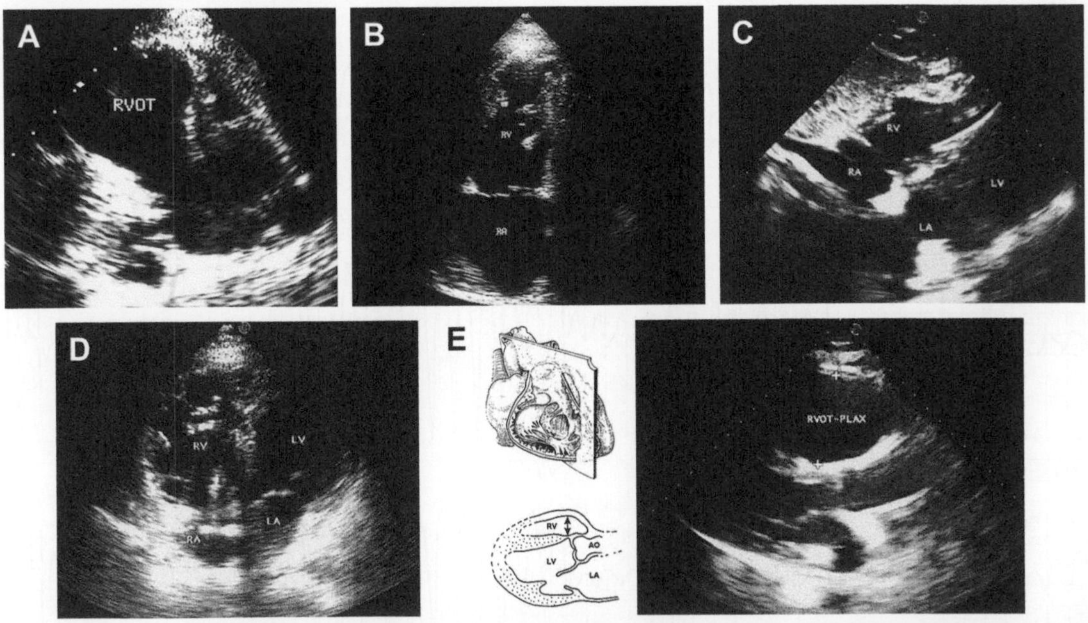

Fig. 5. Two-dimensional echocardiographic images recorded from patients with AC. Right ventricular aneurysms are exhibited on outflow tract by a modified parasternal long axis view (*A*), apex by a modified apical 4-chamber view (*B*), and posterodiaphragmatic wall by subcostal 4-chamber view (*C*). Trabecular derangement and hyperreflective moderator band are shown in right ventricular apical region (*D*). (*E*) Right ventricular outflow tract dilatation on a standard parasternal long axis view; right ventricular outflow tract end-diastolic diameter (RVOT-PLAX) of 51 mm.

of left ventricular involvement to the underlying pathogenic molecular substrate.[6,22,26] Ten percent of patients homozygous for recessive JUP mutation (Naxos disease) develop left ventricular structural/functional abnormalities on 2-dimensional echocardiography by the second decade of life, reaching 60% by the fifth decade.[49] By contrast, in patients homozygous for recessive DSP mutation (Carvajal syndrome) the disease presents earlier, 90% of these patients having severely involved left ventricle by the second decade of life, with a clinical cardiac phenotype close to dilated cardiomyopathy.[49,62] Left-dominant disease has been also observed in carriers of dominant DSP mutations.[63] Preliminary genotype-phenotype assessment increasingly confirms that the left ventricle is predominantly involved when mutations disrupt the cytoskeletal integrity, as with mutations affecting the desmin-binding site at the inner dense plaque of desmosomes.[64,65] Under these conceptions the term "arrhythmogenic cardiomyopathy" is more representative than "arrhythmogenic right ventricular cardiomyopathy" for the broad clinical spectrum of the disease.

SUMMARY

The clinical presentation of AC may vary from concealed to overt and end-stage disease. In the early concealed phase that is common among family members diagnosis is easy to miss, though an electrical substrate might harbor the risk of potentially lethal ventricular arrhythmias. At this stage electrocardiography and cardiac magnetic resonance with late-enhancement imaging seem more sensitive in revealing the disease. In the overt phase, clinical expression and disease evolution vary broadly, depending mostly on structural/functional alterations that range from predominantly right to predominantly left ventricular involvement. Nevertheless, the hallmark of clinical disease presentation is ventricular arrhythmias, so that the term "arrhythmogenic cardiomyopathy" might be more appropriate than "arrhythmogenic right ventricular cardiomyopathy".

REFERENCES

1. Thiene G, Corrado D, Basso C. Arrhythmogenic right ventricular cardiomyopathy/dysplasia. Orphanet J Rare Dis 2007;2:45.
2. Basso C, Thiene G, Corrado D, et al. Arrhythmogenic right ventricular cardiomyopathy. Dysplasia, dystrophy, or myocarditis? Circulation 1996;94: 983–91.
3. Basso C, Corrado D, Marcus FI, et al. Arrhythmogenic right ventricular cardiomyopathy. Lancet 2009;373:1289–300.
4. Basso C, Czarnowska E, Della Barbera M, et al. Ultrastructural evidence of intercalated disc remodelling in arrhythmogenic right ventricular cardiomyopathy: an electron microscopy investigation on endomyocardial biopsies. Eur Heart J 2006;27: 1847–54.
5. McKoy G, Protonotarios N, Crosby A, et al. Identification of a deletion in plakoglobin in arrhythmogenic right ventricular cardiomyopathy with palmoplantar keratoderma and woolly hair (Naxos disease). Lancet 2000;355:2119–24.
6. Norgett EE, Hatsell SJ, Carvajal-Huerta L, et al. Recessive mutation in desmoplakin disrupts desmoplakin-intermediate filament interactions and causes dilated cardiomyopathy, woolly hair and keratoderma. Hum Mol Genet 2000;9:2761–6.
7. Rampazzo A, Nava A, Malacrida S, et al. Mutation in human desmoplakin domain binding to plakoglobin causes a dominant form of arrhythmogenic right ventricular cardiomyopathy. Am J Hum Genet 2002;71:1200–6.
8. Alcalai R, Metzger S, Rosenheck S, et al. A recessive mutation in desmoplakin causes arrhythmogenic right ventricular dysplasia, skin disorder, and woolly hair. J Am Coll Cardiol 2003;42:319–27.
9. Gerull B, Heuser A, Wichter T, et al. Mutations in the desmosomal protein plakophilin-2 are common in arrhythmogenic right ventricular cardiomyopathy. Nat Genet 2004;36:1162–4.
10. Pilichou K, Nava A, Basso C, et al. Mutations in desmoglein-2 gene are associated with arrhythmogenic right ventricular cardiomyopathy. Circulation 2006;113:1171–9.
11. Awad MM, Dalal D, Cho E, et al. DSG2 mutations contribute to arrhythmogenic right ventricular dysplasia/cardiomyopathy. Am J Hum Genet 2006; 79:136–42.
12. Syrris P, Ward D, Evans A, et al. Arrhythmogenic right ventricular dysplasia/cardiomyopathy associated with mutations in the desmosomal gene desmocollin-2. Am J Hum Genet 2006;79:978–84.
13. Heuser A, Plovie ER, Ellinor PT, et al. Mutant desmocollin-2 causes arrhythmogenic right ventricular cardiomyopathy. Am J Hum Genet 2006;79: 1081–8.
14. Asimaki A, Syrris P, Wichter T, et al. A novel dominant mutation in plakoglobin causes arrhythmogenic right ventricular cardiomyopathy. Am J Hum Genet 2007;81:964–73.
15. Den Haan AD, Yew Tan B, Zikusoka MN, et al. Comprehensive desmosome mutation analysis in North Americans with arrhythmogenic right ventricular dysplasia/cardiomyopathy. Circ Cardiovasc Genet 2009;2:428–35.

16. Tsatsopoulou A, Protonotarios N. Desmosomes outside the epidermis. Desmosomes and myocardium: a pivotal role of desmosomes in myocardial degeneration, ventricular arrhythmias and sudden death. In: Cirillo N, Lanza A, Gombos F, editors. Pathophysiology of the desmosomes. Kerala (India): Research Singpost; 2009. p. 105–19.
17. Bauce B, Basso C, Rampazzo A, et al. Clinical profile of four families with arrhythmogenic right ventricular cardiomyopathy caused by dominant desmoplakin mutations. Eur Heart J 2005;16: 1666–75.
18. Syrris P, Ward D, Asimaki A, et al. Clinical expression of plakophilin-2 mutations in familial arrhythmogenic right ventricular cardiomyopathy. Circulation 2006; 113:356–64.
19. Antoniades L, Tsatsopoulou A, Anastasakis A, et al. Arrhythmogenic right ventricular cardiomyopathy caused by deletions in plakophilin-2 and plakoglobin (Naxos disease) in families from Greece and Cyprus: genotype–phenotype relations, diagnostic features and prognosis. Eur Heart J 2006;27: 2008–16.
20. Sen-Chowdhry S, Syrris P, Ward D, et al. Clinical and genetic characterization of families with arrhythmogenic right ventricular dysplasia/cardiomyopathy provides novel insights into patterns of disease expression. Circulation 2007;115:1710–20.
21. Protonotarios N, Tsatsopoulou A. Recessive forms of ARVC/D. In: Marcus FI, Nava A, Thiene G, editors. Arrhythmogenic right ventricular cardiomyopathy/dysplasia. Milano (Italy): Springer; 2007. p. 15–20.
22. Protonotarios N, Tsatsopoulou A, Anastasakis A, et al. Genotype-phenotype assessment in autosomal recessive arrhythmogenic right ventricular cardiomyopathy (Naxos disease) caused by a deletion in plakoglobin. J Am Coll Cardiol 2001;38: 1477–84.
23. Marcus FI, Fontaine GH, Guiraudon G, et al. Right ventricular dysplasia: a report of 24 adult cases. Circulation 1982;65:384–98.
24. Thiene G, Nava A, Corrado D, et al. Right ventricular cardiomyopathy and sudden death in young people. N Engl J Med 1988;318:129–33.
25. Corrado D, Thiene G, Nava A, et al. Sudden death in young competitive athletes: clinicopathologic correlations in 22 cases. Am J Med 1990;89: 588–96.
26. Norman M, Simpson M, Mogensen J, et al. Novel mutation in desmoplakin causes arrhythmogenic left ventricular cardiomyopathy. Circulation 2005; 112:636–42.
27. McKenna WJ, Thiene G, Nava A, et al. Diagnosis of arrhythmogenic right ventricular dysplasia/cardiomyopathy. Task Force of the Working Group Myocardial and Pericardial Disease of the European Society of Cardiology and of the Scientific Council on Cardiomyopathies of the International Society and Federation of Cardiology. Br Heart J 1994;71: 215–8.
28. Hamid MS, Norman M, Quraishi A, et al. Prospective evaluation of relatives for familial arrhythmogenic right ventricular cardiomyopathy/dysplasia reveals a need to broaden diagnostic criteria. J Am Coll Cardiol 2002;40:1445–50.
29. Marcus FI, Sherrill D. Strengths and weaknesses of the task force criteria: proposed modifications in arrhythmogenic right ventricular cardiomyopathy/dysplasia. In: Marcus FI, Nava A, Thiene G, editors. Arrhythmogenic right ventricular cardiomyopathy dysplasia. Milan (Italy): Springer Verlag; 2007. p. 97–104.
30. Marcus FI, McKenna WJ, Sherrill D, et al. Diagnosis of arrhythmogenic right ventricular cardiomyopathy/dysplasia (ARVC/D): proposed modification of the task force criteria. Circulation 2010;121:1133–41; and Eur Heart J 2010;31:806–14.
31. Sen-Chowdhry S, Prasad SK, Syrris P, et al. Cardiovascular magnetic resonance in arrhythmogenic right ventricular cardiomyopathy revisited: comparison with task force criteria and genotype. J Am Coll Cardiol 2006;48:2132–40.
32. Nava A, Thiene G, Canciani B, et al. Familial occurrence of right ventricular dysplasia: a study involving nine families. J Am Coll Cardiol 1988;12:1222–8.
33. Nava A, Bauce B, Basso C, et al. Clinical profile and long-term follow-up of 37 families with arrhythmogenic right ventricular cardiomyopathy. J Am Coll Cardiol 2000;36:2226–33.
34. Protonotarios N, Tsatsopoulou A, Patsourakos P, et al. Cardiac abnormalities in familial palmoplantar keratosis. Br Heart J 1986;56:321–6.
35. Protonotarios N, Tsatsopoulou A. The Naxos disease. In: Nava A, Rossi L, Thiene G, editors. Arrhythmogenic right ventricular dysplasia/cardiomyopathy. Amsterdam: Elsevier Science B.V; 1997. p. 454–62.
36. Tsatsopoulou A, Protonotarios N. Naxos cardiocutaneous syndrome. Eur J Pediatr Dermatol 2008;18: 82–5.
37. Kaplan SR, Gard JJ, Protonotarios N, et al. Remodeling of myocyte gap junctions in arrhythmogenic right ventricular cardiomyopathy due to a deletion in plakoglobin (Naxos disease). Heart Rhythm 2004;1:3–11.
38. Saffitz JE. Dependence of electrical coupling on mechanical coupling in cardiac myocytes: insights gained from cardiomyopathies caused by defects in cell-cell connections. Ann N Y Acad Sci 2005; 1047:336–44.
39. Quarta G, Deidre W, Tomé Esteban MT, et al. Dynamic electrocardiographic changes in patients with arrhythmogenic right ventricular cardiomyopathy. Heart 2010;96:516–22.

40. Fontaine G, Fontaliran F, Frank R. Arrhythmogenic right ventricular cardiomyopathies. Clinical forms and main differential diagnoses. Circulation 1998; 97:1532–5.
41. Fontaine G, Fontaliran F, Hébert JL, et al. Arrhythmogenic right ventricular dysplasia. Annu Rev Med 1999;50:17–35.
42. Corrado D, Basso C, Thiene G, et al. Spectrum of clinicopathologic manifestations of arrhythmogenic right ventricular cardiomyopathy/dysplasia: a multicenter study. J Am Coll Cardiol 1997;30:1512–20.
43. Marcus FI, Zareba W, Calkins H, et al. Arrhythmogenic right ventricular cardiomyopathy/dysplasia, clinical presentation and diagnostic evaluation: results from the North American Multidisciplinary Study. Heart Rhythm 2009;6:984–92.
44. Lazaros G, Anastasakis A, Tsiachris D, et al. Naxos disease presenting with ventricular tachycardia and troponin elevation. Heart Vessels 2009;24:63–5.
45. Protonotarios N, Tsatsopoulou A, Gatzoulis K. Arrhythmogenic right ventricular cardiomyopathy caused by a deletion in plakoglobin (Naxos disease). Card Electrophysiol Rev 2002;6:72–80.
46. Hulot JS, Jouven X, Empana JP, et al. Natural history and risk stratification of arrhythmogenic right ventricular cardiomyopathy. Circulation 2004;110:1879–84.
47. Basso C, Tsatsopoulou A, Thiene G, et al. "Petrified" right ventricle in long-standing Naxos arrhythmogenic right ventricular cardiomyopathy. Circulation 2001;104:E132–3.
48. Vasaiwala SC, Finn R, Delpiore J, et al. Prospective study of cardiac sarcoid mimicking arrhythmogenic right ventricular dysplasia. J Cardiovasc Electrophysiol 2009;20:473–6.
49. Protonotarios N, Tsatsopoulou A. Naxos disease and Carvajal syndrome: cardiocutaneous disorders that highlight the pathogenesis and broaden the spectrum of arrhythmogenic right ventricular cardiomyopathy. Cardiovasc Pathol 2004;13:185–94.
50. Nasir K, Bomma C, Tandri H, et al. Electrocardiographic features of arrhythmogenic right ventricular dysplasia/cardiomyopathy according to disease severity: a need to broaden diagnostic criteria. Circulation 2004;110:1527–34.
51. Cox MG, Nelen MR, Wilde AA, et al. Activation delay and VT parameters in arrhythmogenic right ventricular dysplasia/cardiomyopathy: toward improvement of diagnostic ECG criteria. J Cardiovasc Electrophysiol 2008;19:775–81.
52. Marcus FI. Prevalence of T-wave inversion beyond V1 in young normal individuals and usefulness for the diagnosis of arrhythmogenic right ventricular cardiomyopathy/dysplasia. Am J Cardiol 2005;95:1070–1.
53. Marcus FI, Zareba W, Sherrill D. Evaluation of the normal values for signal-averaged electrocardiogram. J Cardiovasc Electrophysiol 2007;18:231–3.
54. Peters S, Trummel M. Diagnosis of arrhythmogenic right ventricular dysplasia-cardiomyopathy: value of standard ECG revisited. Ann Noninvasive Electrocardiol 2003;8:238–45.
55. Sterlotis AK, Bauce B, Daliento L, et al. Electrocardiographic pattern in arrhythmogenic right ventricular cardiomyopathy. Am J Cardiol 2009;103:1302–8.
56. Tandri H, Saranathan M, Rodriguez R, et al. Noninvasive detection of myocardial fibrosis in arrhythmogenic right ventricular cardiomyopathy using delayed-enhancement magnetic resonance imaging. J Am Coll Cardiol 2005;45:98–103.
57. Bomma C, Rutberg J, Tandri H, et al. Misdiagnosis of arrhythmogenic right ventricular dysplasia/cardiomyopathy. J Cardiovasc Electrophysiol 2004;15:300–6.
58. Blomström-Lundqvist C, Beckman-Suurkula M, Wallentin A, et al. Ventricular dimensions and wall motion assessed by echocardiography in patients with arrhythmogenic right ventricular dysplasia. Eur Heart J 1988;9:1291–302.
59. Yoerger DM, Marcus F, Sherrill D, et al. Echocardiographic findings in patients meeting task force criteria for arrhythmogenic right ventricular dysplasia. J Am Coll Cardiol 2005;45:860–5.
60. Bluemke DA, Krupinski EA, Ovitt T, et al. MRI Imaging of arrhythmogenic right ventricular cardiomyopathy: morphological findings and intraobserver reliability. Cardiology 2003;99:153–62.
61. Pinamonti B, Sinagra GF, Salvi A, et al. Left ventricular involvement in right ventricular dysplasia. Am Heart J 1992;123:711–24.
62. Carvajal-Huerta L. Epidermolytic-palmoplantar keratoderma with woolly hair and dilated cardiomyopathy. J Am Acad Dermatol 1998;39:418–21.
63. Sen-Chowdhry S, Syrris P, Prasad SK, et al. Left-dominant arrhythmogenic cardiomyopathy: an under-recognized clinical entity. J Am Coll Cardiol 2008;52:2175–87.
64. Tsatsopoulou A, Protonotarios N, McKenna WJ. Arrhythmogenic right ventricular dysplasia, a cell-adhesion cardiomyopathy: insights into disease pathogenesis from preliminary genotype-phenotype assessment. Heart 2006;92:1720–3.
65. Delmar M, McKenna WJ. The cardiac desmosome and arrhythmogenic cardiomyopathies: from gene to disease. Circ Res 2010;107:700–14.

Twelve-Lead ECG in Arrhythmogenic Cardiomyopathy

Richard N.W. Hauer, MD, PhD[a,b,*], Moniek G.P.J. Cox, MD[a,b]

KEYWORDS

- Arrhythmogenic right ventricular cardiomyopathy/dysplasia
- Diagnosis • Electrocardiography • Ventricular tachycardia

Arrhythmogenic cardiomyopathy (AC) is a disorder characterized histopathologically by fibrofatty replacement of the myocardium, primarily of the right ventricle (RV), and clinically by ventricular tachyarrhythmias, sudden death, and progressive heart failure.[1–7] Recent molecular genetic observations provide accumulating evidence that this fibrofatty replacement is preceded by mutation-related desmosomal changes.[8–17] Desmosomes are crucial for maintaining mechanical coupling of cardiomyocytes. Several reports have shown that alterations in desmosomal proteins affect expression and distribution of other desmosomal and nondesmosomal proteins, such as Connexin43, responsible for electrical coupling. In this way mechanical uncoupling could give rise to electrical uncoupling.[18–23]

The relationship between uncoupling and fibrofatty replacement is largely unknown. However, the hypothesis that cardiac cellular uncoupling precedes fibrofatty alteration is strongly supported by identification in proven AC patients of an altered distribution of desmosomal proteins and Connexin43, in histologically still unaffected left ventricular and septal tissue.[23] This observation can possibly have diagnostic implications especially in the early concealed phase of the disease, characterized by still absent or minor histopathological tissue alteration, also in the RV. However, sudden death may occur at that stage as first manifestation of AC.[24,25] Both electrical uncoupling and altered tissue architecture due to the fibrofatty infiltration lead to inhomogeneous activation delay by electrical conduction block, lengthening of conduction pathways, load mismatch at pivotal points, and slow conduction. This activation delay and conduction block provide a substrate for reentrant mechanisms and thereby ventricular tachycardia (VT) (**Fig. 1**).[26–29] Previous invasive electrophysiologic studies have confirmed that VT in patients with AC is caused by reentry in areas with abnormal myocardium.[30,31]

Immunohistochemical analysis of intercalated disk proteins have clearly demonstrated that AC is a disorder of both ventricles, at least at a molecular level.[23] Why fibrofatty alteration is usually more prominent in the RV is still unclear. A larger stretch at the thin right RV wall has been suggested as a potentially causative factor. A histologically dominant RV involvement seems to be related to

This work was supported by Grant No. 06901 from the Interuniversity Cardiology Institute of the Netherlands, and Grant No. 2007B139 from the Netherlands Heart Foundation.
The authors have nothing to disclose.

[a] Department of Cardiology, University Medical Center Utrecht, Heidelberglaan 100, 3584CX, Utrecht, The Netherlands
[b] Interuniversity Cardiology Institute of the Netherlands, Catharijnesingel 52, 3501 DG Utrecht, The Netherlands
* Corresponding author. Department of Cardiology, University Medical Center Utrecht, Heidelberglaan 100, 3584CX, Utrecht, The Netherlands.
E-mail address: r.n.w.hauer@umcutrecht.nl

Card Electrophysiol Clin 3 (2011) 237–244
doi:10.1016/j.ccep.2011.02.004
1877-9182/11/$ – see front matter

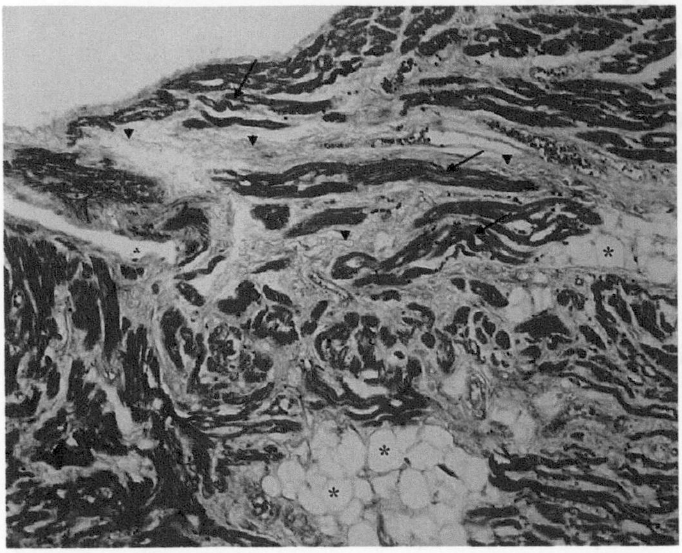

Fig. 1. Histology of RV of a 13-year-old girl who died suddenly during exercise. AZAN staining (original magnification ×400) showing cardiac myocytes (*arrows*), collagen (*arrowheads*), and adipocytes (*asterisks*). Bundles of myocardium are embedded in fibrotic tissue, which reaches the endocardium. These thin bundles may interconnect, giving rise to activation delay and reentrant circuits, the typical electrophysiologic substrate for ventricular arrhythmias in AC. No mutation analysis was possible. (*Reprinted from* Cox MG, Nelen MR, Wilde AA, et al. Activation delay and VT parameters in AC: towards improvement of diagnostic ECG criteria. J Cardiovasc Electrophysiol 2008;19:775–81; with permission.)

an RV origin of specifically monomorphic VT. Systematic studies on the origin of polymorphic VT and ventricular fibrillation are lacking. Finally, the ventricles are not homogeneously affected. Marcus and colleagues[1] described as early as 1982 the so-called triangle of dysplasia, being the RV outflow tract, an area below the tricuspid valve, and the RV apex. However, other areas in the RV, as well as the left ventricle, may also be affected. Histologically and in imaging studies, the interventricular septum is rarely involved.

The gold standard for AC diagnosis is a demonstration of transmural fibrofatty infiltration of the RV. However, for this information autopsy or surgery is required. To facilitate diagnosis in clinical practice, an international Task Force established a set of criteria (TFC) based on electrocardiographic, functional, and morphologic features, as well as family history, in 1994.[32] Since then, these TFC have proven to be highly specific for AC diagnosis and have been universally used. The main drawback, however, is their limited sensitivity. Thus, patients were often not recognized until a late stage of the disease. Research on increasing numbers of index cases and their family members in the following years delivered important insights into the development and behavior of the disease process.[14,15,33] Therefore, recently a new Task Force introduced modifications to the 1994 TFC by implementation of these new insights, based on consensus.[34] Similar to the 1994 TFC, in the new TFC abnormalities were subdivided into major and minor according to the specificity for AC. AC diagnosis was based on the combination of either 2 major criteria, 1 major and 2 minor criteria, or 4 minor criteria. Criteria were derived from: (1) global or regional dysfunction and structural alterations, (2) tissue characterization, (3) depolarization abnormalities, (4) repolarization abnormalities, (5) arrhythmias, and (6) family history.

The 12-lead electrocardiogram (ECG) is one of the most important tools for the diagnosis of AC. Half of the diagnostic criteria items are based on 12-lead ECG recording. In addition, in line with early electrical uncoupling, the consensus report stated that ECG changes and arrhythmias may develop before overt structural abnormalities or clinical evidence of RV dysfunction.[34] This finding means that 12-lead ECG analysis may contribute to early diagnosis of AC.

Activation delay and site of origin of VT are reflected in various characteristics of the surface 12-lead ECG. Because the 12-lead ECG is easy to obtain, this technique is particularly useful not only for AC diagnosis but also for evaluation of progress of the disease during follow-up. In addition, 12-lead ECG recording of VT is crucial in selecting and mapping a specific VT for catheter ablation procedures.

TWELVE-LEAD ECG DURING NORMAL SINUS RHYTHM

Activation Delay (Depolarization) Parameters

Activation delay due to cellular uncoupling and altered tissue architecture by fibrofatty alteration is often visible on the ECG. In the original descriptions and 1994 TFC, typical manifestations are epsilon waves and widening of the QRS complex (>110 ms) in leads V_1 to V_3.[32] Epsilon waves and localized QRS prolongation are major criteria of the 1994 TFC. Epsilon wave was defined

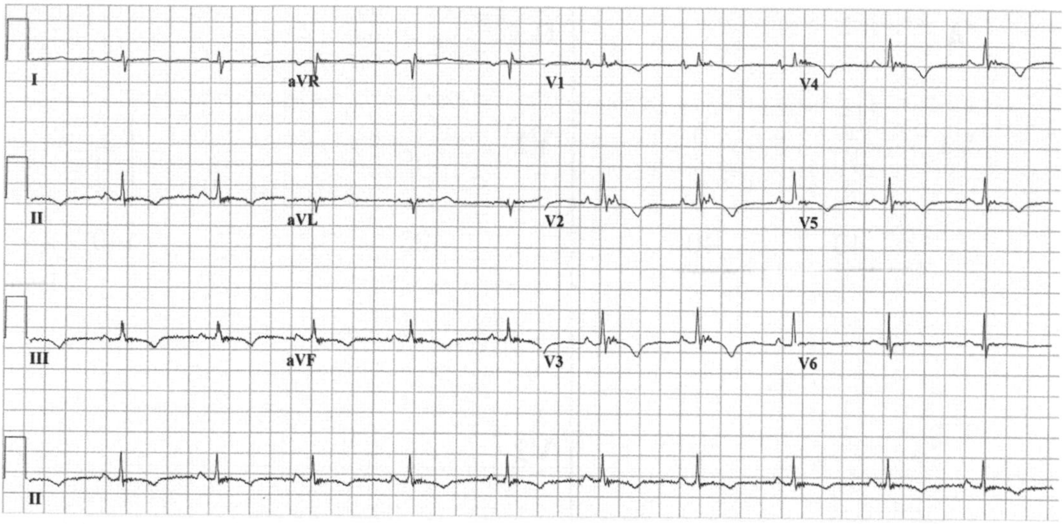

Fig. 2. Epsilon waves in precordial leads V_{1-3} from AC patient with plakophilin2 mutation. Epsilon wave is a distinct deflection clearly separated from QRS complex. Epsilon wave remains a major criterion in the new Task Force criteria.

as a distinct deflection after the end of the QRS complex, that is, after the QRS complex had returned to the isoelectric line (**Fig. 2**).[35] In the new TFC the epsilon wave remained as a major criterion, but the widening of the QRS complex was deleted. This widening may give rise to confusion, because discrimination from right bundle branch block (RBBB) may be difficult. Although the epsilon wave is highly specific for AC, sensitivity is low. Cox and colleagues[7] showed identification of recording in only 4 out of 42 patients (10%) with proven AC according to the 1994 TFC. Because of this limited sensitivity, other parameters have been evaluated.

Peters and Trummel[36] determined increased precordial QRS ratio by $(V_1+V_2+V_3)/(V_4+V_5+V_6) > 1.2$ to solve the problem of discrimination with RBBB. However, this criterion was found in only 35% of patients with proven AC.[7] Nasir and colleagues[37] reported the delayed S-wave upstroke, defined from the nadir of the S wave up to the isoelectric line in V_{1-3}, of 55 milliseconds or more to be a sensitive criterion representing activation delay.

The authors' group[7] introduced prolonged terminal activation duration (TAD). TAD is defined as the longest value in V_{1-3}, from the nadir of the S wave to the end of all depolarization deflections, thereby including not only the S-wave upstroke but also late fractionated signals and epsilon waves (**Fig. 3**). Thus, total activation delay was conveyed by this new parameter. In **Fig. 3**, the difference between S-wave upstroke and TAD is clearly visible. TAD was considered prolonged if 55 milliseconds or more, and only applicable in the absence of complete RBBB. The authors applied the same value as determined for prolonged S-wave upstroke by Nasir and colleagues,[37] because it proved to be a cutoff point with high specificity in the authors' study as well. Prolonged TAD appeared to be the most sensitive activation delay criterion. It was recorded in 30 of 42 AC patients (71%), whereas the criterion of only prolonged S wave was identified in only 52% of these patients. Prolonged TAD was not identified in 26 of 27 patients with idiopathic VT (**Fig. 4**). Because of the superiority in sensitivity and the high specificity of prolonged TAD, this new criterion was included in the newly proposed TFC.[34]

It has to be realized that these diagnostic criteria use only V_{1-3}, which face the RV outflow tract. Therefore, all criteria mentioned might reflect activation delay primarily of this part of the RV. Other still undefined criteria may be needed to reflect alterations in other parts of both right and left ventricles.

Repolarization Parameters

Abnormalities in repolarization in patients with AC are visible as inverted T waves. In the 1994 TFC, inverted (negative) T waves in V_{1-3} or beyond were considered as a minor criterion for AC diagnosis in the absence of RBBB, and only if the patient was older than 12 years (see **Fig. 2**; **Fig. 5**). Because of the high specificity for AC, this criterion was upgraded to a major criterion in the new TFC, for individuals older than 14 years and in the absence of complete RBBB. In the authors' series of 42 AC patients, this criterion was observed in 28 patients (67%) and in none

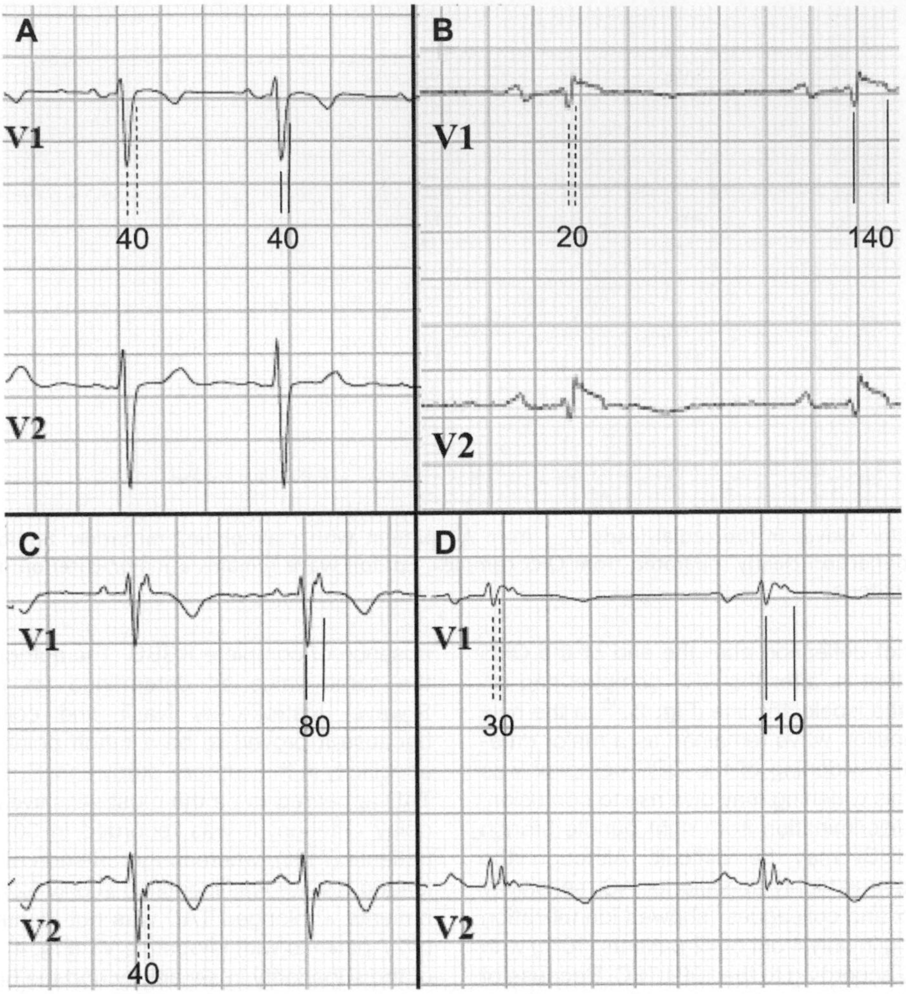

Fig. 3. ECG recordings V_1 and V_2 of 4 patients in sinus rhythm, while off drugs (25 mm/s, low-pass filter 100 Hz). RBBB was absent. Difference in measurement results (in milliseconds) of S-wave upstroke (first complexes, *dashed lines*) and terminal activation duration (TAD; second complexes, *continuous lines*). Panel (*A*) (control patient) shows no differences in S-wave upstroke and TAD, both being normal. By contrast, in panels (*B–D*) (AC patients), S-wave upstroke is less than 55 milliseconds, whereas TAD is prolonged. Prolonged TAD is a minor criterion in the new Task Force criteria. (*Reprinted from* Cox MG, Nelen MR, Wilde AA, et al. Activation delay and VT parameters in AC: towards improvement of diagnostic ECG criteria. J Cardiovasc Electrophysiol 2008;19:775–81; with permission.)

of the patients with idiopathic VT.[7] Thus, sensitivity and specificity are similar to prolonged TAD.

In the new TFC, two additional criteria were included as minor criteria:

1. Inverted T waves *only* in leads V_1 and V_2 in individuals older than 14 years and in the absence of complete RBBB.[34] This criterion was identified in 4 of the authors' 42 patients (10%).[7]
2. Inverted T waves in leads V_{1-4} in individuals older than 14 years in the presence of RBBB.[34] This criterion was added because RBBB may be attributable to local activation delay, and a negative T wave in V_4 and beyond is very unlikely in classic RBBB.

TWELVE-LEAD ECG DURING VT

VT Parameters for Diagnosis and Localization of Site of Origin

Type and number of VT morphologies reflect location and extension of the disease process. In the absence of severe left ventricular and septal structural disease, a VT with left bundle branch block (LBBB) morphology (dominant negativity in V_1) means a site of origin in the RV. This is the reason why AC is associated with monomorphic VT with

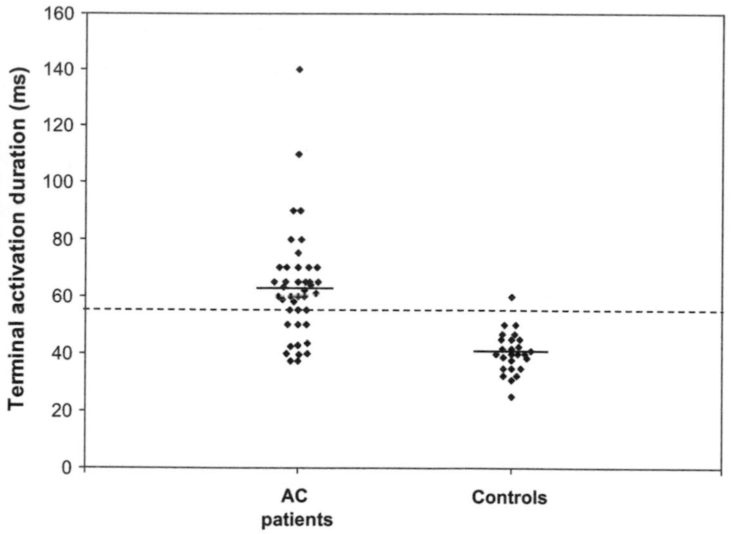

Fig. 4. Results of measurements of TAD from AC patients and idiopathic VT controls. Mean values are indicated by horizontal lines. AC patients had a significantly longer TAD than idiopathic VT control patients (*P*<.001). The dashed line indicates the cutoff point of 55 milliseconds. (*Reprinted from* Cox MG, Nelen MR, Wilde AA, et al. Activation delay and VT parameters in ARVD/C: towards improvement of diagnostic ECG criteria. J Cardiovasc Electrophysiol 2008;19:775–81; with permission.)

LBBB morphology. In the 1994 TFC, recording of this VT morphology was a minor criterion for AC diagnosis.[32]

However, the authors hypothesized that additional information could be obtained if the axis of the VT was taken into account.

Idiopathic VT originating from the RV outflow tract typically shows LBBB morphology with an inferior (vertical) axis. By contrast, in AC, affected areas are also found in other parts of the RV including the so-called triangle of dysplasia.[1] Consequently, VTs originating from these areas can show LBBB morphology with a nonvertical axis as well. The authors evaluated the occurrence of LBBB VT with a superior axis, arbitrarily defined from −30° to −150° (**Fig. 6**).[7]

This morphology was recorded in 27 of 42 patients (64%) with AC diagnosed according to the 1994 TFC. None of the 27 patients with idiopathic VT had this morphology. Thus, this criterion had a similar specificity and sensitivity to that of prolonged TAD. In accordance with the authors' definition, recording of a VT with LBBB morphology and superior axis, defined as negative or indeterminate QRS in leads II, III, and aVF, and positive in lead aVL, became a major criterion in the new TFC.[34] A VT with LBBB morphology and inferior axis remained a minor criterion (**Fig. 7**). The number of premature ventricular complexes on Holter recording required for counting as a minor criterion decreased to 500 per 24 hours.

Because of the variable extension of the disease process in AC, the number of different VT morphologies may vary as well. Thus, multiple VT morphologies may be recorded in a single patient. Previous studies showed mean numbers of different VT morphologies per patient ranging from 1.8 to 3.8.[30,38] The number of different VTs

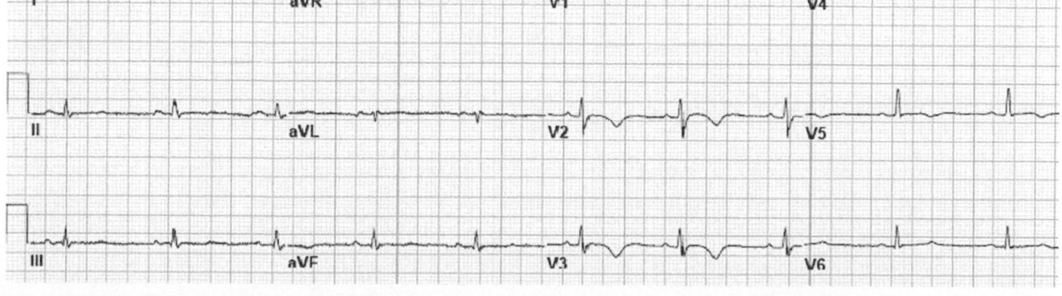

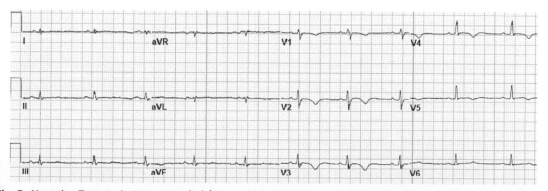

Fig. 5. Negative T waves in V_{1-5}, recorded from an AC patient with both a plakophilin2 mutation and a desmoglein2 mutation. Negative T waves in V_{1-3} and beyond are a major criterion in the new Task Force criteria.

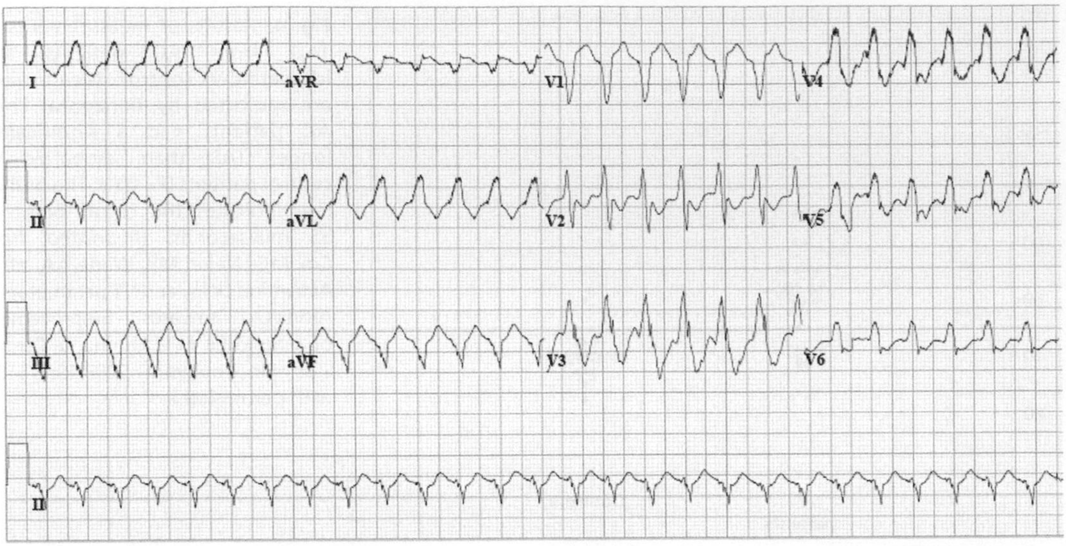

Fig. 6. VT with LBBB morphology and superior axis, recorded from an AC patient with plakophilin2 mutation. This morphology is a major criterion in the new Task Force criteria.

in AC patients was quantified and compared with data from a control group after 8 years of follow-up.[7] Multiple VT morphologies were recorded in 27 of 42 AC patients (64%), whereas the control group with idiopathic VT had only a single morphology. This study confirmed that occurrence of multiple VT morphologies is the rule rather than the exception in AC patients. In the case of only a single VT morphology occurring spontaneously, programmed electrical stimulation (PES) contributed significantly to yield multiple morphologies. In total, 10 additional AC patients or in total 88% fulfilled the multiple VT morphology criterion.[7] Because of significant overlap with the superior axis criterion, the number of VT morphologies was not used in the new TFC.

VALIDATION OF ADDITIONAL ECG CRITERIA

Because sudden death frequently is the first manifestation of AC, even as early as adolescence, the main diagnostic challenge is to identify individuals with disease at an early stage. In a recent study, the authors aimed to establish whether the previously

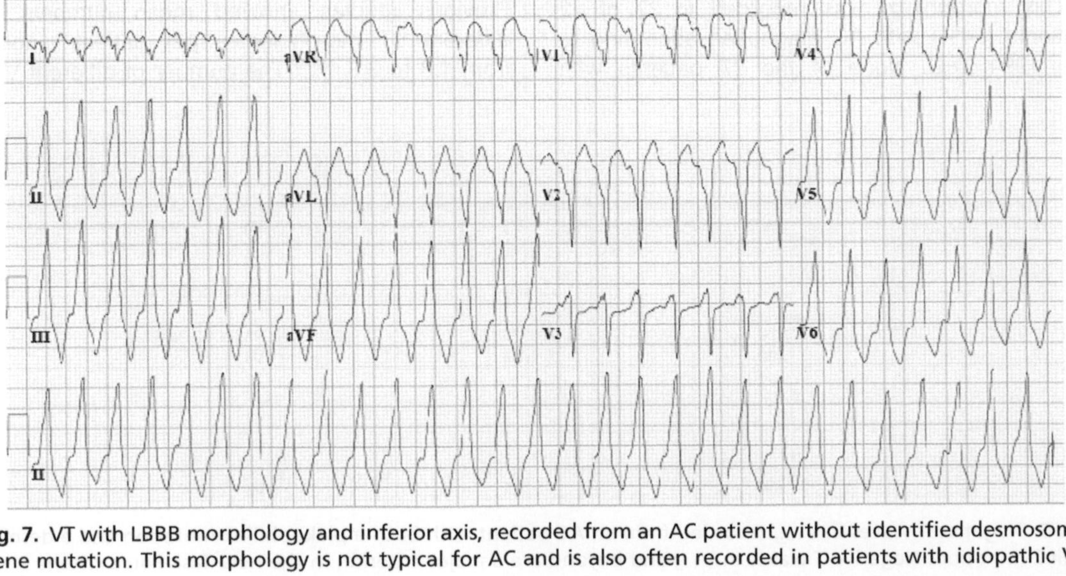

Fig. 7. VT with LBBB morphology and inferior axis, recorded from an AC patient without identified desmosomal gene mutation. This morphology is not typical for AC and is also often recorded in patients with idiopathic VT.

proposed additional ECG criteria would improve diagnosis in patients highly suspected of having AC, but who did not fulfill the 1994 TFC for AC diagnosis.[39] Thereto, presence of those newly proposed additional criteria was studied in so-called probable AC patients because they fulfilled either only 1 major and 1 minor, or only 3 minor criteria. The authors specifically studied the diagnostic contribution of the following proposed additional criteria: (1) prolonged TAD in V_{1-3}, (2) VT with LBBB morphology and superior axis, and (3) recording of multiple different VT morphologies. Two groups were studied: Group A (n = 21) with probable but not proven AC index patients, and Group B (n = 12) consisting of family members of 50 other proven (fulfilling 1994 TFC) AC index patients.

In Group A, none had epsilon waves or QRS greater than 110 ms, whereas prolonged TAD was recorded in 7 (33%) patients, therefore fulfilling AC diagnosis when this criterion was applied in addition to 1994 TFC. In 8 Group A patients (38%), a spontaneously occurring VT with LBBB morphology and superior axis has been recorded. In addition, this morphology was inducible with PES in 4 additional patients. In 4 Group A patients (19%), multiple VT morphologies were recorded during spontaneous episodes, as well as in 5 additional patients during PES.

In total, 16 of 21 Group A index patients did fulfill at least one of the newly proposed criteria.

In Group B, one family member had epsilon waves and 8 had prolonged TAD. Because of both absence of spontaneous VT episode recordings and PES, VT criteria could not contribute to diagnosis in Group B. Thus in total, 7 Group B family members fulfilled newly proposed criteria.

SUMMARY

The 12-lead ECG is one of the most important tools for the diagnosis of AC. In addition, this tool contributes to evaluation of progression of the disease during follow-up. Because in AC ventricular arrhythmias and sudden death are caused by reentrant mechanisms, activation delay is a critical component. Recently a new parameter of activation delay, prolonged TAD, has appeared to be superior in sensitivity to previously defined criteria, without loss of specificity. In addition, repolarization and new VT criteria contribute importantly to AC diagnosis.

REFERENCES

1. Marcus FI, Fontaine GH, Guiraudon G, et al. Right ventricular dysplasia: a report of 24 adult cases. Circulation 1982;65:384–98.
2. Basso C, Thiene G, Corrado D, et al. Arrhythmogenic right ventricular cardiomyopathy: dysplasia, dystrophy, or myocarditis? Circulation 1996;94:983–91.
3. Basso C, Corrado D, Marcus FI, et al. Arrhythmogenic right ventricular cardiomyopathy. Lancet 2009;373:1289–300.
4. Dalal D, Nasir K, Bomma C, et al. Arrhythmogenic right ventricular dysplasia: a United States experience. Circulation 2005;112:3823–32.
5. Roguin A, Bomma CS, Nasir K, et al. Implantable cardioverter-defibrillators in patients with arrhythmogenic right ventricular dysplasia/cardiomyopathy. J Am Coll Cardiol 2004;43:1843–52.
6. Picinni JP, Dalal D, Roguin A, et al. Predictors of appropriate implantable defibrillator therapies in patients with arrhythmogenic right ventricular dysplasia. Heart Rhythm 2005;2:1188–94.
7. Cox MG, Nelen MR, Wilde AA, et al. Activation delay and VT parameters in arrhythmogenic right ventricular dysplasia/cardiomyopathy: towards improvement of diagnostic ECG criteria. J Cardiovasc Electrophysiol 2008;19:775–81.
8. McKoy G, Protonotarios N, Crosby A, et al. Identification of a deletion in plakoglobin in arrhythmogenic right ventricular cardiomyopathy with palmoplantar keratoderma and woolly hair (Naxos disease). Lancet 2000;335:2119–24.
9. Protonotarios N, Tsatsopoulou A, Anastasakis A, et al. Genotype-phenotype assessment in autosomal recessive arrhythmogenic right ventricular cardiomyopathy (Naxos disease) caused by a deletion in plakoglobin. J Am Coll Cardiol 2001;38:1477–84.
10. Rampazzo A, Nava A, Malacrida S, et al. Mutation in human desmoplakin domain binding to plakoglobin causes a dominant form of arrhythmogenic right ventricular cardiomyopathy. Am J Hum Genet 2002;71:1200–6.
11. Gerull B, Heuser A, Wichter T, et al. Mutations in the desmosomal protein plakophilin-2 are common in arrhythmogenic right ventricular cardiomyopathy. Nat Genet 2004;36:1162–4.
12. Syrris P, Ward D, Asimaki A, et al. Clinical expression of plakophilin-2 mutations in familial arrhythmogenic right ventricular cardiomyopathy. Circulation 2006;113:356–64.
13. Pilichou K, Nava A, Basso C, et al. Mutations in desmoglein-2 gene are associated with arrhythmogenic right ventricular cardiomyopathy. Circulation 2006;113:1171–9.
14. Van Tintelen JP, Entius MM, Bhuiyan ZA, et al. Plakophilin-2 mutations are the major determinant of familial arrhythmogenic right ventricular dysplasia/cardiomyopathy. Circulation 2006;113:1650–8.
15. Dalal D, Molin LH, Piccini J, et al. Clinical features of arrhythmogenic right ventricular dysplasia/cardiomyopathy associated with mutations in plakophilin-2. Circulation 2006;113:1641–9.

16. Syrris P, Ward D, Evans A, et al. Arrhythmogenic right ventricular dysplasia/cardiomyopathy associated with mutations in the desmosomal gene desmocollin-2. Am J Hum Genet 2006;79:978–84.
17. Den Haan AD, Tan BY, Zikusoka MN, et al. Comprehensive desmosome mutation analysis in North Americans with arrhythmogenic right ventricular dysplasia/cardiomyopathy. Circ Cardiovasc Genet 2009;(5):428–35.
18. Kaplan SR, Gard JJ, Carvajal-Huerta L, et al. Structural and molecular pathology of the heart in Carvajal syndrome. Cardiovasc Pathol 2004;13:26–32.
19. Kaplan SR, Gard JJ, Protonotarios N, et al. Remodeling of myocyte gap junctions in arrhythmogenic right ventricular cardiomyopathy due to a deletion in plakoglobin (Naxos disease). Heart Rhythm 2004;1:3–11.
20. Oxford EM, Musa H, Maass K, et al. Connexin43 remodeling caused by inhibition of plakophilin-2 expression in cardiac cells. Circ Res 2007;101:703–11.
21. Stein M, van Veen TA, Remme CA, et al. Combined reduction of intercellular coupling and membrane excitability differentially affects transverse and longitudinal cardiac conduction. Cardiovasc Res 2009; 83:52–60.
22. Noorman M, van der Heyden MA, van Veen TA, et al. Cardiac cell-cell junctions in health and disease: electrical versus mechanical coupling. J Mol Cell Cardiol 2009;47:23–31.
23. Asimaki A, Tandri H, Huang H, et al. A new diagnostic test for arrhythmogenic right ventricular cardiomyopathy. N Engl J Med 2009;360:1075–84.
24. Thiene G, Nava A, Corrado D, et al. Right ventricular cardiomyopathy and sudden death in young people. N Engl J Med 1988;318:129–33.
25. Blomstrom-Lundqvist C, Wlodarska EK, Fontaine G, et al. Spectrum of clinicopathologic manifestations of arrhythmogenic right ventricular cardiomyopathy/dysplasia: a multicenter study. J Am Coll Cardiol 1997;30:1512–20.
26. Spear JF, Horowitz LN, Hodess AB, et al. Cellular electrophysiology of human myocardial infarction, I: abnormalities of cellular activation. Circulation 1979;59:247–56.
27. De Bakker JM, van Capelle FJ, Janse MJ, et al. Slow conduction in the infarcted human heart. 'Zigzag' course of activation. Circulation 1993;88:915–26.
28. Cabo C, Pertsov AM, Baxter WT, et al. Wave-front curvature as a cause of slow conduction and block in isolated cardiac muscle. Circ Res 1994;75:1014–28.
29. Fast VG, Kléber AG. Role of wavefront curvature in propagation of cardiac impulse. Cardiovasc Res 1997;33:258–71.
30. Ellison KE, Friedman PL, Ganz LI, et al. Entrainment mapping and radiofrequency catheter ablation of ventricular tachycardia in right ventricular dysplasia. J Am Coll Cardiol 1998;32:724–8.
31. Marchlinski FE, Zado E, Dixit S, et al. Electroanatomic substrate and outcome of catheter ablative therapy for ventricular tachycardia in setting of right ventricular cardiomyopathy. Circulation 2004;110:2293–8.
32. McKenna WJ, Thiene G, Nava A, et al. Diagnosis of arrhythmogenic right ventricular dysplasia/cardiomyopathy. Task Force of the Working Group Myocardial and Pericardial Disease of the European Society of Cardiology and of the Scientific Council on Cardiomyopathies of the International Society and Federation of Cardiology. Br Heart J 1994;71:215–8.
33. Hulot JS, Jouven X, Empana JP, et al. Natural history and risk stratification of arrhythmogenic right ventricular dysplasia/cardiomyopathy. Circulation 2004; 110:1879–84.
34. Marcus FI, McKenna WJ, Sherill D, et al. Diagnosis of arrhythmogenic right ventricular cardiomyopathy/dysplasia (ARVC/D); proposed modifications of the Task Force Criteria. Circulation 2010;121: 1533–41; and Eur Heart J 2010;31:806–14.
35. Fontaine G, Umemura J, Di Donna P, et al. Duration of QRS complexes in arrhythmogenic right ventricular dysplasia. A new non-invasive diagnostic marker. Ann Cardiol Angeiol (Paris) 1993; 42:399–405 [in French].
36. Peters S, Trummel M. Diagnosis of arrhythmogenic right ventricular dysplasia-cardiomyopathy: value of standard ECG revisited. Ann Noninvasive Electrocardiol 2003;8:238–45.
37. Nasir K, Bomma C, Tandri H, et al. Electrocardiographic features of arrhythmogenic right ventricular dysplasia/cardiomyopathy according to disease severity: a need to broaden diagnostic criteria. Circulation 2004;110:1527–34.
38. O'Donnell D, Cox D, Bourke J, et al. Clinical and electrophysiological differences between patients with arrhythmogenic right ventricular dysplasia and right ventricular outflow tract tachycardia. Eur Heart J 2003;24:801–10.
39. Cox MG, Van der Smagt JJ, Wilde AA, et al. New ECG criteria in arrhythmogenic right ventricular dysplasia/cardiomyopathy. Circ Arrhythm Electrophysiol 2009;2:524–30.

Echocardiography in Arrhythmogenic Cardiomyopathy

Danita M.Y. Sanborn, MD*, Michael H. Picard, MD

KEYWORDS

- Arrhythmogenic right ventricular cardiomyopathy/dysplasia
- Cardiac imaging • Diagnosis • Echocardiography

Arrhythmogenic cardiomyopathy (AC) is a cardiomyopathy characterized by fibrofatty replacement of the myocardium of the right ventricle (RV). The disease is often familial and is an important cause of ventricular arrhythmia in the young as well as of RV dilatation and dysfunction.

Echocardiography is an important tool in the initial evaluation of a patient suspected of having AC. It is an ideal modality to assess RV size and function because of its widespread availability, portability, and ease of performance and interpretation. The ability to perform imaging even in patients with AC who have been treated with implantable cardioverter/defibrillators is an important advantage over magnetic resonance imaging (MRI) for following up the affected individuals over time.

Abnormalities of RV structure and function were important components of the diagnostic criteria put forth by the Task Force of the Working Group on Cardiomyopathies in 1994[1]; however, the criteria for major and minor RV structure and function abnormalities developed by this group of experts lacked quantitative cut-points to help clinicians analyze the echocardiographic images of an individual suspected of having AC. At present, there is no single gold standard for the diagnosis, which makes it challenging to correctly categorize individuals at risk for AC. This challenge is most apparent when assessing the family members of the affected individuals or those individuals who may have a subclinical form of the disease.[2,3] Moreover, the echocardiographic natural history of AC has not yet been defined, and a better understanding of disease progression is needed. In 2002, the Multidisciplinary Study of Right Ventricular Dysplasia was initiated in North America to better characterize and quantify the cardiac structural, clinical, and genetic aspects of AC.[4] Recently, modifications to the original task force criteria (TFC) have been proposed by an international working group based on the data collected in this and other studies. These modifications have added quantitative echocardiographic measures to criterion 1 to help improve diagnostic accuracy.[5] The new diagnostic criteria also included cut-points in RV dimensions corrected for body size. **Table 1** summarizes the changes in echocardiographic quantitation in criterion 1 proposed by the working group.

ECHOCARDIOGRAPHIC FINDINGS IN AC

RV Structure

Several structural abnormalities have been noted with increased frequency in individuals with AC. Morphologic abnormalities noted on echocardiography include trabecular prominence and derangement, focal aneurysms or sacculations, and a hyperreflective moderator band (**Fig. 1**).[3,6] The Multidisciplinary Study of Right Ventricular Dysplasia allowed for comparison of a variety of structural and functional echocardiographic parameters between probands with AC and matched controls.[6] In a subgroup of probands from the registry, trabecular derangement was

Cardiology Division, Cardiac Ultrasound Laboratory, Massachusetts General Hospital, Harvard Medical School, 55 Fruit Street, Boston, MA 02114, USA
* Corresponding author. Cardiology Division, Cardiac Ultrasound Laboratory, Massachusetts General Hospital, Harvard Medical School, Yaw 5B-5916, 55 Fruit Street, Boston, MA 02114.
E-mail address: dysanborn@partners.org

Card Electrophysiol Clin 3 (2011) 245–253
doi:10.1016/j.ccep.2011.02.014

Table 1
Quantitative Changes to AC Task Force Criterion 1

Original Task Force Criterion 1: Global and/or Regional Dysfunction and Structural Alterations	Revised Task Force Criterion 1: Global and/or Regional Dysfunction and Structural Alterations
Major	*Major*
Severe dilatation and reduction of RV EF with no (or only mild) LV impairment	RWMA or aneurysm and *1* of the following:
Localized RV aneurysms	PLAX ≥32 mm (≥19 mm/m^2)
Severe segmental RV dilatation	PSAX ≥36 mm (≥21 mm/m^2)
	FAC ≤33%
Minor	*Minor*
Mild global RV dilatation and/or RV EF reduction with normal LV and *1* of the following:	Regional RV akinesia or dyskinesia
Mild segmental dilatation of RV	PLAX 29–32 mm
Regional RV hypokinesia	PSAX 32–36 mm
	RV FAC 33%–40%

Abbreviations: EF, ejection fraction; FAC, fractional area change; LV, left ventricle; PLAX, parasternal long axis; PSAX, parasternal short axis; RWMA, regional wall motion abnormality.

the most frequently noted abnormality, occurring in 54% of the affected individuals and not in any matched controls. In addition, qualitative abnormalities in RV function were frequently noted because 79% of probands demonstrated abnormal regional wall motion. The anterior wall and apex were the most common regions affected in the probands with AC.

The new modifications to the TFC proposed that the finding of localized aneurysm (akinesia and/or dyskinesia) coupled with dilatation or global dysfunction is considered a major criterion for the diagnosis of AC.[5] The presence of aneurysm with only mild dilatation or mild global dysfunction is a minor criterion.

RV dilatation is a common finding in individuals with AC.[3,7,8] The echocardiographic study from the Multidisciplinary Study of Right Ventricular Dysplasia provided potential quantitative parameters to differentiate probands from the matched controls.[6] An enlarged RV outflow tract (RVOT) was found in 100% of probands. The proposed TFC modifications provide quantitative threshold values for RV dimension in the diagnostic criteria for AC and should help improve diagnostic accuracy when the disease is suspected.[5] RVOT dilatation from the parasternal long axis (PLAX) (≥32 mm) or parasternal short axis (PSAX) (≥36 mm) views coupled with depressed RV function or localized aneurysms (akinesia or dyskinesia) is considered a major criterion for the diagnosis of AC. The sensitivity and specificity for the diagnosis of AC are, respectively, 75% and 95% for the PLAX dimension and 62% and 95% for the PSAX dimension (**Fig. 2**).

RV enlargement is of course not specific to AC. The diagnosis of AC in highly trained athletes can be challenging because RV enlargement has been described as an adaptation to endurance sports.[9] In addition, AC with RV enlargement has been associated with sudden death and ventricular arrhythmias in athletes, particularly from the Veneto region of Italy.[10,11] Thus, a careful medical and family history, as well as application of the TFC exclusive of RV structure and function, may help distinguish disease from the normal adaptation to high-intensity exercise. In the future, the use of echocardiography in such patients may be enhanced by the use of newer echocardiographic parameters such as tissue Doppler and speckle imaging for RV myocardial strain and strain rate.

RV Function

Global RV dysfunction is also often noted in individuals with AC. Because of the asymmetric geometry of the RV and difficulty with visualization of the entire RV endocardium in some individuals, estimation of RV volume by conventional 2-dimensional (2D) echocardiography is challenging, thus making accurate estimation of an RV ejection fraction (EF) difficult. The RV fractional area change (FAC) from the apical 4-chamber view has been shown to be a useful correlate of RV function[12] and is decreased in individuals with AC compared with controls (**Fig. 3**).[6] Unfortunately, there have been no large population studies describing normal values for RV FAC with normalization for gender or body size. Recently, using data from the Multidisciplinary Study of AC and a large group (n = 450) of normals, the TFC for diagnosis of AC based on echocardiographic quantitation of RV function have been modified with an RV FAC of 33% or less coupled with localized aneurysm or regional wall motion abnormality being a major criterion. In the presence of regional wall motion abnormality, an FAC of 33% or less has sensitivity of 55% and specificity of 95% for the diagnosis of AC.[5]

NEWER ECHOCARDIOGRAPHIC TECHNIQUES IN AC

In addition to the standard 2D imaging used in the diagnosis of AC, there are new echocardiographic techniques that hold promise. Some of these will enable a more accurate assessment of RV size and some will detect more subtle abnormalities of global or regional RV function.

Three-dimensional (3D) echocardiography is an emerging tool that shows promise for more accurate estimation of RV volumes and RV EF (**Fig. 4**).[13] This technique enables imaging of the entire RV volume from a single transducer position and single image acquisition.[14] Studies have shown that RV volume calculated from 3D echocardiography has less variability than similar calculations by 2D echocardiography.[15–18] One small study demonstrated that RV EFs calculated by 3D echocardiography were decreased in patients with AC compared with normal controls.[19] Another study found that 3D echocardiographic measures could discriminate those with AC from unaffected family members and normal controls; however, variability in this study was higher than that noted in previous RV 3D validation studies.[13] Although this technique can provide improved accuracy in the determination of volume and EF, at present, there are limitations in image quality with 3D transthoracic echocardiography (TTE) and technical considerations of image acquisition, cropping, and measurement that require significant experience with the technique. Normal values and disease cut-points are still being established; thus, at present, the use of this technique is limited to specialized centers with expertise in the use and limitations of 3D echocardiography.

Tissue Doppler echocardiography may aid in the diagnosis of AC. Doppler quantitation of tricuspid valve annular motion can be used as a measure of global RV function (**Fig. 5**). In addition, RV free wall myocardial velocity, strain, and strain rate by either Doppler or feature ("speckle") tracking can precisely quantify global and regional function. Lindstrom and colleagues[8] described reduced systolic (*S*) and early diastolic (E_A) RV annular velocity in subjects with AC compared with unmatched control subjects ($E_{A\ lateral}$ 10.5 ± 3.1 in AC vs 14.6 ± 3.4 in normals). Individuals with AC were found to have a reduced ratio of E_A to the late diastolic (A_A) velocity (0.9 ± 0.3 in AC vs 1.4 ± 0.6 in normals). More recently, systolic strain and systolic strain rate have been shown to be reduced in patients with AC compared with healthy controls.[19–21] RV strain at the base was −6.9 ± 11.9 in an AC group (n = 34) and −24.6 ± 5.8 in a group of normal controls (n = 34).[20] An important limitation of these measures is the angle dependence, requiring that the motion of the wall that is sampled be parallel to the ultrasound beam. Accurate and reproducible measures of RV peak systolic velocity, strain, and strain rate can be challenging even for experienced echocardiographers when the RV becomes significantly enlarged because it is more difficult to line up the distorted RV free wall so that its longitudinal motion is parallel to the ultrasound beam. Thus, the findings described in these small research studies are intriguing, but at present, these measures are best performed at specialized centers experienced in the limitations of the technique. One would expect that quantitation of RV strain and strain rate by feature tracking will be more applicable because it is not based on Doppler and thus is angle independent. Because no studies of patients with AC have been reported with this technique, it remains to be proven as to whether the thinner RV free walls in these patients can be successfully and reproducibly tracked and quantified.

A simple Doppler index of RV function, the RV myocardial performance index (MPI), is independent of geometric assumptions[22] and has been applied in diseases affecting the RV, such as pulmonary hypertension[23] and Ebstein anomaly.[24] Preliminary data regarding the use of this index in AC have demonstrated reduced RV MPI in probands with AC, even when global RV function as assessed by FAC was normal.[25] A more recent small study found this to be a less informative estimate of global RV dysfunction in AC.[21] This index needs to be tested in larger populations to determine its diagnostic use in individuals suspected of having AC.

The RV walls can be difficult to visualize using standard 2D echocardiography; thus, the use of echocardiographic contrast has been described to provide RV opacification and enhanced border detection. Published reports have suggested that the use of intravenous echocardiographic contrast can improve detection of subtle areas of regional dysfunction[26] and have even suggested that abnormalities of RV perfusion can be detected in areas affected by fatty infiltration.[27] Larger populations suspected of having AC need to be studied to define the use of contrast echocardiography in this disease.

The Multidisciplinary Study of Right Ventricular Dysplasia enrolled newly AC diagnosed individuals, and the study protocol included multimodality imaging with TTE, cardiac MRI, and RV

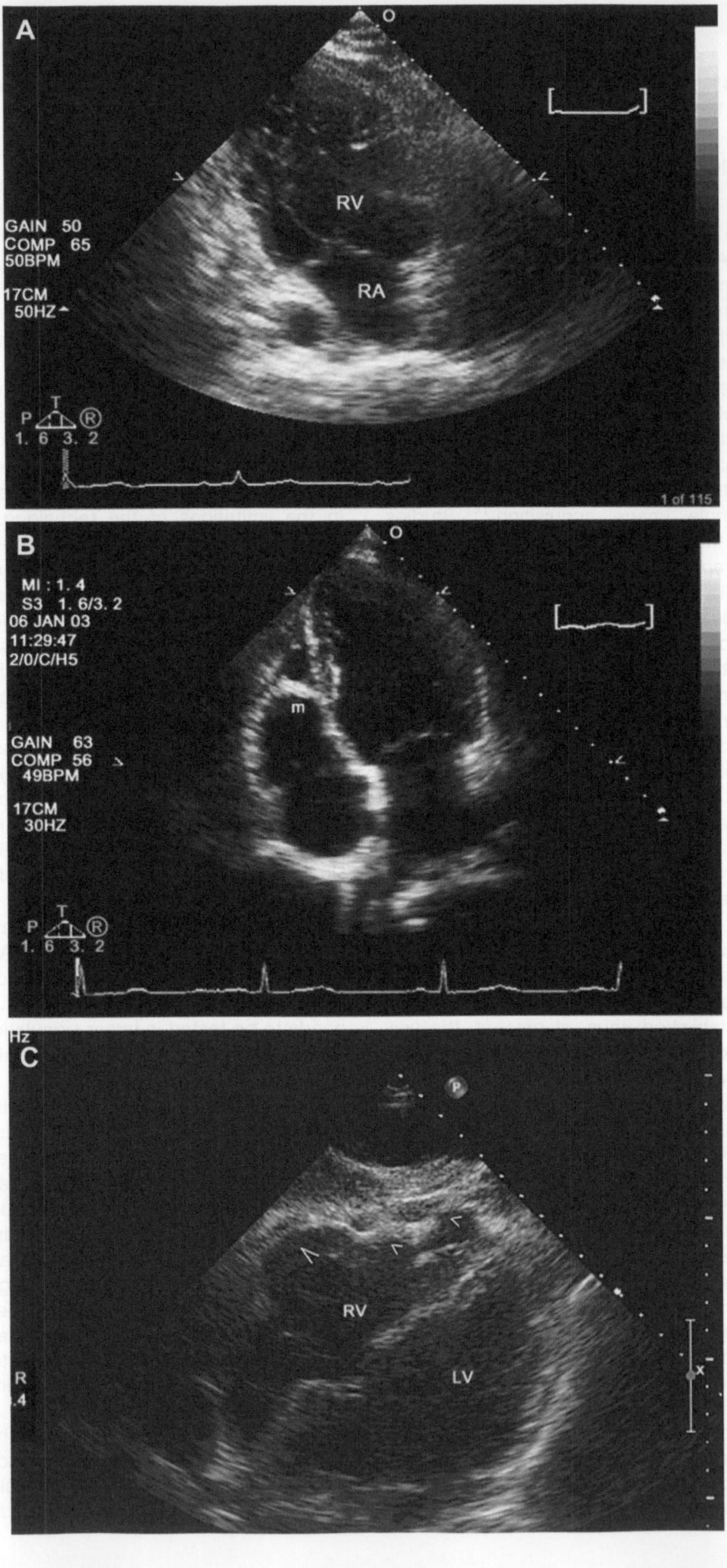
A
O
RV
RA
GAIN 50
COMP 65
50BPM
17CM
50HZ
P T R
1. 6 3. 2
1 of 115
B
O
MI : 1. 4
S3 1. 6/3. 2
06 JAN 03
11:29:47
2/0/C/H5
m
GAIN 63
COMP 56
49BPM
17CM
30HZ
P T R
1. 6 3. 2
Hz
C
P
RV
LV
R
.4
X

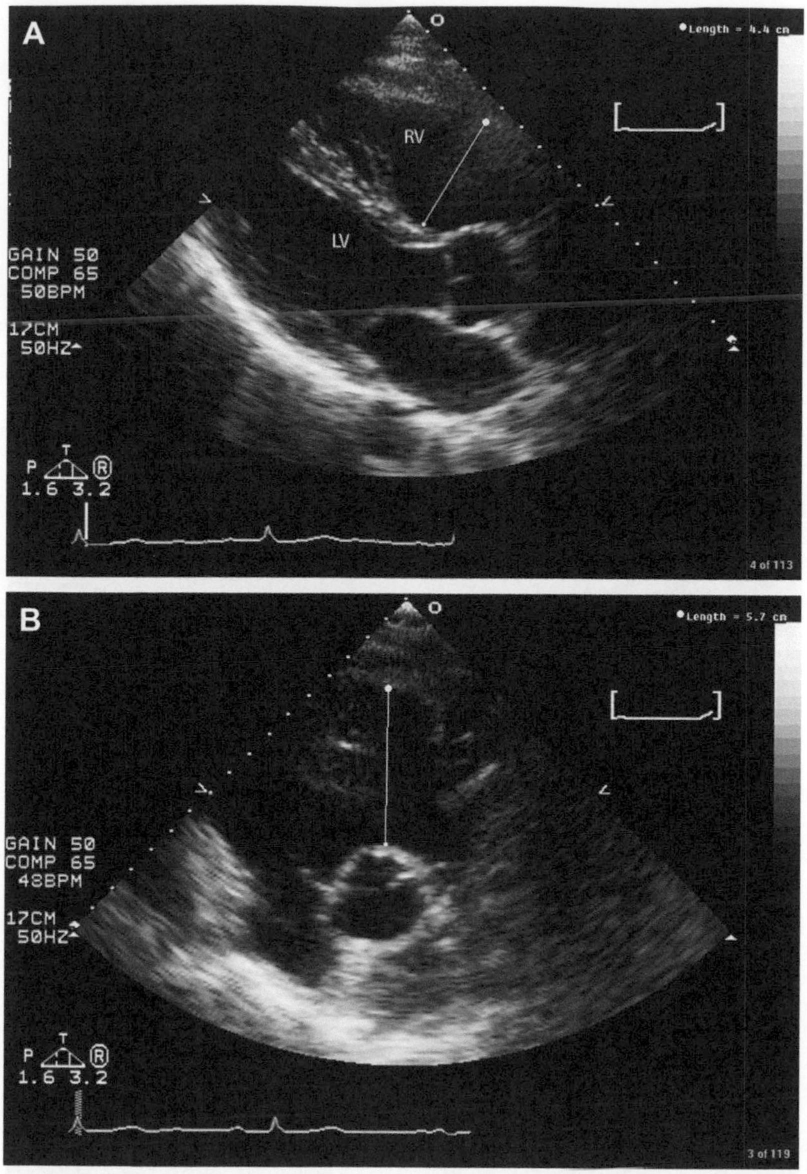

Fig. 2. Measurement of RVOT dimensions on 2-dimensional echocardiography. (*A*) From the parasternal long axis view. (*B*) From the parasternal short axis view. LV, left ventricle; RV, right ventricle.

angiography, all performed at enrolling centers and subsequently interpreted at core laboratories. The diagnostic performance of the tests revealed that echocardiography was superior to MRI with 80% accuracy in affected individuals and 40% accuracy in borderline individuals, compared with 49% accuracy in affected individuals and 15% accuracy in borderline individuals for MRI.[4] Regional wall motion abnormalities were more often identified by echocardiography (73%) than by RV angiography (70%) or MRI (51%).

A multivariable predictive model using 7 variables (MRI, electrocardiography [ECG], echocardiography, signal-averaged ECG, RV biopsy, Holter monitor, and RV angiography) was tested removing 1 variable at a time to determine which

Fig. 1. Structural alternations noted on 2-dimensional echocardiography with increased frequency in AC. (*A*) Trabecular derangement. (*B*) Reflective moderator band. (*C*) Localized aneurysms (*arrowheads*) in the RV free wall. RA, right atrium; m, RV moderator band.

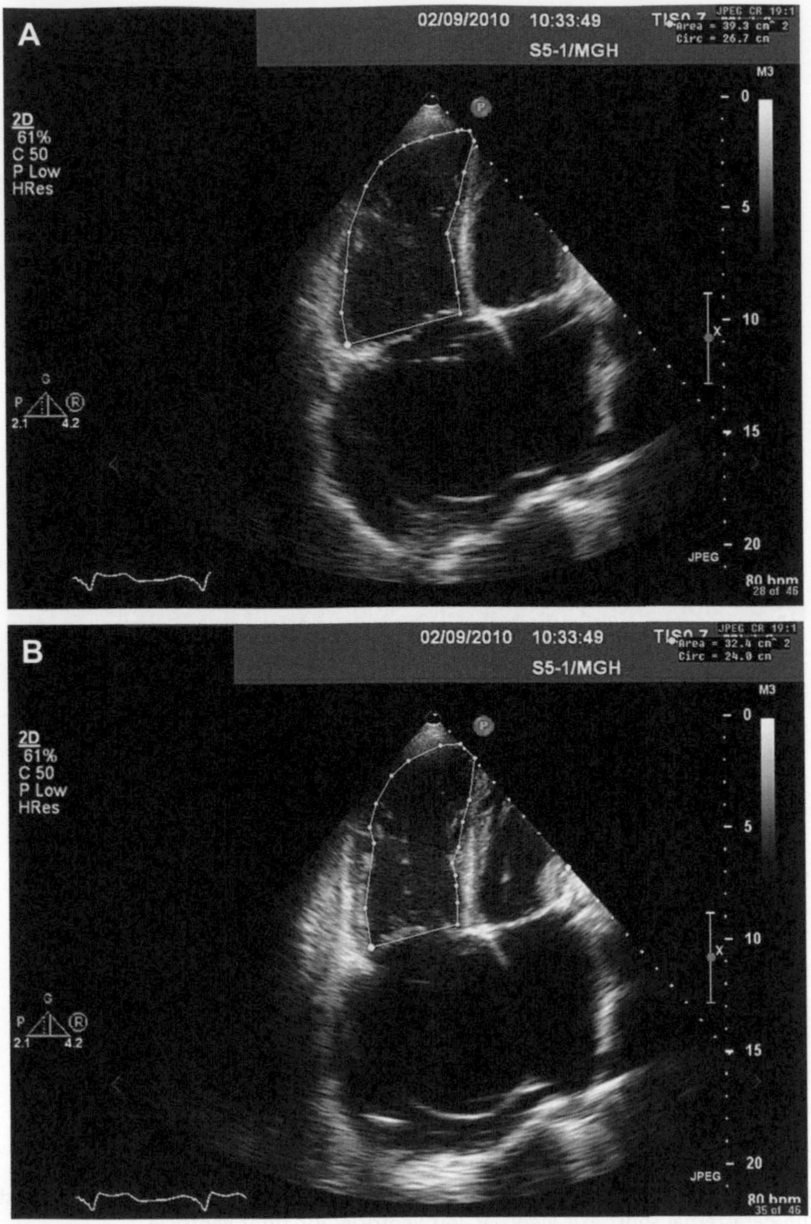

Fig. 3. Example of RV FAC measurement from the apical 4-chamber view. (*A*) RV area at end diastole. (*B*) RV area at end systole.

tests would cause the most decline in diagnostic accuracy. The largest decline occurred when echocardiography was removed from the model, suggesting that echocardiography is an important imaging method in the diagnosis of AC.

GENETICS OF AC AND ECHOCARDIOGRAPHY

A variety of mutations in genes encoding desmosomal proteins have been found in families and individuals with AC. The pattern of inheritance seems mostly autosomal dominant with incomplete penetrance, although recessive forms have also been described.[28,29] Plakophilin-2 mutations have been associated with RV structural abnormalities in 68% of patients with AC.[30] Certain genetic mutations seem associated with a biventricular form of the disease, with left ventricular (LV) dilatation and dysfunction in conjunction with RV abnormalities.[31] Desmoplakin mutations

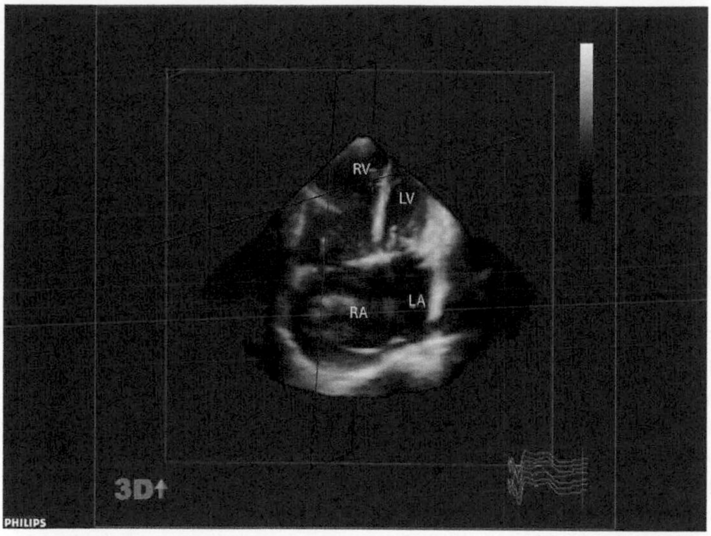

Fig. 4. 3D echocardiography of AC from the apical 4-chamber perspective. LA, left atrium; LV, left ventricle; RA, right atrium; RV, right ventricle.

have been associated with RV echocardiographic abnormalities in 54% and LV involvement in half of those with RV involvement.[32] In the Multidisciplinary Study of Right Ventricular Dysplasia, a similar frequency of desmosomal abnormalities was noted in those phenotyped as borderline and those phenotyped as affected, thus supporting the hypothesis that probands phenotyped as borderline have an early form of the disease.

SUMMARY

Echocardiography is a useful tool for clinicians treating an individual suspected of having AC. Dilatation of the RV (and in particular the RVOT) is the most frequently observed echocardiographic abnormality. RV dilatation (PLAX $\geq$32 mm or PSAX $\geq$36 mm) coupled with localized aneurysm (akinesia or dyskinesia) or global RV dysfunction (FAC $\leq$33%) is now considered

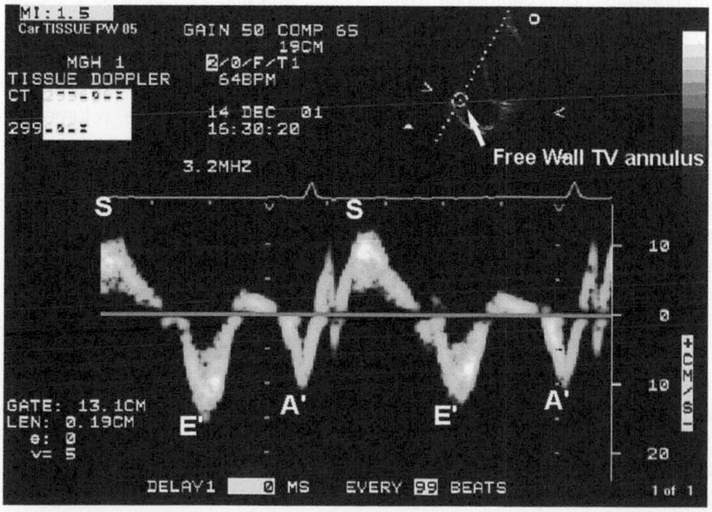

Fig. 5. Tissue Doppler echocardiography of RV from the apical 4-chamber view. Doppler sample volume is placed on the tricuspid valve (TV) annulus at the free wall. E′, early TV annular peak diastolic velocity; A′, late TV annular peak diastolic velocity; S, TV annular peak systolic velocity.

a major criterion for the diagnosis of AC. Morphologic abnormalities are also often noted in individuals with AC and may provide useful supporting evidence when AC is suspected. Echocardiography has a high diagnostic accuracy for the disease compared with MRI.

REFERENCES

1. McKenna WJ, Thiene G, Nava A, et al. Diagnosis of arrhythmogenic right ventricular dysplasia/cardiomyopathy. Task Force of the Working Group Myocardial and Pericardial Disease of the European Society of Cardiology and of the Scientific Council on Cardiomyopathies of the International Society and Federation of Cardiology. Br Heart J 1994;71:215–8.
2. Nava A, Bauce B, Basso C, et al. Clinical profile and long-term follow-up of 37 families with arrhythmogenic right ventricular cardiomyopathy. J Am Coll Cardiol 2000;36:2226–33.
3. Scognamiglio R, Fasoli G, Nava A, et al. Contribution of cross-sectional echocardiography to the diagnosis of right ventricular dysplasia at the asymptomatic stage. Eur Heart J 1989;10:538–42.
4. Marcus FI, Zareba W, Calkins H, et al. Arrhythmogenic right ventricular cardiomyopathy/dysplasia clinical presentation and diagnostic evaluation: results from the North American multidisciplinary study. Heart Rhythm 2009;6:984–92.
5. Marcus FI, McKenna WJ, Sherrill D, et al. Diagnosis of arrhythmogenic right ventricular cardiomyopathy/dysplasia: proposed modification of the task force criteria. Circulation 2010;121:1533–41; and Eur Heart J 2010;31:806–14.
6. Yoerger DM, Marcus F, Sherrill D, et al. Echocardiographic findings in patients meeting task force criteria for arrhythmogenic right ventricular dysplasia: new insights from the multidisciplinary study of right ventricular dysplasia. J Am Coll Cardiol 2005;45:860–5.
7. Blomstrom-Lundqvist C, Beckman-Suurkula M, Wallentin I, et al. Ventricular dimensions and wall motion assessed by echocardiography in patients with arrhythmogenic right ventricular dysplasia. Eur Heart J 1988;9:1291–302.
8. Lindstrom L, Wilkenshoff UM, Larsson H, et al. Echocardiographic assessment of arrhythmogenic right ventricular cardiomyopathy. Heart 2001;86:31–8.
9. Henriksen E, Kangro T, Jonason T, et al. An echocardiographic study of right ventricular adaptation to physical exercise in elite male orienteers. Clin Physiol 1998;18:498–503.
10. Corrado D, Fontaine G, Marcus FI, et al. Arrhythmogenic right ventricular dysplasia/cardiomyopathy: need for an international registry. Study Group on Arrhythmogenic Right Ventricular Dysplasia/Cardiomyopathy of the Working Groups on Myocardial and Pericardial Disease and Arrhythmias of the European Society of Cardiology and of the Scientific Council on Cardiomyopathies of the World Heart Federation. Circulation 2000;101:E101–6.
11. Thiene G, Nava A, Corrado D, et al. Right ventricular cardiomyopathy and sudden death in young people. N Engl J Med 1988;318:129–33.
12. Lang RM, Bierig M, Devereux RB, et al. Recommendations for chamber quantification: a report from the American Society of Echocardiography's Guidelines and Standards Committee and the Chamber Quantification Writing Group, developed in conjunction with the European Association of Echocardiography, a branch of the European Society of Cardiology. J Am Soc Echocardiogr 2005;18:1440–63.
13. Prakasa KR, Dalal D, Wang J, et al. Feasibility and variability of three dimensional echocardiography in arrhythmogenic right ventricular dysplasia/cardiomyopathy. Am J Cardiol 2006;97:703–9.
14. Picard MH. Three dimensional echocardiography. In: Otto CM, editor. The practice of clinical echocardiography. Philadelphia: Elsevier; 2007. p. 86–114.
15. Jiang L, Handschumacher MD, Hibberd MG, et al. Three-dimensional echocardiographic reconstruction of right ventricular volume: in vitro comparison with two-dimensional methods. J Am Soc Echocardiogr 1994;7:150–8.
16. Jiang L, Siu SC, Handschumacher MD, et al. Three-dimensional echocardiography. In vivo validation for right ventricular volume and function. Circulation 1994;89:2342–50.
17. Leibundgut G, Rohner A, Grize L, et al. Dynamic assessment of right ventricular volumes and function by real-time three-dimensional echocardiography: a comparison study with magnetic resonance imaging in 100 adult patients. J Am Soc Echocardiogr 2010;23:116–26.
18. Shiota T, Jones M, Chikada M, et al. Real-time three-dimensional echocardiography for determining right ventricular stroke volume in an animal model of chronic right ventricular volume overload. Circulation 1998;97:1897–900.
19. Kjaergaard J, Hastrup Svendsen J, Sogaard P, et al. Advanced quantitative echocardiography in arrhythmogenic right ventricular cardiomyopathy. J Am Soc Echocardiogr 2007;20:27–35.
20. Teske AJ, Cox MG, De Boeck BW, et al. Echocardiographic tissue deformation imaging quantifies abnormal regional right ventricular function in arrhythmogenic right ventricular dysplasia/cardiomyopathy. J Am Soc Echocardiogr 2009;22:920–7.
21. Wang J, Prakasa K, Bomma C, et al. Comparison of novel echocardiographic parameters of right ventricular function with ejection fraction by cardiac magnetic resonance. J Am Soc Echocardiogr 2007;20:1058–64.

22. Tei C, Dujardin KS, Hodge DO, et al. Doppler echocardiographic index for assessment of global right ventricular function. J Am Soc Echocardiogr 1996; 9:838–47.
23. Sebbag I, Rudski LG, Therrien J, et al. Effect of chronic infusion of epoprostenol on echocardiographic right ventricular myocardial performance index and its relation to clinical outcome in patients with primary pulmonary hypertension. Am J Cardiol 2001;88:1060–3.
24. Eidem BW, Tei C, O'Leary PW, et al. Nongeometric quantitative assessment of right and left ventricular function: myocardial performance index in normal children and patients with Ebstein anomaly. J Am Soc Echocardiogr 1998;11:849–56.
25. Yoerger DM, Marcus F, Sherrill D, et al. Right ventricular myocardial performance index in probands from the multicenter study of arrhythmogenic right ventricular dysplasia. J Am Coll Cardiol 2005; 45(3 Suppl A):147A.
26. Lopez-Fernandez T, Garcia-Fernandez MA, Perez David E, et al. Usefulness of contrast echocardiography in arrhythmogenic right ventricular dysplasia. J Am Soc Echocardiogr 2004;17:391–3.
27. Nemes A, Vletter WB, Scholten MF, et al. Contrast echocardiography for perfusion in right ventricular cardiomyopathy. Eur J Echocardiogr 2005;6:470–2.
28. Alcalai R, Metzger S, Rosenheck S, et al. A recessive mutation in desmoplakin causes arrhythmogenic right ventricular dysplasia, skin disorder, and woolly hair. J Am Coll Cardiol 2003;42:319–27.
29. McKoy G, Protonotarios N, Crosby A, et al. Identification of a deletion in plakoglobin in arrhythmogenic right ventricular cardiomyopathy with palmoplantar keratoderma and woolly hair (Naxos disease). Lancet 2000;355:2119–24.
30. Syrris P, Ward D, Asimaki A, et al. Clinical expression of plakophilin-2 mutations in familial arrhythmogenic right ventricular cardiomyopathy. Circulation 2006; 113:356–64.
31. Bauce B, Nava A, Beffagna G, et al. Multiple mutations in desmosomal proteins encoding genes in arrhythmogenic right ventricular cardiomyopathy/ dysplasia. Heart Rhythm 2010;7:22–9.
32. Bauce B, Basso C, Rampazzo A, et al. Clinical profile of four families with arrhythmogenic right ventricular cardiomyopathy caused by dominant desmoplakin mutations. Eur Heart J 2005;26:1666–75.

Ventricular Angiography in Arrhythmogenic Cardiomyopathy

Thomas Wichter, MD[a,*], Julia H. Indik, MD, PhD[b], Matthias Paul, MD[c]

KEYWORDS

- Angiography
- Arrhythmogenic right ventricular cardiomyopathy/dysplasia
- Cardiac imaging • Diagnosis

Arrhythmogenic cardiomyopathy (AC) is characterized by regional or global abnormalities of right ventricular (RV) structure and function and ventricular tachyarrhythmias, including sudden death.[1,2] Progressive atrophy and loss of myocytes with subsequent fatty and/or fibrous tissue replacement and interspersed surviving myocyte fibers provide the morphologic substrate for reentrant arrhythmias and regional (segmental) or global abnormalities of RV structure and function. In the early phase of AC, the myocardium of the RV free wall is predominantly involved, whereas the trabecular as well as septal and left ventricular myocardium are usually spared. In advanced disease stages, clinical signs of right or global heart failure and left ventricular involvement may develop.[3,4]

AC is inheritable, with an autosomal dominant trait, mainly involving mutations in genes encoding for desmosomal proteins.[5] However, incomplete penetrance and variable expressivity account for different clinical disease manifestations and the occurrence of asymptomatic silent gene carriers without clinical signs or symptoms of AC.

PATHOPHYSIOLOGY

Current pathophysiologic concepts hypothesize that a genetic disposition of (latent) dysfunction of desmosomal cell contacts may lead to mechanical disruption of cell-to-cell adhesion and loss of intercellular signaling functions. This course may be triggered or aggravated by inflammatory processes (superimposed myocarditis), autonomic dysfunction, or mechanical stretch of the myocardium and leads to myocyte atrophy and fibrofatty replacement, ultimately resulting in the clinically dominant propensity for ventricular arrhythmias and heart failure. Although not proven, this concept is attractive and plausible because it explains the high prevalence of AC among athletes and the predominant manifestation in the RV free wall, which is more prone to myocardial stretch during physical activity, training, and sports. On

This work was partly supported by grants from the European Commission, Brussels, Belgium (QLG1-CT-2000-01,091); National Institutes of Health, Bethesda, MD, USA (1 UO1 HL65594-01); and Deutsche Forschungsgemeinschaft, Bonn, Germany (SFB-556; project C4).

[a] Department of Internal Medicine and Cardiology, Heart Center Osnabrück–Bad Rothenfelde, Niels Stensen Kliniken, Marienhospital Osnabrück, Bischofsstr. 1, D-49074, Osnabrück, Germany
[b] Section of Cardiology, Sarver Heart Center, University of Arizona College of Medicine, 1501 North Campbell Avenue, Tucson, AZ 85724-5037, USA
[c] Department of Cardiology and Angiology, Medizinische Klinik und Poliklinik C (Kardiologie und Angiologie), Universitätsklinikum Münster, Albert-Schweitzer-Strasse 33, D-48149, Münster, Germany
* Corresponding author. Klinik für Innere Medizin/Kardiologie, Niels Stensen Kliniken, Marienhospital Osnabrück, Herzzentrum Osnabrück-Bad Rothenfelde, Bischofsstr. 1, D-49074, Osnabrück, Germany.
E-mail address: thomas.wichter@mho.de

Card Electrophysiol Clin 3 (2011) 255–267
doi:10.1016/j.ccep.2011.02.008
1877-9182/11/$ – see front matter © 2011 Published by Elsevier Inc.

the other hand, the concept explains the compensatory hypertrophy of RV trabeculae and the late involvement of septal and left ventricular myocardium, which are less exposed to myocardial stretch.[6,7]

STRUCTURAL ABNORMALITIES IN AC

Fibrofatty replacement of RV myocardium results in abnormal structure, morphology, geometry, and wall motion of the RV. In AC, the major structural abnormality consists in the regional loss (atrophy) of myocardium with subsequent replacement by fibrofatty tissue (**Fig. 1**A).

This abnormality results in localized RV wall thinning, aneurysms, bulgings, and abnormal systolic motion, which predominantly occur in RV free wall areas. Predilection sites are located in the outflow tract, the apex, and the inferobasal (subtricuspid) areas of the RV (see **Fig. 1**B). These sites were already recognized in the early clinical description of AC by Marcus and colleagues[1] who introduced the term triangle of dysplasia.

In contrast, the interventricular septum and the left ventricle are usually spared in the early stage of AC. RV trabeculae are also not primarily affected by the atrophic process and tend to show a compensatory hypertrophy, resulting in an aspect of increased trabeculation and fissuring of the RV walls. In more advanced stages of AC, the RV may develop global dilatation and dysfunction with subsequent tricuspid regurgitation caused by dilatation of the tricuspid annulus, which may cause clinical signs of right heart failure.

Left ventricular involvement can frequently be detected by postmortem histology[8] but is rarely

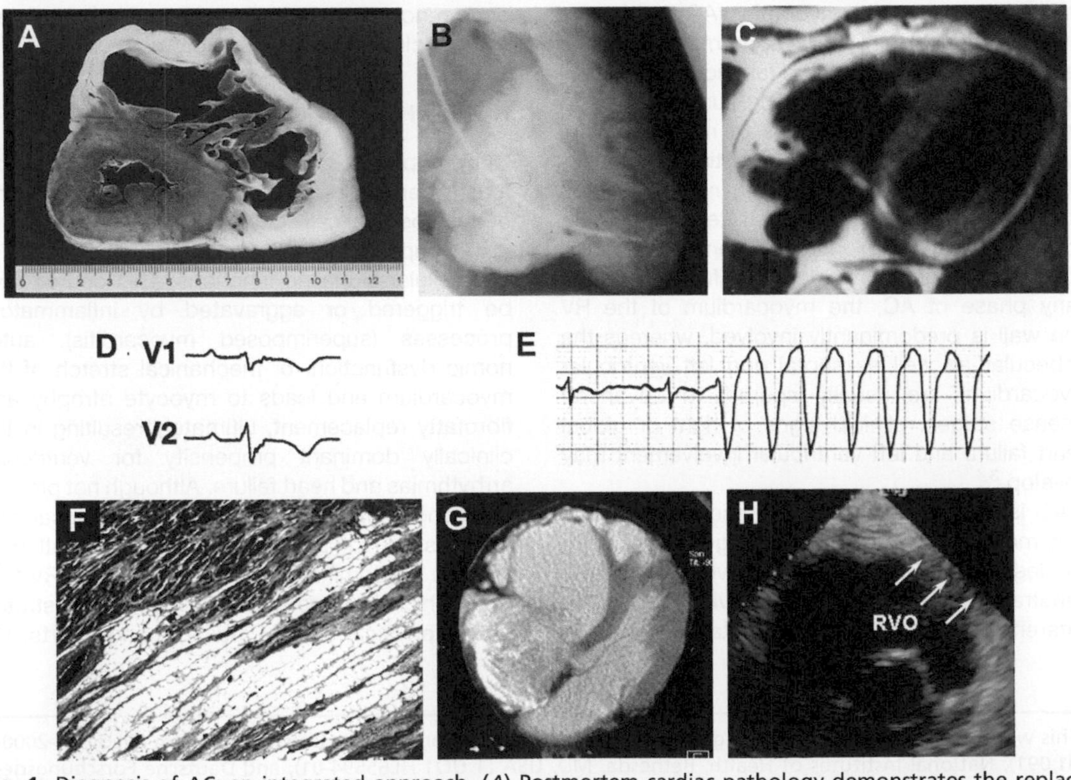

Fig. 1. Diagnosis of AC: an integrated approach. (*A*) Postmortem cardiac pathology demonstrates the replacement of RV free wall myocardium by fatty and fibrous tissues in a patient with classical and advanced stage of AC. (*B*) RV angiogram with global dilatation and regional dyskinesia in the outflow tract, apex, and subtricuspid area (triangle of dysplasia) of the RV. (*C*) Magnetic resonance image showing transmurally increased signal intensity, indicating fatty replacement of the RV free wall. (*D*) Right precordial electrocardiography recording demonstrating T-wave inversion, QRS prolongation, broad S wave, and ϵ potential. (*E*) Onset of monomorphic ventricular tachycardia. (*F*) Typical histologic finding in a patient with AC: RV myocardial atrophy and subsequent replacement by fibrofatty tissue with single surviving strands of myocytes. (*G*) Cardiac multislice computed tomographic image demonstrating severe RV enlargement and fatty replacement of the anterior RV free wall myocardium. (*H*) Echocardiography (parasternal short axis view) demonstrating an aneurysm in the RV outflow tract (*arrows*). (*From* Wichter T, Paul M, Breithardt G. Arrhythmogene rechtsventrikuläre Kardiomyopathie: sportmedizinische Aspekte. Deutsche Zeitschrift für Sportmedizin 2005;56:122 [in German]; with permission.)

an early or dominant clinical manifestation. However, if left ventricular involvement is detectable by clinical signs or cardiac imaging, it usually indicates an advanced, progressive, or longstanding disease and may become clinically relevant by progression to global heart failure.

DIAGNOSIS OF AC

The structural abnormalities of the RV myocardium provide the basis for the main clinical and diagnostic features of AC. Apart from the ventricular tachyarrhythmias that are frequently the first clinical manifestation of AC, these abnormalities also result in characteristic features in the electrocardiography (ECG) and imaging.

However, the clinical diagnosis of AC may be difficult because there is no easily obtained single test or finding with high diagnostic accuracy.[9,10] Therefore, the diagnosis of AC usually requires an integrated approach with assessment of electrical, anatomic, and functional abnormalities (see **Fig. 1**). In the recent prospective North American Multidisciplinary Study on AC,[10] a 5-variable model including echocardiography, RV angiography, ECG, signal-averaged ECG, and Holter monitoring resulted in good diagnostic performance. Additionally performing magnetic resonance imaging (MRI) and endomyocardial biopsy (EMB) added only marginally to the diagnostic accuracy.[10]

ROLE OF VENTRICULAR ANGIOGRAPHY IN AC

General Aspects

Invasive contrast RV cine angiocardiography was the first imaging modality to be used for the diagnosis of AC. Subsequently, several imaging techniques were introduced into routine diagnostic workup for the detection and characterization of abnormal structure and motion of ventricular walls. Among these techniques are echocardiography, radionuclide angiography, MRI, multislice computed tomography, and the electroanatomic mapping of the right and left ventricles. However, none of these techniques are ideal as a single diagnostic test because they all have individual advantages and limitations in the diagnosis and characterization of AC.[9–13]

In particular, the role of MRI remains a matter of controversy because of the technical limitations to depict the RV free wall with high resolution and the considerable interobserver variability, which result in significant overdiagnosing, underdiagnosing, and misdiagnosing.[14] However, under optimal conditions of expert interpretation, the various imaging modalities employed in the diagnostic evaluation of AC should be considered and used complementarily rather than competitively.[9–13]

RV Angiography

Despite its invasiveness, RV cine angiography still remains a reference imaging technique in the diagnosis of AC mainly because selective angiography displays not only the entire cavity but also the contours of the RV better than other techniques. However, because of its complex shape and geometry, the angiographic definition of the normal RV is difficult because variable morphologic and functional findings produce a wide range of normality.

Angiographic features of RV structure and function in AC include global and regional dilatations or aneurysms with abnormalities of wall structure and motion. Additional aspects refer to trabecular size and structure as well as delayed ventricular contrast evacuation (dye persistence). Although many of these angiographic signs and features are frequently found in AC, only few are specific for the diagnosis. Furthermore, such findings are mainly dependent on the subjective interpretation of an experienced investigator because objective criteria or quantitative (cutoff) measures for evaluation have not been available in the past.

In addition, the specificity of angiographic findings in AC requires further definition, particularly in relation to normal subjects and patients with other diseases affecting the RV. It is therefore important that cine angiography of the RV is performed under optimal conditions according to a standardized protocol.

HOW TO PERFORM VENTRICULAR ANGIOGRAPHY IN AC

The following recommendations were developed and proposed by Wichter[15] for the core laboratory of RV angiography within the National Institutes of Health–funded North American Multidisciplinary Study of Right Ventricular Dysplasia[10,12] and the European Union–funded European Registry of Arrhythmogenic Right Ventricular Cardiomyopathy.[13] The protocol was designed to perform RV angiograms of best quality to assess structural and functional RV abnormalities in AC and to allow quantitative measurements of RV volumes, ejection fraction, and regional contraction and relaxation.

Right Heart Catheterization

After jugular or femoral venous puncture, right heart catheterization should be performed before RV angiography to assess RV and pulmonary vascular hemodynamics. Pressures are recorded in the pulmonary capillary wedge position, pulmonary artery, RV, and right atrium. Cardiac output is determined by oximetry and/or thermodilution. Cardiac index, stroke volume, and pulmonary vascular resistance are calculated from these measures.[15] Additional RV EMB may be performed for histologic, ultrastructural, or molecular biology investigations if clinically indicated or if part of a research program.

Calibration Reference

Volume calculations from right ventricular angiograms require calibration for reference. Usually, catheters with defined distance markers are used for calibration reference. As alternatives, a metal ball with defined diameter or a ruler with defined distances may be used as reference tools (**Fig. 2**). A simple way is to use a 20-cm ruler with staples at each 2-cm distance. The external calibration reference tool (ball or ruler) should be placed 10 cm below and horizontal to the amplifier tube and recorded by cine. The height of the table and the distance of the amplifier tube to the patient chest should not be changed during the following angiograms.[15]

Right Ventricular Contrast Cine Angiography

For selective RV angiography, a pigtail catheter (5F or larger) or a Berman catheter (6F or larger) may be used for contrast injection. The catheter should be positioned approximately 1 cm above the midinferior RV wall without direct contact with the RV wall or trabeculae to avoid mechanical induction of extrasystoles and to allow homogeneous opacification of the RV cavity during contrast injection. At least 3 standard projections are recommended: 30° right anterior oblique (RAO), anteroposterior (AP), and straight lateral ([LAT] sagittal).[15] An additional 30° RAO projection with 20° to 30° caudocranial angulation may be used to better visualize wall motion abnormalities confined to the inferior and inferobasal RV walls.

Cine angiograms should be acquired during deep inspiration and breath holding and recorded at 25 or 30 images per second. Cine angiogram is useful to film a long sequence to allow analysis of regional contrast persistence, lung passage, as well as left atrial and ventricular size and function. Depending on the global size of the RV, 40 to 50 mL of low-toxicity contrast medium should be injected with a flow rate (velocity) of 12 to 15 mL/s.[15]

Optimizing Image Quality

To optimize the image quality of RV cine angiograms, the investigator should make sure that the entire RV is depicted in the field of view during breath holding in all projections. Patient and table movements should be avoided during contrast injection.

Artificial wall motion abnormalities resulting from ventricular extrasystoles or mechanical catheter wall contact or pressure as well as tricuspid regurgitation during contrast injection and image recording

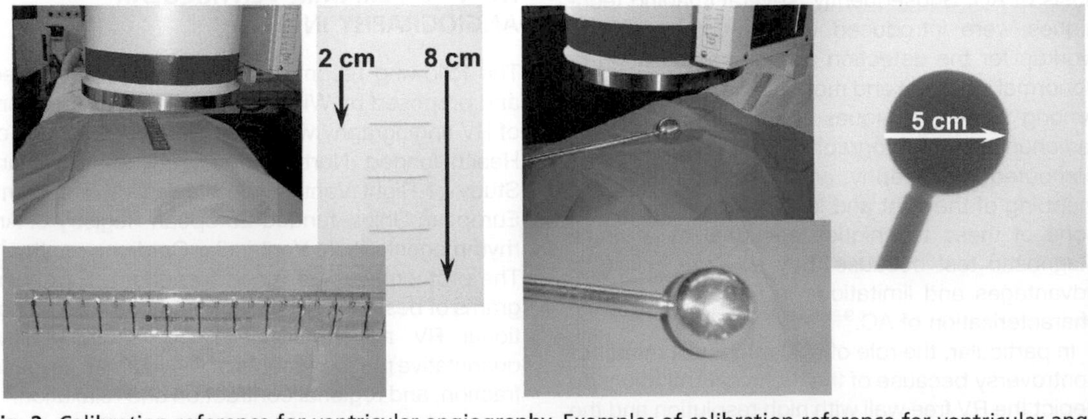

Fig. 2. Calibration reference for ventricular angiography. Examples of calibration reference for ventricular angiography. A ruler with staples placed at defined distances (ie, 2 cm) (*A*) or a metal ball with a defined diameter (ie, 5 cm) (*B*) may be used as simple tools for calibration. As an alternative, catheters with calibration markers may be used for reference. (*From* Wichter T, Indik JH, Daliento L. Diagnostic role of angiography. In: Marcus FI, Nava A, Thiene G, editors. Arrhythmogenic RV cardiomyopathy/dysplasia: recent advances. Milan (Italy): Springer; 2007. p. 149. Chapter 16. Fig. 16.3; with permission.)

may impair visual and quantitative assessment of RV motion and volumes.

Both ventricular extrasystoles and catheter contact to the RV walls can be avoided by optimal catheter position and limitation of contrast injection velocity. Catheter-induced artificial tricuspid regurgitation can be avoided by smooth catheter passage of the tricuspid valve without mechanical distension of valvular structures.[14]

Left Ventricular Contrast Cine Angiography

Left ventricular angiography should be performed according to common practice and guidelines with biplane 30° RAO and 60° left anterior oblique (LAO) projections and 30 to 40 mL of low-toxicity contrast medium at a flow rate (velocity) of 10 to 12 mL/s.

ANGIOGRAPHIC FEATURES IN AC

A variety of morphologic and structural RV angiographic features have been reported to be suggestive or diagnostic of AC. These features include global and regional dilatation, dilatation of the outflow tract, localized akinetic or dyskinetic bulges and outpouchings, polycyclic contours (cauliflower aspect), and trabecular hypertrophy and/or disarray with deep horizontal fissures (pile d'assiettes) of the RV as well as contrast persistence caused by delayed evacuation in abnormal ventricular areas.[16]

RV WALL STRUCTURE

Trabecular Hypertrophy

Transverse orientation of hypertrophic trabeculae, mainly located in the anterior and anteroseptal RV areas, separated by deep horizontal fissures create the so-called pile d'assiettes image (**Fig. 3**) that is considered a frequent but not very specific finding in AC.[17,18]

The diagnostic value of trabecular hypertrophy is controversial[17] because of the difficulty to define and to distinguish abnormal from normal RV trabeculation. Therefore, and probably because of the large variability of normality and the subjective assessment and interpretation, this feature was not included as a diagnostic angiographic finding in the Task Force criteria for the diagnosis of AC.[9,11]

However, in the association with trabecular hypertrophy (≥4 mm) and the presence of deep fissures or so-called Y-shaped giant trabeculae, transverse trabecular arrangement (see **Fig. 3**) is considered to be of much higher diagnostic value. This higher diagnostic value is particularly true when these angiographic features are located in the apical and supra-apical RV areas where they are considered to reflect abnormal hypertrophy of the papillary muscles and the moderator band.

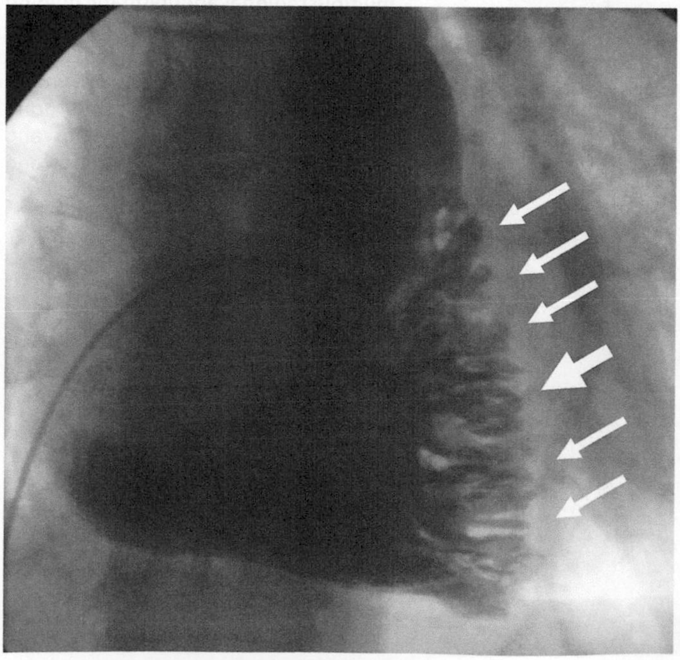

Fig. 3. Transverse trabecular hypertrophy. RV angiogram (30° RAO view) demonstrating transverse trabecular hypertrophy (*arrows*) with horizontal fissures (pile d'assiettes) and Y-shaped giant trabecula (*big arrow*) in the anteroseptal, apical, and outflow tract areas of the RV in a patient with AC. (*From* Wichter T, Indik JH, Daliento L. Diagnostic role of angiography. In: Marcus FI, Nava A, Thiene G, editors. Arrhythmogenic RV cardiomyopathy/dysplasia: recent advances. Milan (Italy): Springer; 2007. p. 151. Chapter 16. Fig. 16.4; with permission.)

Polycyclic Contours

In areas of more severe structural remodeling, multiple sacculations or round opacified areas merge to produce a polycyclic contour of the RV wall, also described as a cauliflower aspect (**Figs. 4** and **5**). This finding is considered a specific and diagnostic angiographic feature strongly suggestive of AC. However, this feature is not very sensitive because it mainly occurs in more advanced disease stages.

Contrast Persistence

Regionally delayed contrast evacuation (dye persistence) in the RV is a frequent angiographic finding in AC. However, this feature also occurs in normal control subjects, particularly in the inferobasal area, and therefore lacks specificity. In such cases, the finding appears to be related to the physiologic asynchronous contraction of the RV wall. Therefore, localized contrast persistence should only be considered as a finding indicative for AC if it occurs in an area of abnormal RV structure or function.

RV WALL MOTION

Regional Hypokinesia

In contrast to the homogeneous and uniform contraction of the normal left ventricle, the normal RV shows regional differences in contraction. These regional differences were clearly demonstrated in the quantitative analyses of regional RV wall motion in normal control subjects and patients with AC in a study by Indik and colleagues.[19,20] These studies showed significant differences of wall motion in the various regions of the RV. RV inflow tract areas contributed much more to systolic contraction than midanterior and outflow tract areas as measured by the normalized change in total contour area of RV angiograms (**Fig. 6**).[19,20]

Furthermore, the relative timing of contraction was inhomogeneous. Strain as another measure of nonuniform contraction was also found to vary significantly in different locations, thus also reflecting the heterogeneous motion of the RV wall. One study also demonstrated no differences in RV wall motion between normal control subjects and patients with idiopathic RV outflow tract (RVOT) tachycardia.[19]

Therefore, mild hypokinesia in the apical, anterior, or outflow tract region is not a pathologic but rather a normal finding of RV wall motion. This wide overlap with normality makes it particularly difficult to differentiate mild forms of localized AC from normal RV wall motion. Therefore, more detailed quantification of regional RV wall motion is required to evaluate and correctly diagnose such patients.

Bulgings and Aneurysms

In contrast to regional hypokinesia, localized akinetic or dyskinetic areas (aneurysms, bulgings,

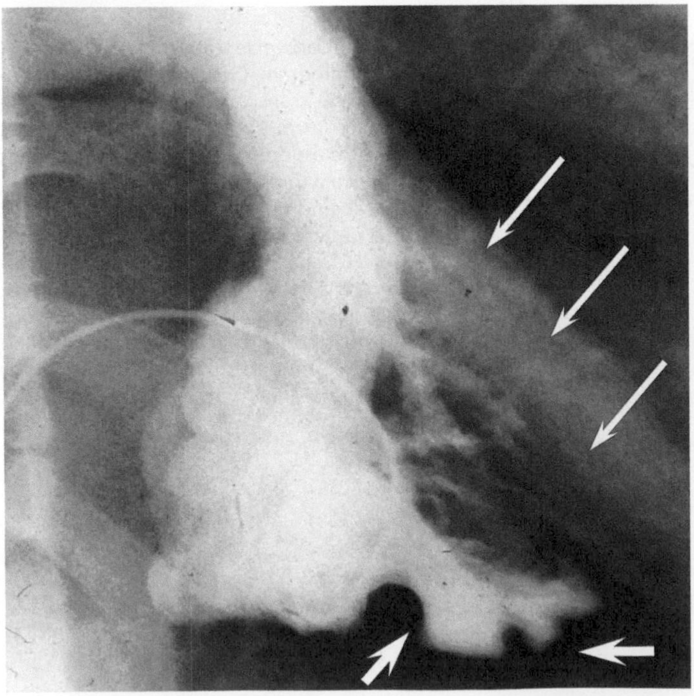

Fig. 4. Trabecular hypertrophy and multiple regional aneurysmatic bulging and outpouchings in AC. RV angiogram (30° RAO view) in a patient with AC showing trabecular hypertrophy in the anteroseptal and supra-apical RV (*long arrows*) as well as outpouchings and polycyclic contours in the inferior and apical RV walls (*short arrows*).

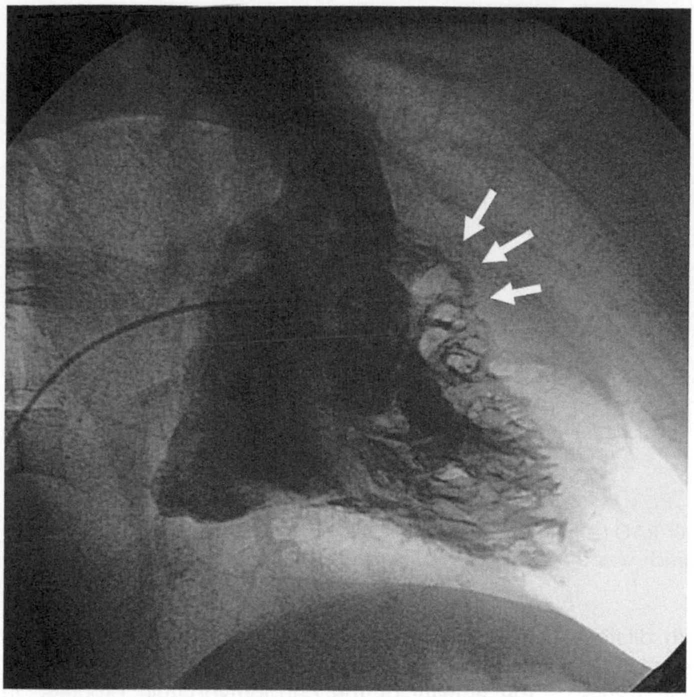

Fig. 5. Regional hypokinesia and polycyclic contours in the RV outflow tract in AC. RV angiography (30° RAO view, end systole) in a patient with AC showing polycyclic contours (*arrows*) and moderate hypokinesia in the RV outflow tract. (*From* Wichter T, Indik JH, Daliento L. Diagnostic role of angiography. In: Marcus FI, Nava A, Thiene G, editors. Arrhythmogenic RV cardiomyopathy/dysplasia: recent advances. Milan (Italy): Springer; 2007. p. 152. Chapter 16. Fig. 16.6; with permission.)

outpouchings, or sacculations; **Fig. 7**) have not been found in normal control subjects and are rare angiographic findings in other diseases affecting the RV. Therefore, these features are specific and diagnostic for AC and are mainly located in the triangle of dysplasia (see **Fig. 1**B).

Daliento and colleagues[17] compared the diagnostic value of RV angiographic features in

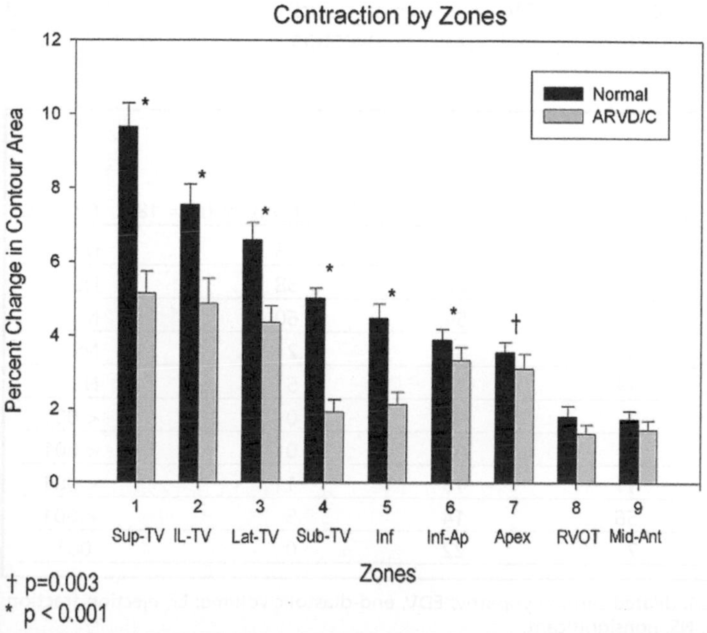

Fig. 6. RV regional systolic contraction. Regional systolic RV wall motion in patients with AC versus normal control subjects. Comparison of mean contour area and movement in patients with AC and in normal subjects in 9 RV zones (mean ± SEM) (**Fig. 11**). Mean wall motion is significantly reduced in those with AC in the tricuspid valve regions (superior tricuspid valve [Sup-TV], inferolateral tricuspid valve [IL-TV], LAT tricuspid valve [Lat-TV], and subtricuspid valve [Sub-TV]; $P<.001$), as well as in inferior wall (Inf, $P<.001$), inferior apical (Inf-Ap, $P<.001$), and apical (Apex, $P = .003$) regions. Wall motion in the RV outflow tract and midanterior (Mid-Ant) wall is minimal in normal subjects and not significantly reduced in AC. (*From* Indik JH, Wichter T, Gear K et al. Quantitative assessment of angiographic right ventricular wall motion in arrhythmogenic right ventricular dysplasia/cardiomyopathy (ARVD/C). J Cardiovasc Electrophysiol 2008;19:40; with permission.)

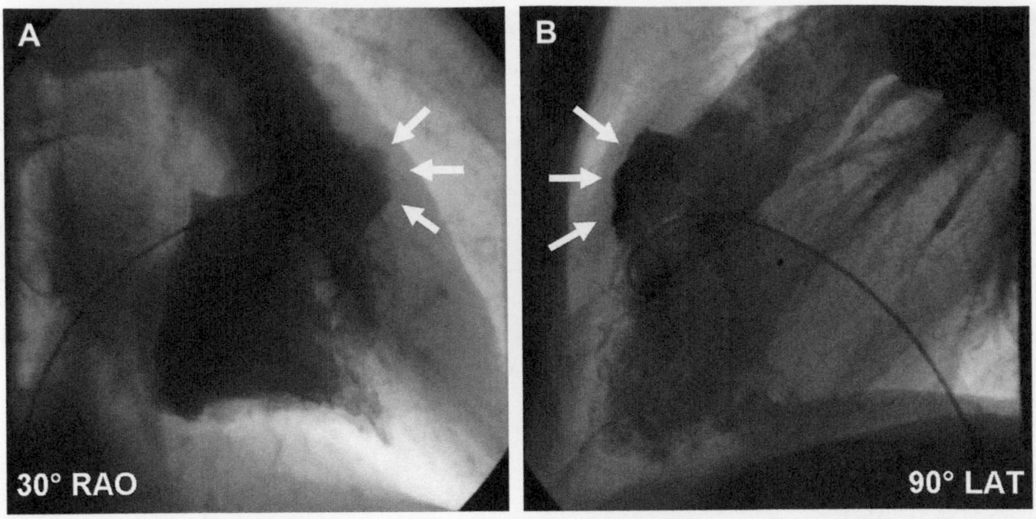

Fig. 7. RVOT aneurysm. RV angiograms in 30° RAO (*A*) and 90° LAT (*B*) views in a patient with AC. Note the large aneurysm in the anterior RVOT (*arrows*), which was the origin of recurrent ventricular tachycardia.

patients with AC with that in those with dilated cardiomyopathy and atrial septal defect and normal controls. In a discriminate analysis, transverse oriented hypertrophic trabeculae as well as bulgings of the anterior, infundibular (RVOT) and inferobasal (subtricuspid) regions were the only other independent variables indicative of AC. Coexistence of these signs was associated with a sensitivity of 88% and a specificity of 96% for the correct diagnosis of AC (**Table 1**).[17]

However, no correlation was demonstrated between RV wall motion and histologic abnormalities. In particular, aneurysms were associated with fibrous as well as adipose tissues. However, histologic findings provided useful information in confirming the diagnosis of AC and in assessing the activity of the cardiomyopathic process. In a stable phase of AC, fibrofatty replacement is the predominant finding, whereas in phases of active disease and progression, histologic signs of subacute necrosis, apoptosis, and inflammation as well as electrical instability may be present.[21]

Tricuspid Annulus Plane Systolic Excursion

RV base-to-apex shortening plays a key role in RV contraction and emptying. Hebert and colleagues[22] investigated 85 patients with AC

Table 1
Diagnostic accuracy of RV angiography in AC

	AC (n = 32)	DCM (n = 27)	ASD (n = 28)	Control (n = 18)	*P* Value
EDV-RV (mL/m^2)	131	165	141	95	NS
ESV-RV (mL/m^2)	62	104	66	38	NS
EF-RV (%)	53	38	54	60	NS
RVOT Diameter (cm)	5	6	5	2	NS
Long Axis RV (cm)	12	14	12	5	NS
Dyskinesia RV-Apex (%)	41	7	0	0	<.001
Dyskinesia RV-Inferior (%)	28	7	0	0	<.001
Bulging RVOT (%)	75	11	18	11	<.001
Bulging Inferobasal (%)	91	56	14	5	<.001
Tricuspid Prolapse (%)	41	7	22	0	.001

Abbreviations: ASD, atrial septal defect; DCM, dilated cardiomyopathy; EDV, end-diastolic volume; EF, ejection fraction; ESV, end-systolic volume; RV, right ventricle; NS, nonsignificant.

Data from Daliento L, Rizzoli G, Thiene G, et al. Diagnostic accuracy of right ventriculography in arrhythmogenic right ventricular cardiomyopathy. Am J Cardiol 1990;66:741–5.

and demonstrated a strong relationship between the tricuspid annulus plane systolic excursion (TAPSE) and RV ejection fraction. The sensitivity and specificity of TAPSE less than 12 mm in identifying patients with a RV ejection fraction less than 35% were 96% and 78%, respectively. Decreased TAPSE less than 12 mm and a diffuse RVOT aneurysm were sensitive and specific indicators of RV ejection fraction less than 35% and left ventricular ejection fraction less than 40%, respectively.

Tricuspid Regurgitation

In AC, tricuspid regurgitation results from 2 potential mechanisms: (1) dilated tricuspid annulus secondary to RV enlargement and (2) fibrotic involvement of tricuspid papillary muscles. Therefore, clinically relevant tricuspid regurgitation mainly occurs in patients with advanced stages of AC (**Fig. 8**).

LEFT VENTRICULAR WALL STRUCTURE AND MOTION

Left ventricular involvement of AC has been reported to be more frequently present than clinically diagnosed.[3,8,21] The main findings are localized abnormalities of wall motion (hypokinesia, localized dyskinesia) in the anterior, inferobasal, and apical walls (**Fig. 9**). However, global left ventricular function is rarely impaired.

A review of left ventricular cine angiograms from the group in Padua, Italy[23] showed unusual aspects of parietal motion in at least 60% of cases. Left ventricular end-diastolic volumes (90 $\pm$ 29 mL/m^2) and ejection fractions (60 $\pm$ 6%) as well as stress to end-systolic volume ratios (5.4 $\pm$ 2) and mass to volume ratios (0.8 $\pm$ 0.1) were normal in a group of patients with AC who were younger than 20 years. In an older group (38 $\pm$ 13 years), only the end-diastolic volume was slightly increased (93 $\pm$ 36 mL/m^2). Statistical analysis demonstrated an overlap of the functional indices in the young and adult groups.[23] However, an increase of dyskinetic areas was observed in the adult group.

These findings are consistent with the experience in Münster, Germany, in which left ventricular involvement of AC was mainly detected in patients with a long history of and advanced stages of RV dysfunction.

QUANTITATIVE ANALYSIS OF VENTRICULAR WALL MOTION

In normal individuals, RV volumes are usually higher than left ventricular volumes. There is an increase of RV volume indices (normalized to the body surface area) with age. Considerable interindividual differences of normal RV volumes, geometry, and contraction indicate the variability of RV performance and the wide range of normality.

In addition, RV wall motion is not homogeneous. Contractions are greatest at the inferior, inferolateral, and tricuspid wall areas and least at the anterior and anteroseptal regions.[19,20]

The complex and variable shape and geometry of the RV hinder simple and correct measurements of RV volumes and ejection fractions. The greatest error in estimating RV volumes from angiograms is probably because of the need for geometric assumptions, when only 2-dimensional data are available.

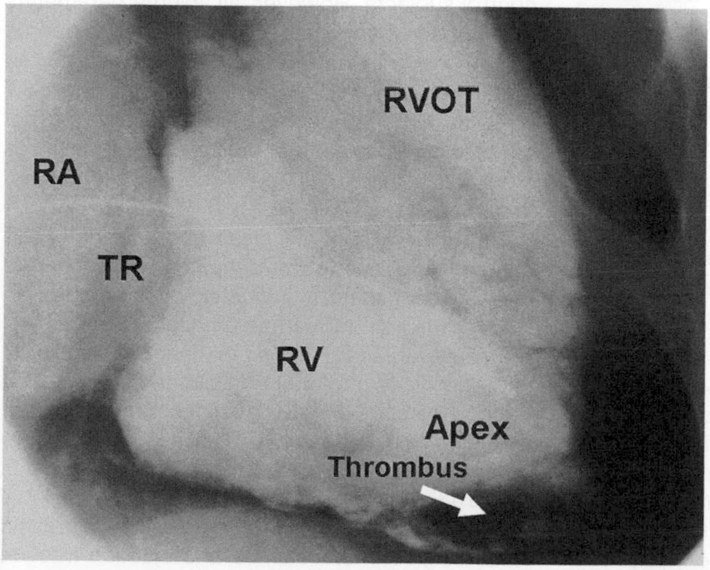

Fig. 8. Severe RV dilatation and dysfunction with apical thrombus. RV angiography (30° RAO view) in a patient with AC and severe RV dilatation and global systolic dysfunction. Also note the significant dilatation of the RVOT and the thrombus in the RV apex (*arrow*). In addition, there is severe tricuspid regurgitation (TR) as a result of dilatation of tricuspid annulus with subsequent enlargement of the right atrium (RA).

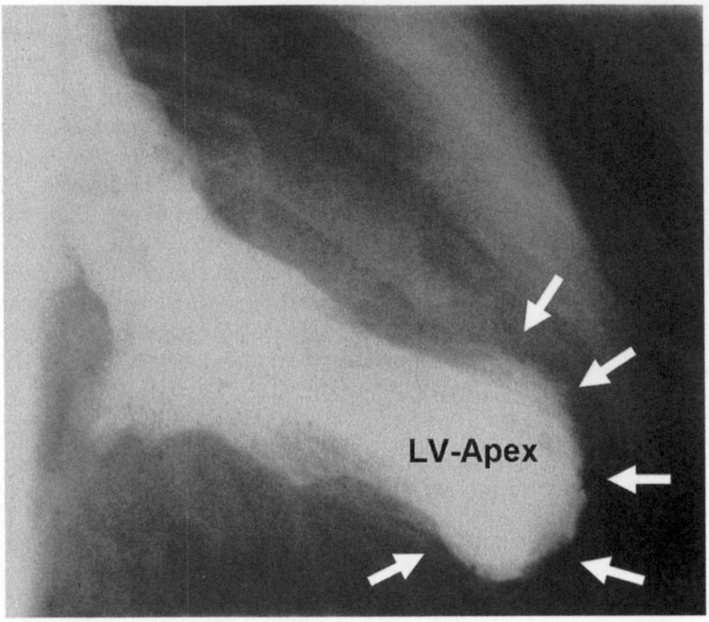

Fig. 9. Left ventricular involvement in progressive AC. Left ventricular angiogram (30° RAO view, end systole) showing left ventricular involvement with anteroapical and inferoapical akinesias (*arrows*) in a patient with a long history of progressive AC and severe global RV enlargement and dysfunction. (*From* Wichter T, Indik JH, Daliento L. Diagnostic role of angiography. In: Marcus FI, Nava A, Thiene G, editors. Arrhythmogenic RV cardiomyopathy/dysplasia: recent advances. Milan (Italy): Springer; 2007. p. 154. Chapter 16. Fig. 16.10; with permission.)

Methods for Quantitative Assessment

Several methods have been described using geometric models and formulas to determine end-diastolic and end-systolic volumes from RV angiograms. Most of these techniques rely on a surface-length method based on Simpson rule and using biplane models and computer-assisted analysis.

Peters and colleagues[24] tested 6 different geometric models for the calculation of RV volumes in 20 patients and also found that Boak formula[25] and a parallelepiped model produced the most reliable results with a high correlation factor and low systemic error when biplane views (30° RAO and 60° LAO) were used.

The accuracy of any RV volume calculation by contrast angiocardiography depends on how contours are defined. Although both manual and semiautomated methods have similar precision and variability, each method requires a different calibration. However, only few of the proposed methods were validated by correlation of the calculated RV volumes with measurements from casts of human hearts.

RV Volumes

Most studies investigating RV volumes in AC used cutoff values of the mean plus 2 standard deviations in the control group to define abnormal RV volumes. To correct for differences in body size, it is crucial to calculate volumes indexed for body surface area (mL/m^2). In addition, physical activity (ie, trained athlete) should be taken into account when RV volumes are assessed and interpreted.

Most of the early angiographic studies on AC[17,18,26] demonstrated increased RV volumes and diameters and reduced global ejection fraction. However, these results were in part due to a selection bias because these studies mainly included patients with advanced manifestations of AC and clearly enlarged RV.

The systematic study by Daliento and colleagues[17] also showed increased RV volumes in those with AC when compared with normal control subjects. However, all volume parameters overlapped when patients with AC were compared with those with atrial septal defect and dilated cardiomyopathy. Thus, increased global RV volumes and reduced ejection fractions are not specific for AC but rather indicate RV dilatation as a result of volume overload or reduced pump function of any cause.

Therefore, global RV sizes and volumes have only limited value in the detection and diagnosis of AC. This finding is indicated by data showing that in mild or moderate manifestations of AC with only regional RV dysfunction, the sensitivity and specificity of global RV volumes and ejection fraction remain low because of the significant overlap with normality. These results were confirmed in more recent and larger studies in which 68% of patients with AC had a normal global RV ejection fraction.[22] In addition, the diagnostic value of global RV volumes and ejection fraction

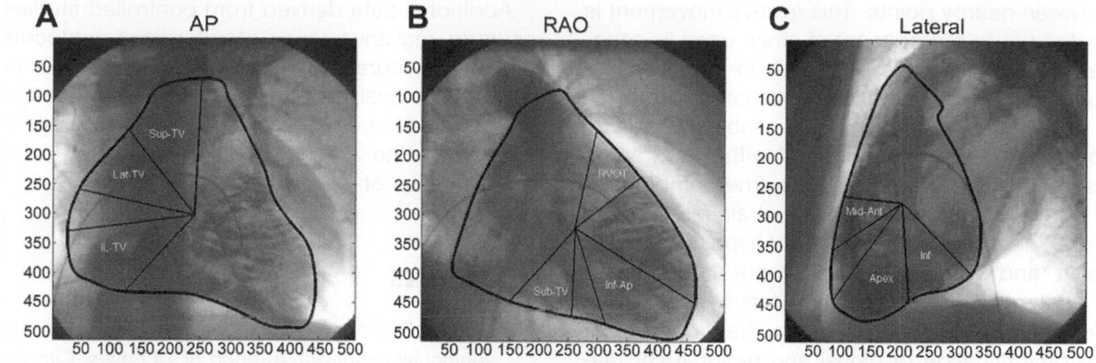

Fig. 10. Quantitative analysis of RV angiograms. Contours are drawn around the angiographic images in the AP (*A*), RAO (*B*), and LAT (*C*) views. In each view, zones subtending 40° are analyzed for contour movement. In the AP projection, the zones are the superior tricuspid valve (Sup-TV), LAT tricuspid valve (Lat-TV), and inferolateral tricuspid valve (IL-TV) regions. In the RAO projection, the zones are the RVOT, inferoapical (Inf-Ap), and subtricuspid valve (Sub-TV) regions. In the LAT projection, the midanterior (Mid-Ant), apex (Apex), and inferior (Inf) wall regions are analyzed. (*From* Indik JH, Wichter T, Gear K et al. Quantitative assessment of angiographic right ventricular wall motion in arrhythmogenic right ventricular dysplasia/cardiomyopathy (ARVD/C). J Cardiovasc Electrophysiol 2008;19:40; with permission.)

is also reduced when AC is compared with many other conditions that may underlie mild or moderate RV enlargement.

Computer Software

Quantitative analyses of regional RV size, volume, structure, and systolic as well as diastolic wall motions from RV angiograms are required to improve the diagnostic evaluation, particularly in mild forms of regionally reduced RV function.

To meet this requirement of regional quantification of RV function, a new computer software for frame-by-frame evaluation of RV wall motion in systole and diastole has been developed at the University of Arizona (http://www.dallas.radiology.arizona.edu/Imaging.htm).

This software program for quantitative analysis of RV function is expected to significantly improve the detection and evaluation of localized mild to moderate abnormalities of RV wall motion, particularly in AC.[19,20] This software compares the contour movement through the contraction (systolic) phase at any specified region in the 30° RAO, AP, and LAT views (**Fig. 10**). In addition, the program can also compare contour movement

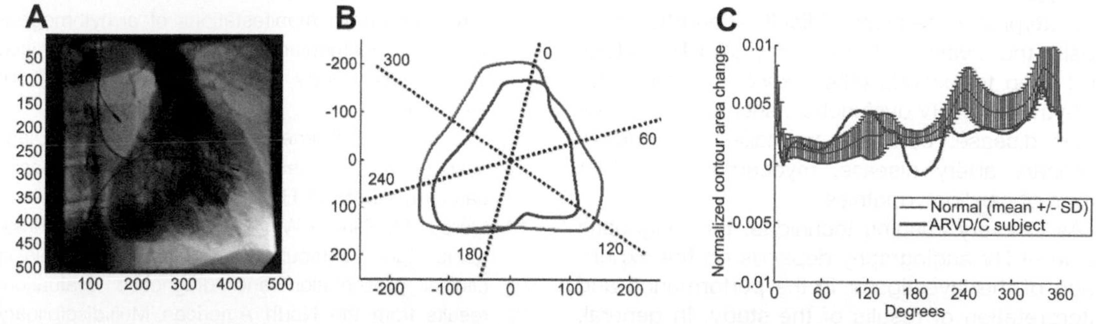

Fig. 11. Quantitative analysis of RV function from angiography. Illustration of analysis of RV contour in an individual with AC. The end-diastolic frame of the contrast ventriculogram in the AP view (*A*). Contours are then drawn around the RV border in a clockwise direction starting at the pulmonic valve; contours are drawn for all frames during systole. Position along a contour is specified by the number of degrees in the clockwise direction with 0 defined at the right edge of the pulmonic valve. The end-diastolic and end-systolic contours are superimposed (*B*). Contour movement is then assessed every 3° and displayed as a function of angle (*C*; *blue*), with a comparison to the mean and standard deviation of contour movement in normal subjects (*red*). The patient with AC has markedly depressed wall motion in the subtricuspid region (160°–210°) that falls well below 2 standard deviations from the normal database. (*From* Indik JH, Wichter T, Gear K et al. Quantitative assessment of angiographic right ventricular wall motion in arrhythmogenic right ventricular dysplasia/cardiomyopathy (ARVD/C). J Cardiovasc Electrophysiol 2008;19:40; with permission.)

between nearby points. This relative movement is analogous to the concept of strain used in echocardiography and is analyzed to quantify the nonuniformity of contour movement. Strain in a given region for the test subject can be computed and then compared with the strain in that region for normal subjects. The combination of contour area movement and strain may help to better identify areas of subtle RV hypokinesia, akinesia, and dyskinesia. Furthermore, the software provides tools for the quantitative analysis of global RV volumes and ejection fraction and for the quantification of global and regional RV diastolic relaxations.[20]

An example of the quantitative analysis of RV contour area movement is illustrated in **Fig. 11**.

SUMMARY

RV angiography remains an integral imaging modality and reference technique in the diagnosis and evaluation of patients with AC and is complementary to ECG and other imaging modalities. This technique should be performed in all patients with suspected or definite AC who undergo an initial diagnostic evaluation and may be combined with an electrophysiological study and/or RV EMB. During the right heart catheterization, additional hemodynamic parameters (pressures, cardiac output) should be measured.

During follow-up, RV angiography is mainly indicated in inconclusive situations of suspected progression of AC or in combination with otherwise indicated invasive cardiac diagnostic procedures.

In atypical cases with difficult differential diagnosis, the invasive strategy may also be helpful and used to exclude other causes of ventricular arrhythmias or RV dysfunction, such as congenital heart disease, coronary anomalies, obstructive coronary artery disease, myocarditis, or other types of cardiomyopathies.

As in every imaging technique, the diagnostic value of RV angiography depends on the experience of the investigator in the performance and interpretation of results of the study. In general, the angiographic diagnosis of AC is based on segmental abnormalities rather than diffuse RV enlargement or hypokinesia.

Dedicated computer softwares for the evaluation of RV volumes and regional wall motion provide a convenient and reproducible method for quantitative assessment of global and (probably more important) regional RV contraction and relaxation in comparison with a database of normal control subjects.

Additional data derived from controlled studies or large registries using standardized protocols for RV angiography and qualitative as well as quantitative analysis of RV structure and function are required to better define the best angiographic criteria for the diagnosis, characterization, and quantification of AC.

REFERENCES

1. Marcus FI, Fontaine G, Guiraudon G, et al. Right ventricular dysplasia: a report of 24 cases. Circulation 1982;65:384–99.
2. Thiene G, Nava A, Corrado D, et al. Right ventricular cardiomyopathy and sudden death in young people. N Engl J Med 1988;318:129–33.
3. Pinamonti B, Sinagra G, Salvi A, et al. Left ventricular involvement in right ventricular dysplasia. Am Heart J 1992;123:711–24.
4. Sen-Chowdhry S, Morgan RD, Chambers JC, et al. Arrhythmogenic cardiomyopathy: etiology, diagnosis, and treatment. Annu Rev Med 2010;61:233–53.
5. Fressart D, Duthoit G, Donal E, et al. Desmosomal gene analysis in arrhythmogenic right ventricular dysplasia/cardiomyopathy: spectrum of mutations and clinical impact in practice. Europace 2010;12:861–8.
6. Wichter T, Schulze-Bahr E, Eckardt L, et al. Molecular mechanisms of inherited ventricular arrhythmias. Herz 2002;27:712–39.
7. Kirchhof P, Fabritz L, Zwiener M, et al. Age- and training-dependent development of arrhythmogenic right ventricular cardiomyopathy in heterozygous plakoglobin-deficient mice. Circulation 2006;114:1799–806.
8. Corrado D, Basso C, Thiene G, et al. Spectrum of clinicopathologic manifestations of arrhythmogenic right ventricular cardiomyopathy/dysplasia: a multicenter study. J Am Coll Cardiol 1997;30:1512–20.
9. McKenna WJ, Thiene G, Fontaliran F, et al. Diagnosis of arrhythmogenic right ventricular dysplasia/cardiomyopathy. Br Heart J 1994;71:215–8.
10. Marcus FI, Zareba W, Calkins H, et al. Arrhythmogenic right ventricular cardiomyopathy/dysplasia clinical presentation and diagnostic evaluation: results from the North American Multidisciplinary Study. Heart Rhythm 2009;6:984–92.
11. Marcus FI, McKenna WJ, Sherrill D, et al. Diagnosis of arrhythmogenic right ventricular cardiomyopathy/dysplasia: proposed modifications of the task force criteria. Circulation 2010;121:1533–41; and Eur Heart J 2010;31:806–14.
12. Marcus FI, Towbin JA, Zareba W, et al. Arrhythmogenic right ventricular dysplasia/cardiomyopathy (ARVD/C). A multidisciplinary study: design and protocol. Circulation 2003;107:2975–8.

13. Basso C, Wichter T, Danieli GA, et al. Arrhythmogenic right ventricular cardiomyopathy: clinical registry and database, evaluation of therapies, pathology registry, DNA banking. Eur Heart J 2004;25:531–4.
14. Bluemke DA, Krupinski EA, Ovitt T, et al. MR imaging of arrhythmogenic right ventricular cardiomyopathy: morphologic findings and interobserver reliability. Cardiology 2003;99:153–62.
15. Wichter T. Standardized protocol for right ventricular angiography in ARVC within the North American Multidisciplinary Study of ARVD and the European ARVC Clinical Registry and Database. Available at: http://www.arvd.org and http://www.anpat.unipd.it/ARVC/protocols/Index.htm. Accessed March 1, 2011.
16. Wichter T, Indik J, Daliento L. Diagnostic role of angiography. In: Marcus FI, Nava A, Thiene G, editors. Arrhythmogenic RV cardiomyopathy/dysplasia: recent advances. Milan (Italy): Springer; 2007. p. 147–58.
17. Daliento L, Rizzoli G, Thiene G, et al. Diagnostic accuracy of right ventriculography in arrhythmogenic right ventricular cardiomyopathy. Am J Cardiol 1990;66:741–5.
18. Daubert JC, Descaves C, Foulgoc JL, et al. Critical analysis of cineangiographic criteria for diagnosis of arrhythmogenic right ventricular dysplasia. Am Heart J 1988;115:448–54.
19. Indik JH, Dallas WJ, Ovitt T, et al. Do patients with right ventricular outflow tract ventricular arrhythmias have normal right ventricular wall motion? A quantitative analysis compared to normal subjects. Cardiology 2005;104:10–5.
20. Indik JH, Wichter T, Gear K, et al. Quantitative assessment of angiographic right ventricular wall motion in arrhythmogenic right ventricular dysplasia/cardiomyopathy (ARVD/C). J Cardiovasc Electrophysiol 2008;19:39–45.
21. Basso C, Thiene G, Corrado D, et al. Arrhythmogenic right ventricular cardiomyopathy: dysplasia, dystrophy or myocarditis? Circulation 1996;94:983–91.
22. Hebert JL, Chemla D, Gerard O, et al. Angiographic right and left ventricular function in arrhythmogenic right ventricular dysplasia. Am J Cardiol 2004;93:728–33.
23. Daliento L, Turrini P, Nava A, et al. Arrhythmogenic right ventricular cardiomyopathy in young versus adult patients: similarities and differences. J Am Coll Cardiol 1995;25:655–64.
24. Peters S, Hartwig CA, Reil GH. Value of different geometric models for determination of right ventricular volume. Herz/Kreisl 1991;23:145–8.
25. Boak JG, Bove AA, Kreulen T, et al. A geometric basis for calculation of right ventricular volume in man. Cathet Cardiovasc Diagn 1977;3:217–30.
26. Blomström-Lundqvist C, Selin K, Jonsson R, et al. Cardioangiographic findings in patients with arrhythmogenic right ventricular dysplasia. Br Heart J 1988;59:556–63.

Magnetic Resonance and Computed Tomographic Imaging in Arrhythmogenic Cardiomyopathy

Harikrishna Tandri, MD*, Hugh Calkins, MD

KEYWORDS

- Arrhythmogenic right ventricular cardiomyopathy/dysplasia
- Cardiac imaging • Computed tomography • Diagnosis
- Magnetic resonance imaging

Right ventricular (RV) structure and functional alterations are important criteria for the diagnosis of arrhythmogenic cardiomyopathy (AC). As such, accurate and reliable evaluation of RV is desirable both for establishing the diagnosis and for follow-up evaluation of AC. The RV has a unique 3-dimensional geometry and complex contraction pattern.[1] Thus, conventional noninvasive imaging modalities, such as echocardiography and radionuclide ventriculography, are limited in their assessment. Magnetic resonance imaging (MRI) and computed tomography (CT) have emerged as robust tools to evaluate the RV in patients with suspected AC.[2–6] The noninvasive nature of these investigations, multiplanar capability, and unique ability to provide tissue characterization are ideal for the assessment of AC. Both the imaging modalities have the ability to provide direct evidence of fatty infiltration and structural alterations of the RV. This article discusses the current status, strengths, and limitations of MRI and cardiac CT in the evaluation of AC.

MRI IN AC

Over the last decade, there have been significant improvements in the MRI hardware, such as dedicated cardiac coils, faster imaging, and excellent blood pool contrast using steady-state free precession (SSFP) imaging, which have made MRI the imaging modality of choice for cardiac applications. Electrocardiographic (ECG) gating and breath-hold imaging have reduced motion artifacts, and improved tissue contrast is achieved by inversion recovery black-blood imaging techniques.[7] SSFP imaging pulse sequence has resulted in better delineation of endocardial borders, enabling accurate and reproducible volumetric measurements.[8] MRI is now routinely used for quantitative and qualitative assessment of cardiac function. Among the current cardiac MRI applications in cardiomyopathies, the greatest potential and the biggest challenges are in the diagnosis of AC. Routinely used imaging planes are suboptimal for RV evaluation, and the technique of AC imaging

The authors wish to acknowledge funding from the National Heart, Lung, and Blood Institute (K23HL093350, to H.T.) and the St Jude Medical Foundation, Medtronic Inc, and Boston Scientific Corp. The Johns Hopkins ARVD Program is supported by the Bogle Foundation, the Healing Hearts Foundation, the Campanella family, and the Wilmerding Endowments. The authors are grateful to the patients with ARVD and their families who have made this work possible.
Division of Cardiology, The Johns Hopkins University, Baltimore, MD, USA
* Corresponding author. Carnegie 565 D, The Johns Hopkins Hospital, 600 North Wolfe Street, Baltimore, MD 21287.
E-mail address: htandri1@jhmi.edu

Card Electrophysiol Clin 3 (2011) 269–280
doi:10.1016/j.ccep.2011.02.002
1877-9182/11/$ – see front matter

involves unconventional imaging planes. Furthermore, the lack of familiarity of the MR image readers with the RV contraction pattern and the normal epicardial fat distribution pose challenges for accurate and reproducible reporting.

Despite these limitations, MRI is uniquely suited for the evaluation of AC. It has the ability to noninvasively provide tissue characterization for the detection of fat infiltration and fibrosis in the RV, which are the histopathologic hallmarks of AC.[9–11] Quantitative and reproducible data on RV volumes and function are useful not only in establishing the diagnosis but also for follow-up of patients with AC. Finally, the multiplanar depiction of RV wall motion is invaluable in assessing RV regional contraction abnormalities, which are often the earliest manifestation of AC.

MRI Protocol

The MRI protocol in AC is aimed at recognizing 2 important aspects of the disease process: (1) fibrofatty infiltration of the RV and (2) global and regional RV dysfunction. Hence, the protocol includes (1) black-blood imaging to identify intramyocardial fatty infiltration, (2) bright-blood cine imaging to visualize RV global and regional dysfunction, and (3) myocardial delayed enhancement images. **Table 1** shows the MRI protocol used at the authors' center. Typically, axial and short-axis black-blood images are acquired for detecting fat infiltration. Axial, short-axis, and 4-chamber images are acquired for assessing RV and left ventricle (LV) wall motion. Delayed enhanced images are obtained in the same views as the functional images. For black-blood imaging, breath-hold imaging with double inversion recovery fast-spin echo (FSE) techniques are preferred to traditional spin echo (SE) imaging. These techniques substantially shorten the imaging time and are devoid of respiratory motion artifacts. Black-blood inversion prepared half-Fourier acquisition single-shot turbo spin echo (HASTE) imaging has not been systematically evaluated but is not recommended at present because of the blurring of detail with this sequence. For bright-blood imaging, SSFP imaging is the most preferred technique (fast imaging employing steady-state acquisition [FIESTA], true fast imaging with steady-state precession [FISP], and balanced fast field echo). If these cine sequences are not available, segmented k-space cine gradient echo imaging (eg, fast low angle shot [FLASH] and fast cardiac gated gradient echo [FASTCARD]) can be used. All techniques are optimally performed during end expiratory breath hold. Delayed enhanced images are obtained at the authors' center using 2-dimensional inversion recovery prepared gradient echo imaging or phase sensitive inversion recovery sequences. It is important to use a dedicated cardiac coil for imaging and to use the anterior coil alone while obtaining black-blood images. Using anterior coil alone prevents wraparound artifacts. Also, not infrequently, patients with AC present with frequent ventricular premature beats that cause blurring of the image because of inadequate gating. For patients with known frequent ventricular ectopy, the authors recommend the use of oral metoprolol, 50 mg, at least 1 hour before the procedure, provided the patient has no contraindications. If ventricular arrhythmias are frequent, then the resulting scan quality is poor and the test becomes uninterpretable.

MRI FINDINGS IN AC

Broadly, MRI abnormalities in AC can be grouped into 2 major categories: morphologic and functional.

Table 1
MRI protocol for AC

Imaging Sequence	Imaging Plane	Remarks
Black-blood imaging	Axial Short axis	Assess for RV and LV fat infiltration
Bright-blood imaging	Axial 4 chamber Short axis	Assess for RV regional function RV size and LV function estimation Optimal for quantification of RV volumes
Myocardial delayed enhancement	Axial 4 chamber Short axis	Assess for fibrosis

MRI protocol is geared to provide information related to the various pathologic manifestations of AC, namely, abnormal RV morphology, global and regional dysfunction, fat infiltration, and fibrosis of the RV. Black-blood images should be obtained with and without fat suppression using fast-spin echo or turbo spin echo technique.

Abbreviation: LV, left ventricle.

Morphologic abnormalities include intramyocardial fat deposits, focal fibrosis, wall thinning, wall hypertrophy, trabecular disarray, and RV outflow tract (RVOT) enlargement. Functional abnormalities include regional contraction abnormalities, aneurysms, RV global dilation and dysfunction, and RV diastolic dysfunction. The sites of involvement of these abnormalities include the "triangle of dysplasia," which is constituted by the inferior subtricuspid area, RV apex, and RV infundibulum (**Fig. 1**). The goal of MRI in AC is to accurately assess the RV for the presence or absence of these abnormalities and to aid in the diagnosis and follow-up of patients.

Intramyocardial Fat

Abundant epicardial and intrapericardial fat is commonly found over the RV, but intramyocardial fat infiltration in the RV is rare. A clear line of demarcation exists between the epicardial fat and the RV myocardium in normal subjects (**Fig. 2**), and disruption of this line is often seen in patients with AC. Shown in **Fig. 3** is a classic example of fat infiltration in AC. The fingerlike projections of the epicardial fat (see **Fig. 3**A) create a signal void in the myocardium in the fat-suppressed images (see **Fig. 3**B).

The prevalence of intramyocardial fat in AC on T1-weighted SE imaging ranges from 22% to 100% in different studies.[2,10,12–14] The authors used breath-hold double inversion recovery FSE technique to evaluate intramyocardial fat in AC

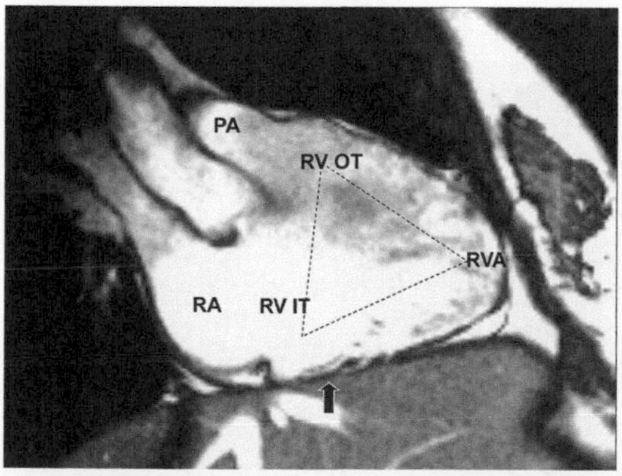

Fig. 1. Bright-blood diastolic MR image of the RV long-axis view (similar to right anterior oblique view on cine angiography) from a normal volunteer obtained with SSFP MRI. The RV can be divided anatomically into an RV inflow region (RVIT), body of the RV, outflow tract (RVOT), and the RV apex (RVA). Cardiac structures visualized in this view include RV, right atrium (RA), RVOT, and the pulmonary artery (PA). AC most commonly affects the subtricuspid region (*arrow*), the apex, and the RVOT; hence, these regions are collectively termed as the triangle of dysplasia.

and found a high intramyocardial T1 signal (fat) in 9 of 12 patients (75%) who were prospectively diagnosed using the current Task Force criteria.[10] The differences in the incidence of fat signal among various studies in AC are largely based on differences in patient selection, the different imaging techniques used, and most importantly, the definition of abnormal intramyocardial fat. It is known from the autopsy studies that the degree of fat infiltration is associated with the stage of the disease. Advanced AC is often associated with a greater degree of fat infiltration, and there may be no evidence of macroscopic fat infiltration on imaging in the early stages of the disease.[15] Current MRI resolution, however, is insufficient to diagnose early stages of the disease, even when there is clear evidence of fat infiltration on histopathologic examination.

Fat infiltration, when present, is predominantly seen in the RVOT, the anterior RV free wall, and the basal RV especially close to the RV inlet. Detection of fat infiltration close to the apex, however, is challenging because this region is usually very thin (2–4 mm) and there is abundant fat close to the cardiac apex. In any case, the use of spectrally selective fat suppression with the black-blood sequences provides additional evidence of fat infiltration because of the high contrast between the epicardial fat and the RV myocardium. The accurate delineation of the underlying RV free wall increases the confidence of diagnosis for the MR physician.

Although detection of fat infiltration on MRI is moderately sensitive to the disease process, the specificity of this finding is unclear. Detection of intramyocardial fat on MRI requires considerable experience, and overreliance on this finding alone often leads to misdiagnosis of AC. Excessive epicardial fat can often masquerade as fat replacement of the RV (**Fig. 4**). In some cases, this disguise also distorts RV regional wall motion, thus further confusing the issue. Steroid use, alcoholism, obesity, and old age have all been associated with fat infiltration.[16–18] Nevertheless, the classic appearance of segmental fat infiltration seems to be unique to AC. However, it cannot be underscored that reliable interpretation of this finding requires considerable expertise, which is often difficult to establish in this rare disease.

Wall Thinning and Wall Hypertrophy

RV wall thinning is defined as focal abrupt reduction in wall thickness to less than 2 mm, surrounded by regions of normal wall thickness. This finding is uncommon in AC and is often overcalled especially close to the RV apex where the

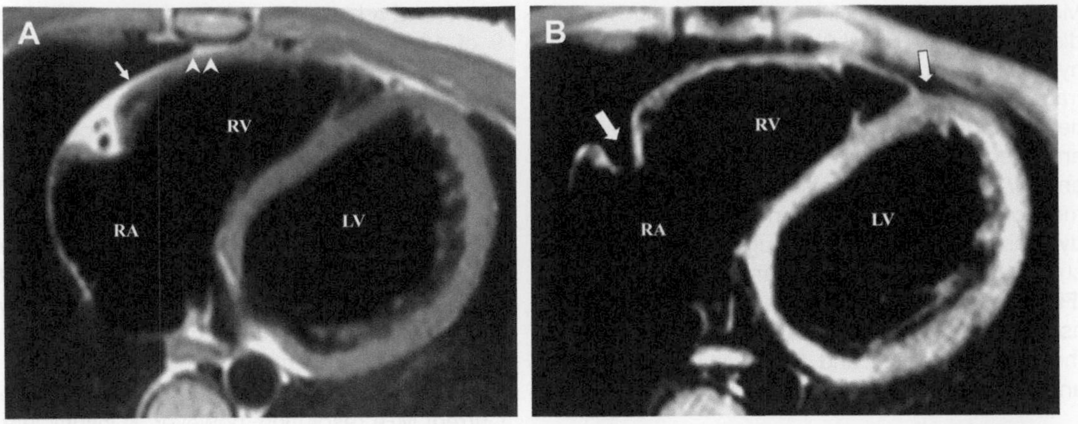

Fig. 2. (*A*) Midventricular axial black-blood MR image of the heart of a normal volunteer, obtained with FSE pulse sequence. In this image, fat appears as a high-intensity signal, myocardium is gray (intermediate signal), and blood appears black. Cardiac chambers visualized in this view include the RV, right atrium (RA), and LV. The RV free wall is thin and normally measures 3 to 4 mm in thickness. Epicardial fat (*arrow*) overlies the RV free wall and is usually abundant at the apex and at the atrioventricular groove. A clear line of demarcation (*arrowheads*) is often seen between the RV epicardial fat and the RV myocardium. Disruption of this line of demarcation with hyperintense signals is observed within the gray RV myocardium and is suggestive of intramyocardial fat infiltration, which is seen in patients with AC. (*B*) Fat-suppressed image of the same in Fig. 3A. The hyperintense signal in the atrioventricular groove and the RV apex is replaced by signal void (*arrows*), and the RV wall has a uniform contour without intramyocardial signal voids suggestive of fat.

RV tends to be normally very thin. Wall thinning is caused by progressive loss of epicardial and myocardial layers that leaves a thin rim of subendocardial myocytes, which are usually not involved until late in the disease process. In the authors' series, wall thinning was found in less than 25% of patients who met the Task Force criteria. In the authors' experience, wall thickness is often difficult to assess because of adjacent high epicardial fat signal and motion artifacts.

Wall hypertrophy, defined as a RV wall thickness of more than 8 mm, is usually an MRI appearance, wherein it is impossible to differentiate the true RV wall from the overlying epicardial fat because the line of separation is completely disrupted. This finding is seldom observed in pathologic

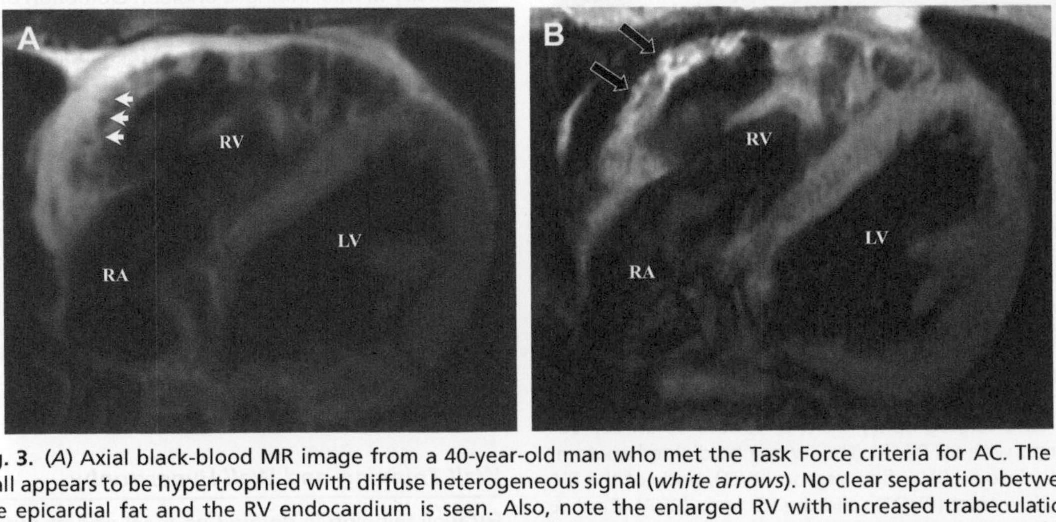

Fig. 3. (*A*) Axial black-blood MR image from a 40-year-old man who met the Task Force criteria for AC. The RV wall appears to be hypertrophied with diffuse heterogeneous signal (*white arrows*). No clear separation between the epicardial fat and the RV endocardium is seen. Also, note the enlarged RV with increased trabeculations within the RV. Morphologic changes, such as global and regional dilation, and functional changes, such as regional wall motion abnormalities, often accompany fat infiltration. The presence of regional contraction abnormalities corresponding to the region of fat infiltration is more suggestive of the diagnosis than fat infiltration alone. (*B*) Fat-suppressed image at the same location shows several signal voids (*black arrows*) within the RV corresponding to the regions of hyperintense signals in the non–fat-suppressed image. RA, right atrium.

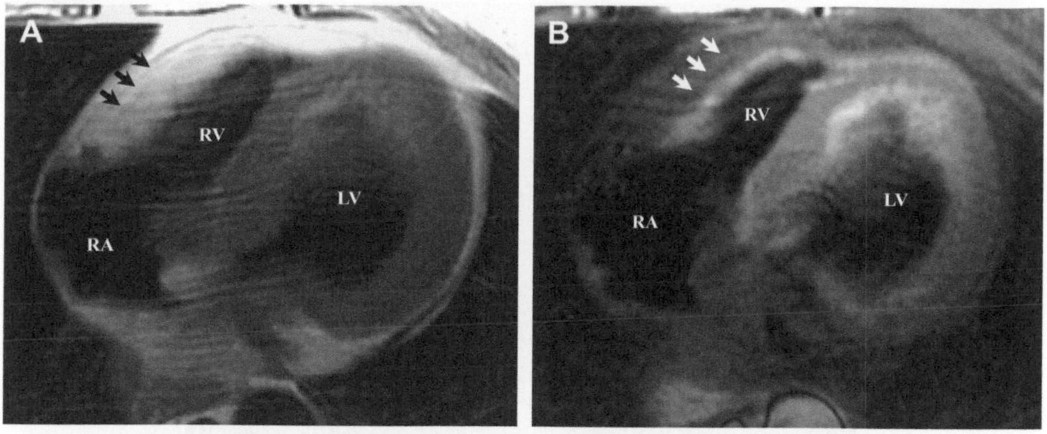

Fig. 4. (*A*) Adiposity of the RV wall on MRI is not unique to AC and can also be seen in obese individuals, elderly, and patients undergoing chronic steroid therapy. An example of excessive epicardial fat is shown in this axial black-blood MR image of a 42-year-old woman who was evaluated for presyncope. Note the abundance of epicardial fat that replaces the entire RV myocardium (*black arrows*). RV function was normal in this patient. (*B*) A fat-suppressed image at the same location reveals the underlying RV myocardial wall (*white arrows*). RA, right atrium.

specimens because the true RV myocardium is measured exclusive of the epicardial fat.[19] In vivo, this differentiation is sometimes not possible because of extensive fibrofatty infiltration with loss of distinction between epicardial fat and the true myocardium. In such cases, the RV wall appears hypertrophied with MR images showing islands of gray muscle surrounded by bright signals compatible with fat. Fat-suppressed image reveals multiple signal voids within the RV myocardium in locations that showed hyperintense signals in the non–fat-suppressed images (see **Fig. 3**B).

Trabecular Disarray

Heavy trabeculation of the RV is frequently observed in AC, more so in patients with RV dysfunction. Hypertrophy of the trabeculae and the RV subendocardium, which compensate for the subepicardial myocyte loss, is thought to result in this appearance. Occasionally, giant Y-shaped trabeculae and hypertrophy of the moderator band are observed in patients with AC. These features have been equated to the angiographic finding of deep fissures with a "pile d'assiettes" (stack of plates) appearance. RV trabecular disarray is a finding that is not specific for AC and may be present in any condition that results in RV hypertrophy or enlargement.

RVOT Enlargement

In the authors' experience, the RVOT is the most common location for localized AC. The RV OT is usually equal to or marginally smaller than the aortic outflow tract at the level of the aortic valve. An exception to this rule is observed in pediatric patients in whom the RVOT may be larger than the LV outflow. Presence of an enlarged RVOT after adolescence is uncommon. More important than a simple enlargement is a dysmorphic appearance of the RVOT (**Fig. 5**). Abnormal appearance of the RVOT, which is dyskinetic in systole, is highly suggestive of AC in the absence of pulmonary hypertension.

MRI Fibrosis in AC

One of the pathologic hallmarks of AC is fibrosis of the RV that accompanies fatty infiltration. Myocardial delayed enhancement MRI allows for noninvasive detection of fibrosis in the RV. Delayed enhancement detected by MRI shows excellent correlation with histopathologic findings and an inverse correlation with global RV function.[20] Further, areas of delayed enhancement often show wall motion abnormalities on cine imaging. Common sites for delayed enhancement are the basal subtricuspid region, the acute angle of the RV, and the RVOT (**Fig. 6**). Presence of delayed enhancement also predicts inducibility of reentrant ventricular tachycardia in AC. One of the most important uses of delayed enhancement imaging is its role in differential diagnosis. Presence of extensive biventricular delayed enhancement in a patient being evaluated for AC should suggest alternative diagnosis such as sarcoidosis or myocarditis. The myocardium of the interventricular septum is rarely involved in AC and frequently involved in sarcoidosis (**Fig. 7**). The differentiation of AC from isolated RV

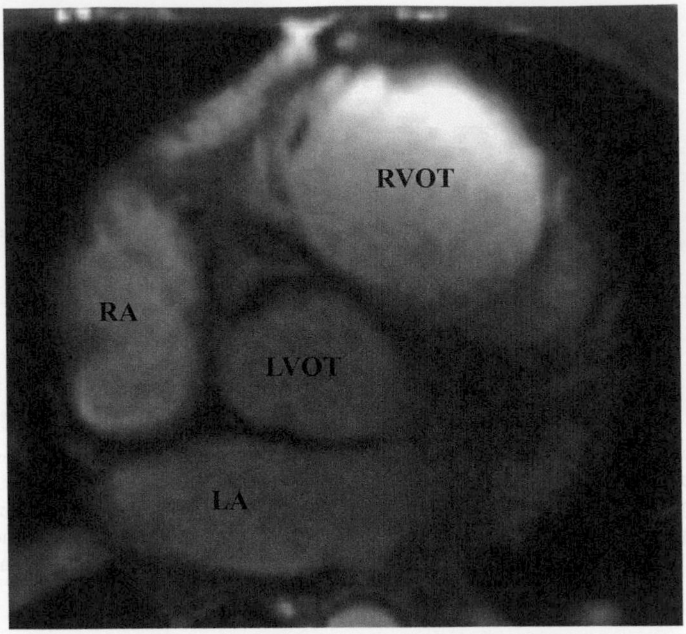

Fig. 5. Axial black-blood MR image from a patient with AC. Note the dysmorphic appearance of the RVOT, which is clearly bigger than the LVOT. LA, left atrium, LVOT, LV outflow tract, RA, right atrium.

myocarditis and sarcoidosis is often difficult using MRI alone. Both sarcoidosis and myocarditis can show patchy involvement of the LV, and fat infiltration is strikingly absent. Clinical findings such as conduction disease, multisystem involvement, and hilar lymphadenopathy suggest a diagnosis of sarcoidosis even when the MRI findings are indistinguishable.

LV INVOLVEMENT IN AC

Desmosomal mutations affect both ventricles; hence, it has been argued that AC is a biventricular disease with predominant involvement of the RV. Studies to date suggest that LV involvement may depend on the underlying mutation. Mutations in desmoplakin and plakoglobin have been associated with biventricular AC or, in some cases,

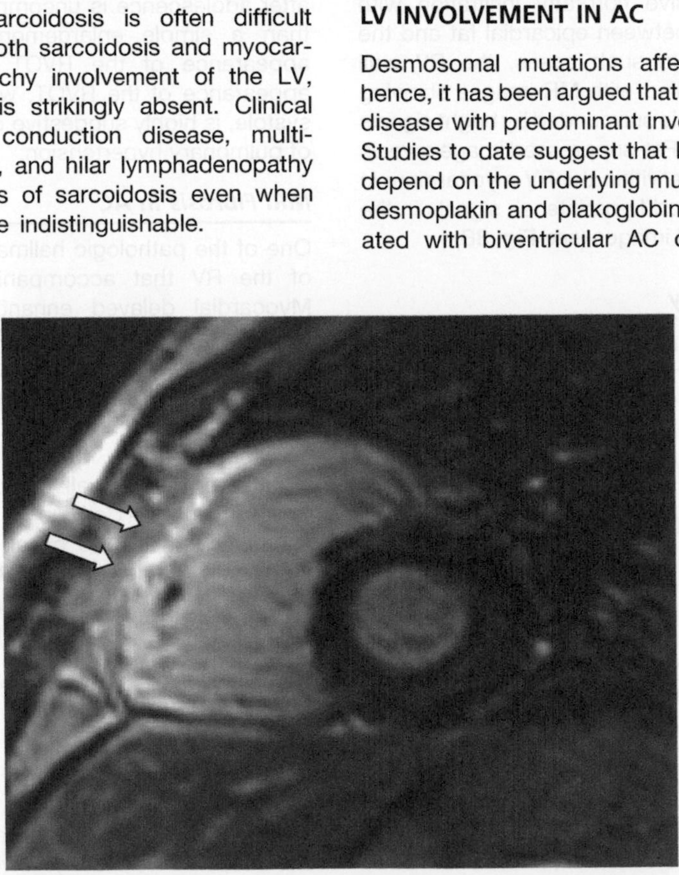

Fig. 6. An example of delayed enhanced MRI in a 33-year-old woman who presented with ventricular tachycardia. Note the diffuse enhancement of the anterior RV wall (*arrows*) suggestive of fibrosis.

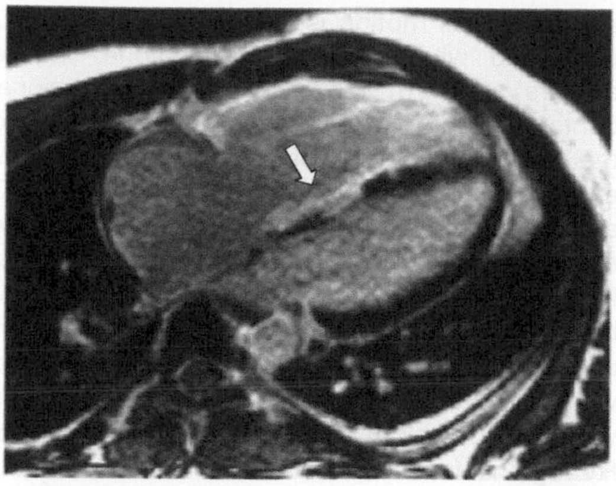

Fig. 7. Delayed enhanced MR image of a patient with cardiac sarcoidosis. Note the enhancement of the basal septum (*arrow*). Also seen is RV enlargement with extensive RV wall enhancement.

left-dominant AC.[21] On the other hand, mutations in Plakophilin 2 (PKP2) result in the classic form of AC with minimal LV involvement, at least minimal global functional involvement.[22] Histologic studies, however, have reported LV involvement in up to 70% of patients, but these are typically autopsy data, and the extent of disease is unknown.[23]

LV MRI findings in AC are unique and are mostly localized to the basal inferior and inferolateral LV (**Fig. 8**). This localization is typically in the form of fat infiltration that extends from the epicardium to the myocardium, sparing the endocardium. Fat infiltration in this location is not seen in any other disease, thus making this a finding that is unique to AC. Even with extensive amount of fat, global LV function is not affected, possibly because this infiltration is localized and well compensated by the remainder of the LV. The same site may show delayed enhancement; however, this finding may be difficult to reconcile from fat infiltration, unless a fat-suppressed delayed enhanced sequence is performed. LV dysfunction and LV arrhythmias are rare in PKP2-related AC, whereas they are commonly reported in desmoplakin mutation carriers (21).

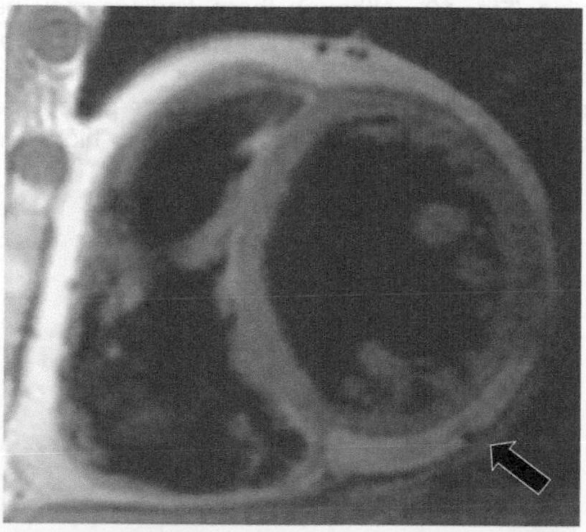

Fig. 8. LV involvement in AC is characteristically located in the inferolateral wall. A short-axis black-blood MR image of the base of the heart in a 30-year-old man with AC. Fat replacement of the inferior and posterolateral walls of the LV (*arrow*) is seen extending from the epicardial surface. Note the decreased thickness of the LV wall in the region of fat infiltration. Other diagnostic features in this image include the diffuse fat infiltration of the RV wall.

MRI ASSESSMENT OF CARDIAC FUNCTION IN AC

The techniques used to image cardiac function are called bright-blood techniques, derived from the appearance of intracavitary blood. Consecutive images acquired with a high temporal resolution can be viewed dynamically to generate functional information. Although several sequences exist for bright-blood imaging, SSFP imaging is the most preferred technique (FIESTA, true FISP, balanced fast field echo). SSFP sequences result in improved contrast between the blood pool and the myocardium compared with segmented k-space cine gradient echo images. If SSFP imaging is not available, segmented k-space cine gradient echo images (eg, FLASH and FAST-CARD) can be used. Conventional gradient-recalled echo (GRE) imaging sequences rely on flowing blood to generate bright blood. In the dysfunctional RV, blood velocities are reduced and signal intensity decreases with conventional GRE imaging. With SSFP imaging, the signal intensity remains high because the signal intensity is proportional to T2 time.

Using bright-blood imaging, ventricular volumes and mass have been shown to be accurate and reproducible, and MRI is considered the standard of reference.[24,25] Thus, MRI is ideal for noninvasive assessment of global RV function in patients with suspected AC and their first-degree relatives.

FUNCTIONAL ABNORMALITIES IN AC

Global RV Dilation and Dysfunction

Fibrofatty replacement of the RV in AC eventually leads to RV dilation and dysfunction. Moderate to severe RV dysfunction constitutes one of the major Task Force criteria for AC. Recent refinements to the Task Force criteria have resulted in the introduction of quantitative cutoffs for global RV volumes and function for the diagnosis of

AC.[26] RV dysfunction is often present in most patients who meet the Task Force criteria, especially in the absence of a family history of AC. Also, there is a linear correlation between the RV end-diastolic volumes and the duration of symptoms, suggesting the progressive nature of the disease. However, asymptomatic first-degree relatives who are diagnosed solely by virtue of their family history or by the presence of a pathogenic mutation often tend to have preserved RV function. Serial quantitative volumetric assessment of RV may play an important role in assessing RV function in first-degree relatives.

Regional Dysfunction

MRI has replaced RV angiography in RV regional function assessment because the former technique is noninvasive and is devoid of ionizing radiation. Regional RV dysfunction is generally thought to be caused by focal fibrofatty infiltration, which precedes changes in global ventricular function. As such, regional dysfunction is seen in the same areas as fat infiltration, which include the RVOT, the anterior RV, and the basal RV inlet. Shown in **Fig. 9** is a basal aneurysm in a patient with advanced AC. Regional functional abnormalities of the RV described in AC include focal hypokinesis (wall thickening of <40%), akinesis (systolic wall thickening of <10%), dyskinesis (myocardial segment, which moves outward in systole), and aneurysms (segments with persistent bulging in diastole and are dyskinetic in systole). Studies have consistently reported high incidence of regional dysfunction in AC. The areas of dysfunction corresponded to the areas of signal abnormality observed on black-blood MRI. The presence of signal abnormality associated with abnormal wall motion is more suggestive of AC compared with either of them alone. In the authors' series, 67% of the patients had regional contraction abnormalities, which correlated to the area of adipose replacement on MRI.[10] RV aneurysmal dilation is often seen in advanced AC and coexists with global RV dysfunction. Care should be taken while interpreting RV regional function from axial views because the axial plane is not orthogonal to the inherent axis of the heart and systolic bulging can be seen even in normal volunteers. Correlation with horizontal long-axis view may be helpful to avoid misinterpretation of RV regional function.

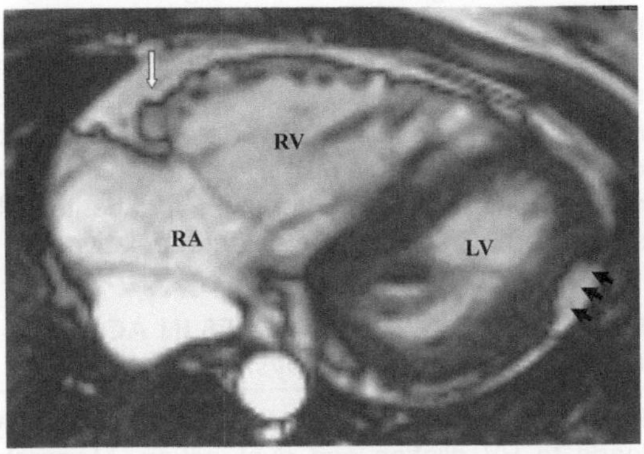

Fig. 9. Regional dysfunction. A systolic axial cine image of a patient with AC. Note the discrete aneurysmal outpouching in the anterior wall close to the diaphragm in systole (*white arrow*). Also, note the LV fat infiltration with thinning of the LV free wall (*black arrows*). RA, right atrium.

Genotype-Phenotype Correlation

Genotype-phenotype correlations suggest that mutations in PKP2 usually present with the classic right-dominant disease,[27] whereas in another series, patients with a relatively higher prevalence of mutations in desmoplakin showed a more-diverse phenotype, including the so-called left-dominant AC.[21] Further, the presence of the mutation is associated with a higher prevalence of LV fat infiltration than in patients with AC in whom no mutation is found. In mutation-positive first-degree relatives, minor contraction abnormalities limited to the RVOT and the RV basal region have been observed.[27] These regional contraction abnormalities are best described as a focal crinkle in the RV during a systole, resembling an accordion (**Fig. 10**). Although these findings may be sensitive, they have reduced specificity and poor reproducibility limiting their use in the diagnosis of AC. Finally, preliminary genotype-phenotype data suggest that disease severity is higher in

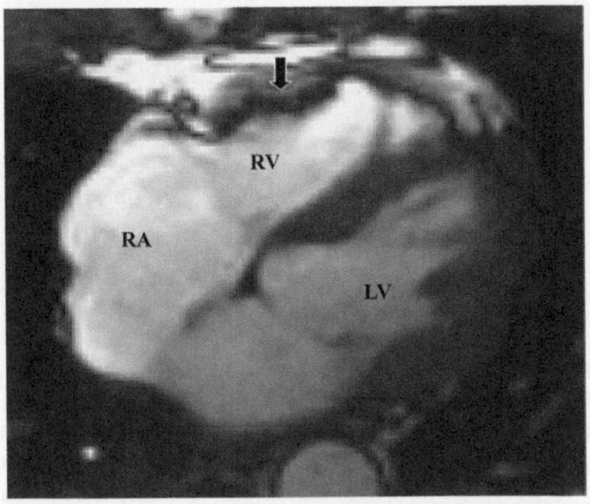

Fig. 10. A cine axial MR image of a 32-year-old first-degree relative of a patient with AC with a mutation in PKP2. Focal wall motion abnormality, resembling an accordion, limited to the peritricuspid region is seen in systole (*arrow*). RA, right atrium.

double mutation carriers, further emphasizing the need to screen all known disease-causing genes even after isolation of a pathogenic mutation.

ROLE OF MRI IN THE DIAGNOSIS OF AC

Diagnosis of AC is challenging especially in the early stages of the disease. The lack of diagnostic gold standard makes it difficult to define the sensitivity and specificity of any single modality in diagnosing AC. Benign arrhythmias arising from the RVOT are frequently encountered in clinical practice, and the presence of characteristic structural abnormalities differentiates AC from benign idiopathic ventricular tachycardia.[28] As such, the role of MRI in accurate phenotyping is invaluable. However, qualitative findings, such as intramyocardial fat infiltration and subtle wall motion abnormalities, need considerable expertise for interpretation. Isolated areas of fat replacement are not specific to AC and have been reported in elderly patients, patients taking long-term steroids, and in other cardiomyopathies. Recently, marked lipomatous infiltration of the RV has been observed in young nonobese individuals who were evaluated for nonsustained ventricular arrhythmias.[18] None of these patients had global or regional functional abnormalities and thus they seemed to be a distinct group of patients defined by MRI who should be differentiated from patients with AC. Overreliance on the presence of intramyocardial fat has in fact resulted in a high frequency of misdiagnosis of AC.[29] In the authors' experience, this finding alone is neither sensitive nor specific for the diagnosis. The authors' experience with MRI of hearts after autopsy led to the conclusion that the achievable spatial resolution in the current state-of-the-art clinical protocols substantially limits the capability to detect subtle RV intramyocardial fatty changes. Because the disease is so rare, most imaging centers have little or no experience with diagnosis of AC. Technical problems in imaging patients with arrhythmias, lack of a standardized protocol for AC, and lack of experienced imaging physicians suggest that MRI should only be one part of a comprehensive evaluation for these patients. According to the Task Force criteria, MRI provides information related to RV size, global and regional function, and aneurysm formation. Quantitative cutoffs are now a part of the Task Force criteria, and relying on quantitative evaluation of RV size and function is advisable and avoids the risk of overdiagnosis of AC.

One of the most important roles of MRI is to reliably identify patients who require additional invasive testing. A completely normal MRI study in a patient with no abnormalities on ECG or echocardiography is reassuring, and such patients may not need invasive testing (angiography/biopsy) in the absence of other clinical criteria. If signal abnormalities and wall motion abnormalities coexist, invasive testing should be performed to confirm the findings. Minor structural abnormalities (ie, signal abnormalities) in the absence of wall motion changes present a challenge because further evaluation of such patients is unclear. Adherence to Task Force criteria is recommended, and these minor criteria may not necessitate invasive testing. Further, it must be recognized that at present, the AC Task Force criteria do not recognize fat signal on MRI (or CT) as well as delayed enhancement as a diagnostic criterion for the disease.

Finally, when evaluating RV structure, special attention should be paid to the RV inflow, RV apex, and the outflow tract because these are the commonly involved sites in AC. The authors recommend assessing RV function from the axial bright-blood cine images. The RV on axial images starts off as a large triangle in diastole, which becomes a smaller triangle in systole. Most of the contraction occurs in the long axis of the RV from the movement of the tricuspid valve toward the RV apex. The RV anterior wall should be examined for bulging and aneurysms because these are morphologic abnormalities associated with AC. Quantification of RV volumes and ejection fraction should be performed routinely because these are more reproducible than qualitative estimates and can easily be applied using the current criteria for the purpose of diagnosis.

CT OF AC

Following a similar trajectory to MRI, there has been a continuous and accelerated development of CT technology, particularly the last 10 years focused toward cardiac imaging. Currently available multidetector CT (MDCT) imaging provides excellent spatial resolution and allows for accurate high-resolution assessment of the morphologic detail of both the cardiac chambers.[6,30,31] The use of a nonionic contrast agent provides excellent contrast resolution with clear delineation of the ventricular endocardium. Multiple cardiac phases can be extracted, with animated movies of the beating heart made available for visual assessment of global and regional function.[32,33] Quantitative determinations of ventricular mass, RV and LV volumes, and global ventricular function can be performed in a variety of cardiac pathologic states.

The main advantages of CT over MRI are that it is fast, is easy to perform, and has more reliable image quality. Although images are acquired only in the axial plane, the acquisition of a 3-dimensional data set allows reformatting in any desirable plane. For these reasons, CT is considered a clinically valuable noninvasive tool for the assessment of myocardial abnormality.

CT imaging has been used to evaluate AC and has the ability to depict the characteristic abnormalities in AC, such as abnormal RV morphology and fat infiltration. The ability of conventional CT to detect intramyocardial fat in AC was first reported by Villa and colleagues[34] in a series of 7 patients with AC, and subsequently, Sotozono and colleagues[35] provided biopsy confirmation of CT findings. Other investigators have shown the utility of CT in AC, including the assessment of LV abnormalities, particularly LV fat infiltration. Intramyocardial fat appears as a hypointense signal on CT, and this signal is particularly prominent in the LV wall (**Fig. 11**). Intramyocardial fat is defined based on tissue attenuation values. The attenuation value for epicardial adipose tissue is around -65 ± 10 Hounsfield units, and 5 to -17 Hounsfield units for intramyocardial fat, which is far less than that of myocardium. Using these values, Tada and colleagues[36] showed high specificity for AC because none of the control subjects and no patient without AC showed any evidence of intramyocardial fat or any other qualitative features of AC. Further, there is a good correlation between areas of fat detected on CT and abnormal RV endocardial voltage on electroanatomic mapping.

Hamada and colleagues[37] imaged 4 patients with AC with RV arrhythmias, who were found to have abnormalities on ECG and angiography using electron beam CT. Quantification of ventricular volumes was performed on cine mode scanning, which showed regional dysfunction and depressed global RV function. Recently, a case of AC was evaluated with 64-detector CT, and with contrast-enhanced volume mode scanning, it was possible to demonstrate morphologic abnormalities consistent with AC, such as RV enlargement, excessive trabeculation, fatty infiltration, and marked RV hypokinesis.[38]

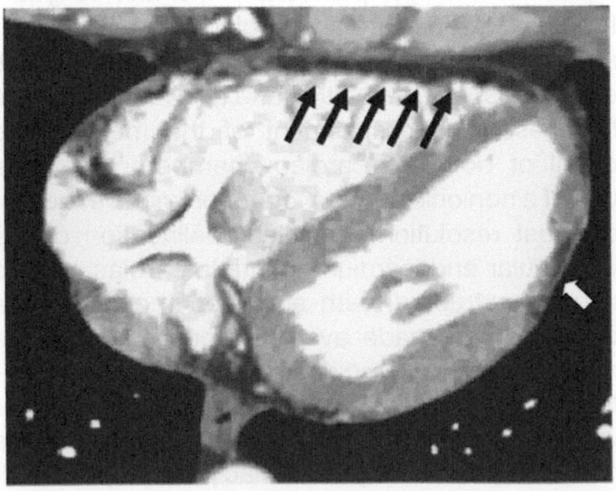

Fig. 11. Multidetector CT image of a patient with AC, showing RV (*black arrows*) and LV (*white arrow*) fat infiltration.

Volumetric assessment of the RV is suboptimal using CT imaging. Problems with using MDCT include artifacts due to implantable cardioverter-defibrillator leads, misregistration of slices, and problems with reformatting the short-axis data from axial images, all of which undermine the accuracy and reproducibility of the data. Most of the patients who were evaluated using CT imaging at the authors' center had implantable defibrillator hardware, which precluded MRI. Nevertheless, all the morphologic features are well depicted by CT, and chamber dimensions can easily be obtained using the current-generation CT imaging.

Role of CT in AC

At present, most of the centers, including the authors', rely on MRI instead of CT imaging for evaluating patients with suspected AC mainly because the former is devoid of radiation. The temporal resolution of CT imaging is suboptimal to allow accurate quantification of volumes. However, most patients who are diagnosed with AC receive implantable defibrillators for prevention of sudden death. In this cohort, CT remains the only imaging technique to assess RV structure and function for serial morphologic evaluation. An additional use of CT imaging is to assess the mediastinum for the presence of lymphadenopathy, a marker of sarcoidosis, which occasionally mimics AC.[39] CT imaging also has the ability to assess the lung fields for nodules or granulomas suggestive of sarcoid involvement of the lung. CT is useful in the occasional patient who has frequent premature beats resulting in arrhythmic artifacts on MRI and also in patients who are claustrophobic.

MDCT radiation dose can be quite high, exceeding that of conventional angiography by a factor of 2 when performing retrospective gating.[40] Thus, MDCT may not be optional for screening of AC in first-degree relatives. Despite these limitations, CT does provide certain advantages over MRI, including consistency in image quality, scan time, and operator dependency. With increase in familiarity of radiologists with the use of helical CT for AC and with the advances in both the temporal and spatial resolution, CT imaging may play an important role both in the diagnosis and in the follow-up of patients with AC.

SUMMARY

Accurate and reliable evaluation of RV is desirable both for establishing diagnosis and for follow-up evaluation of AC. Conventional noninvasive imaging modalities are limited in their assessment. MRI and CT have emerged as robust tools to evaluate the RV in patients with suspected AC. Their noninvasive nature, multiplanar capability, and unique ability to provide tissue characterization are ideal for the assessment of AC. Current status, strengths, and limitations of MRI and CT in the evaluation of AC have been discussed.

REFERENCES

1. Boxt LM. Radiology of the right ventricle. Radiol Clin North Am 1999;37:379–400.
2. Bluemke DA, Krupinski EA, Ovitt T, et al. Imaging of arrhythmogenic right ventricular cardiomyopathy: morphologic findings and interobserver reliability. Cardiology 2003;99:153–62.
3. Araoz PA, Mulvagh SL, Tazelaar HD, et al. CT and MR imaging of benign primary cardiac neoplasms with echocardiographic correlation. Radiographics 2000;20:1303–19.
4. Higgins CB, Caputo GR. Role of MR imaging in acquired and congenital cardiovascular disease. AJR Am J Roentgenol 1993;161:13–22.
5. Rist C, Johnson TR, Becker CR, et al. New applications for noninvasive cardiac imaging: dual-source computed tomography. Eur Radiol 2007;17 (Suppl 6):F16–25.
6. Becker CR, Ohnesorge BM, Schoepf UJ, et al. Current development of cardiac imaging with multidetector-row CT. Eur J Radiol 2000;36:97–103.
7. Simonetti OP, Finn JP, White RD, et al. "Black blood" T2-weighted inversion-recovery MR imaging of the heart. Radiology 1996;199:49–57.
8. Bloomer TN, Plein S, Radjenovic A, et al. Cine MRI using steady state free precession in the radial long axis orientation is a fast accurate method for obtaining volumetric data of the left ventricle. J Magn Reson Imaging 2001;14:685–92.
9. Tandri H, Bomma C, Calkins H, et al. Magnetic resonance and computed tomography imaging of arrhythmogenic right ventricular dysplasia. J Magn Reson Imaging 2004;19:848–58.
10. Tandri H, Calkins H, Nasir K, et al. Magnetic resonance imaging findings in patients meeting task force criteria for arrhythmogenic right ventricular dysplasia. J Cardiovasc Electrophysiol 2003;14: 476–82.
11. Tandri H, Friedrich MG, Calkins H, et al. MRI of arrhythmogenic right ventricular cardiomyopathy/dysplasia. J Cardiovasc Magn Reson 2004;6: 557–63.
12. Midiri M, Finazzo M, Brancato M, et al. Arrhythmogenic right ventricular dysplasia: MR features. Eur Radiol 1997;7:307–12.
13. Kayser HW, de Roos A, Schalij MJ, et al. Usefulness of magnetic resonance imaging in diagnosis of arrhythmogenic right ventricular dysplasia and agreement with electrocardiographic criteria. Am J Cardiol 2003;91:365–7.
14. van der Wall EE, Kayser HW, Bootsma MM, et al. Arrhythmogenic right ventricular dysplasia: MRI findings. Herz 2000;25:356–64.
15. Castillo E, Tandri H, Rodriguez ER, et al. Arrhythmogenic right ventricular dysplasia: ex vivo and in vivo fat detection with black-blood MR imaging. Radiology 2004;232:38–48.
16. Vikhert AM, Tsiplenkova VG, Cherpachenko NM. Alcoholic cardiomyopathy and sudden cardiac death. J Am Coll Cardiol 1986;8(1 Suppl A):3A–11A.
17. Hasumi M, Sekiguchi M, Hiroe M, et al. Endomyocardial biopsy approach to patients with ventricular tachycardia with special reference to arrhythmogenic right ventricular dysplasia. Jpn Circ J 1987;51: 242–9.
18. Macedo R, Prakasa K, Tichnell C, et al. Marked lipomatous infiltration of the right ventricle: MRI findings in relation to arrhythmogenic right ventricular dysplasia. AJR Am J Roentgenol 2007;188:W423–7.
19. Burke AP, Farb A, Tashko G, et al. Arrhythmogenic right ventricular cardiomyopathy and fatty replacement of the right ventricular myocardium: are they different diseases? Circulation 1998;97:1571–80.
20. Tandri H, Saranathan M, Rodriguez ER, et al. Noninvasive detection of myocardial fibrosis in arrhythmogenic right ventricular cardiomyopathy using delayed-enhancement magnetic resonance imaging. J Am Coll Cardiol 2005;45:98–103.
21. Sen-Chowdhry S, Syrris P, Prasad SK, et al. Left-dominant arrhythmogenic cardiomyopathy: an under-recognized clinical entity. J Am Coll Cardiol 2008;52:2175–87.
22. Jain A, Shehata ML, Stuber M, et al. Prevalence of left ventricular regional dysfunction in arrhythmogenic right ventricular dysplasia: a tagged MRI study. Circ Cardiovasc Imaging 2010;3:290–7.
23. Basso C, Corrado D, Marcus FI, et al. Arrhythmogenic right ventricular cardiomyopathy. Lancet 2009;373:1289–300.
24. Bloomgarden DC, Fayad ZA, Ferrari VA, et al. Global cardiac function using fast breath-hold MRI: validation of new acquisition and analysis techniques. Magn Reson Med 1997;37:683–92.
25. Sakuma H, Fujita N, Foo TK, et al. Evaluation of left ventricular volume and mass with breath-hold cine MR imaging. Radiology 1993;188:377–80.
26. Marcus FI, McKenna WJ, Sherrill D, et al. Diagnosis of arrhythmogenic right ventricular cardiomyopathy/dysplasia: proposed modification of the task force

criteria. Circulation 2010;121:1533–41 and Eur Heart J 2010;31:806–14.
27. Dalal D, Tandri H, Judge DP, et al. Morphologic variants of familial arrhythmogenic right ventricular dysplasia/cardiomyopathy a genetics-magnetic resonance imaging correlation study. J Am Coll Cardiol 2009;53:1289–99.
28. Tandri H, Bluemke DA, Ferrari VA, et al. Findings on magnetic resonance imaging of idiopathic right ventricular outflow tachycardia. Am J Cardiol 2004; 94:1441–5.
29. Bomma C, Rutberg J, Tandri H, et al. Misdiagnosis of arrhythmogenic right ventricular dysplasia/cardiomyopathy. J Cardiovasc Electrophysiol 2004;15:300–6.
30. Garcia MJ. Cardiac CT: understanding and adopting a new diagnostic modality. Cardiol Clin 2009;27: 555–62.
31. Sparrow PJ, Merchant N, Provost YL, et al. CT and MR imaging findings in patients with acquired heart disease at risk for sudden cardiac death. Radiographics 2009;29:805–23.
32. Joemai RM, Geleijns J, Veldkamp WJ, et al. Clinical evaluation of 64-slice CT assessment of global left ventricular function using automated cardiac phase selection. Circ J 2008;72:641–6.
33. Muhlenbruch G, Das M, Hohl C, et al. Global left ventricular function in cardiac CT. Evaluation of an automated 3D region-growing segmentation algorithm. Eur Radiol 2006;16:1117–23.
34. Villa A, Di Guglielmo L, Salerno J, et al. Arrhythmogenic dysplasia of the right ventricle. Evaluation of 7 cases using computerized tomography. Radiol Med 1988;75:28–35 [in Italian].
35. Sotozono K, Imahara S, Masuda H, et al. Detection of fatty tissue in the myocardium by using computerized tomography in a patient with arrhythmogenic right ventricular dysplasia. Heart Vessels Suppl 1990;5:59–61.
36. Tada H, Shimizu W, Ohe T, et al. Usefulness of electron-beam computed tomography in arrhythmogenic right ventricular dysplasia. Relationship to electrophysiological abnormalities and left ventricular involvement. Circulation 1996;94:437–44.
37. Hamada S, Takamiya M, Ohe T, et al. Arrhythmogenic right ventricular dysplasia: evaluation with electron-beam CT. Radiology 1993;187:723–7.
38. Soh EK, Villines TC, Feuerstein IM. Sixty-four-multislice computed tomography in a patient with arrhythmogenic right ventricular dysplasia. J Cardiovasc Comput Tomogr 2008;2:191–2.
39. Vasaiwala SC, Finn C, Delpriore J, et al. Prospective study of cardiac sarcoid mimicking arrhythmogenic right ventricular dysplasia. J Cardiovasc Electrophysiol 2009;20:473–6.
40. Hunold P, Vogt FM, Schmermund A, et al. Radiation exposure during cardiac CT: effective doses at multi-detector row CT and electron-beam CT. Radiology 2003;226:145–52.

Arrhythmogenic Cardiomyopathy: Natural History and Risk Stratification

Federico Migliore, MD[a], Anna Baritussio, MD[a], Ilaria Rigato, MD, PhD[a], Martina Perazzolo Marra, MD, PhD[a], Barbara Bauce, MD, PhD[a], Cristina Basso, MD, PhD[b], Sabino Iliceto, MD[a], Domenico Corrado, MD, PhD[a,*]

KEYWORDS

- Arrhythmogenic right ventricular cardiomyopathy/dysplasia
- Natural history • Risk stratification
- Sudden arrhythmic death

Arrhythmogenic cardiomyopathy (AC) is an inherited heart muscle disease. Clinical manifestations are related to ventricular electrical instability which may lead to sudden cardiac death (SCD), mostly in young people.[1–4] Later in the disease history, the right ventricle (RV) becomes more diffusely affected and the involvement of the left ventricle (LV) may result in biventricular heart failure.[1,2]

This article addresses the disease natural history and analyzes the clinical predictors of sudden arrhythmic death and clinical outcome of patients with AC.

NATURAL HISTORY

Based on clinicopathologic and follow-up studies, 4 clinical phases of the disease have been identified: (1) the concealed form is the subclinical and asymptomatic phase, which is characterized by subtle structural abnormalities. In this disease stage, SCD might occur as the first disease manifestation in previously asymptomatic young people, mostly during physical exercise or competitive sports activity.[2,3] Early/minor disease expression is usually observed in family members who are identified during family screening. The electrocardiogram (ECG) may either be normal or show right precordial repolarization abnormalities with no, or only regional, RV wall motion abnormalities. Differential diagnosis with idiopathic RV outflow tract tachycardia is often not achieved by means of conventional clinical testing and may depend on demonstration of underlying fibrofatty replacement of RV myocardium by endomyocardial biopsy,[5] RV delayed enhancement by contrast-enhanced cardiac magnetic resonance (CMR),[6] or electroanatomic scar by endocardial voltage mapping.[7] (2) The overt arrhythmic form is the classic clinical presentation (**Fig. 1**). Ventricular arrhythmias dominate the clinical scenario in the form of frequent premature ventricular beats, short runs of ventricular tachycardia (VT), or sustained monomorphic VT, with a left bundle branch block (LBBB) morphology. Such arrhythmias may provoke syncope, especially during physical exercise, and may degenerate into ventricular fibrillation (VF) leading to cardiac arrest. Common ECG abnormalities consist of T wave inversion and prolongation of QRS interval (≥110 milliseconds) in the precordial leads that explore the RV (ie, V1–V2/V3). The spectrum of RV morphofunctional alterations ranges from global dilatation/

[a] Division of Cardiology, Department of Cardiac, Thoracic and Vascular Sciences, University of Padua Medical School, Via Giustiniani, 2-35121 Padua, Italy
[b] Cardiovascular Pathology, Department of Medical-Diagnostic Sciences and Special Therapies, University of Padua Medical School, Via A. Gabelli, 35121 Padua, Italy
* Corresponding author.
E-mail address: domenico.corrado@unipd.it

Card Electrophysiol Clin 3 (2011) 281–291
doi:10.1016/j.ccep.2011.02.012

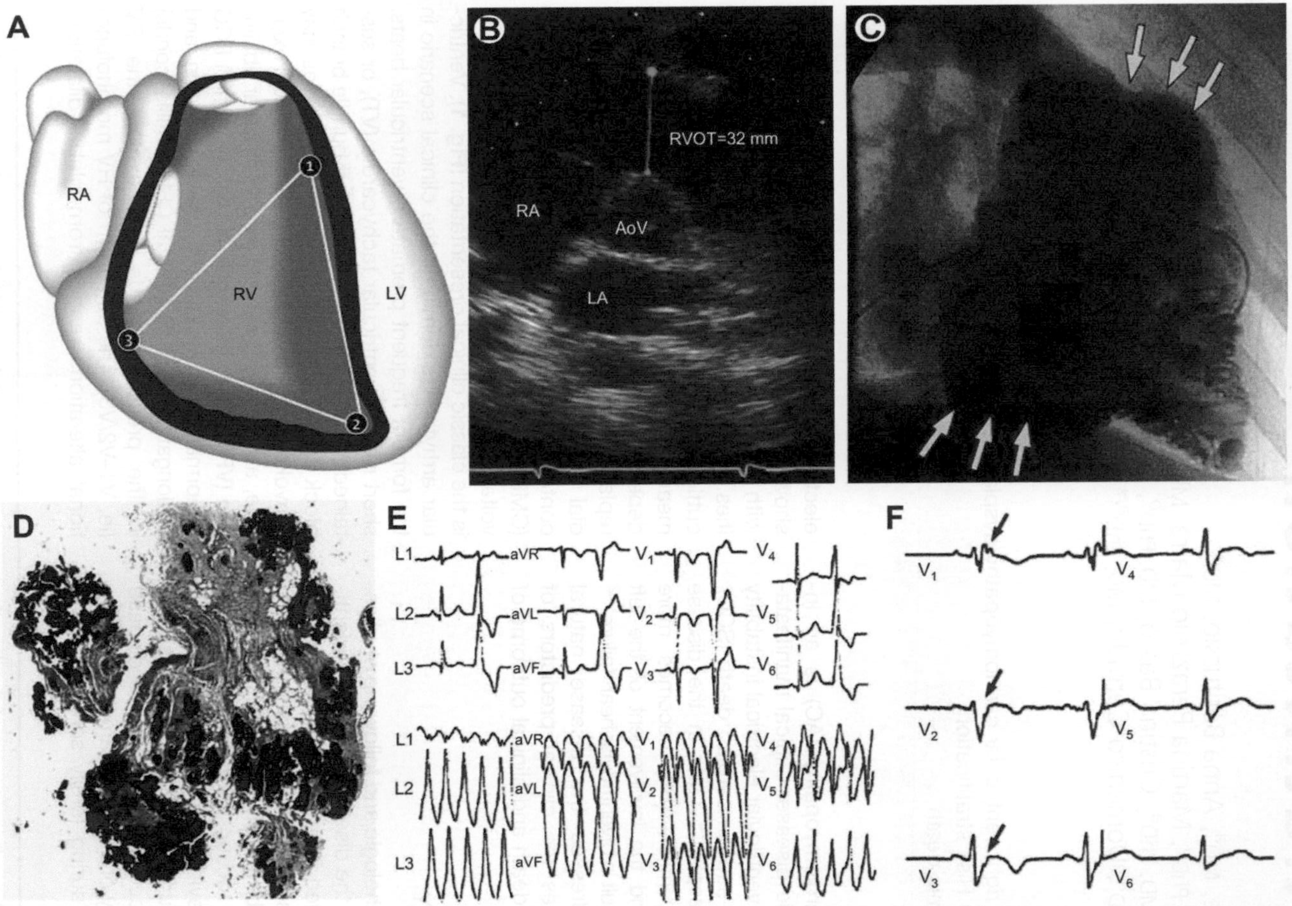

Fig. 1. Morphofunctional, electrocardiographic, and tissue characterization diagnostic features of AC. (*A*) The triangle of dysplasia, showing the characteristic areas for structural and functional abnormalities of the RV. (*B*) Two-dimensional echocardiography showing RV outflow tract enlargement from the parasternal short-axis view. (*C*) RV contrast angiography (30° right anterior-oblique view) showing a localized RV outflow tract aneurysm (*arrows*) as well as inferobasal akinesia (*arrows*) with mild tricuspid regurgitation. (*D*) Endomyocardial biopsy sample with extensive myocardial atrophy and fibrofatty replacement (trichrome; ×6). (*E*) Twelve-lead ECG with inverted T waves (V1, V2, V3), with LBBB morphology, premature ventricular beats, and VT. (*F*) ECG tracing showing postexcitation epsilon wave in precordial leads V1, V2, V3 (*arrows*). AoV, aortic valve; LA, left atrium; LV, left ventricle; RA, right atrium; RV, right ventricle; RVOT, RV ventricle outflow tract. (*Modified from* Basso C, Corrado D, Marcus F, et al. Arrhythmogenic right ventricular cardiomyopathy. Lancet 2009;373:1292; with permission.)

dysfunction to regional wall motion abnormalities and diastolic bulging typically localized in the triangle of dysplasia (see **Fig. 1**). The LV and the septum are usually involved to a lesser extent, whereas biventricular or left-dominant variants of disease have been reported.[6] Ventricular structural abnormalities are clearly detected by current imaging techniques such as echocardiography, angiography, and CMR (see **Fig. 1; Fig. 2**). In patients experiencing severe arrhythmic symptoms/events, implantable cardioverter defibrillator (ICD) has proved to represent a life-saving therapy. (3) RV failure caused by progressive loss of myocardium with severe RV dilatation and systolic dysfunction, in the presence of preserved LV function (or mild dysfunction). (4) Biventricular heart failure with significant LV involvement, which mimics dilated cardiomyopathy of other causes with progressive heart failure and related complications, such as atrial fibrillation, thromboembolic events,[8] requiring anticoagulation therapy, ICD, and, in the most severe cases, cardiac transplantation.[9–12]

More recent studies on genotype-phenotype correlations have shown common and early LV involvement in carriers of desmoplakin mutations (**Fig. 3**).[13,14] In contrast with the original idea of an almost exclusive RV involvement, 3 distinct AC phenotypes are currently recognized: the RV phenotype, either isolated or associated with mild LV involvement; the left dominant phenotype, with early and prominent LV manifestations; and the biventricular phenotype, characterized by equal involvement of both ventricles.[8] Therefore, the old view that LV involvement occurs secondarily in advanced disease has evolved into the current perspective that AC is a genetically determined myocardial disease affecting the whole heart.

Incidence of SCD and Heart Failure

The mortality of patients with AC is currently estimated to be around 1% per year. Most deaths are related to life-threatening ventricular arrhythmias that may occur at any time during the disease course. Progressive ventricular dysfunction leading to heart failure and embolic stroke may cause death in a smaller proportion of patients.[3] The overall incidence of SCD caused by VF varies between 0.1% and 3% per year in adults with diagnosed and treated AC, although it is unknown and expected to be higher in adolescents and young adults, in whom the disease is clinically silent until sudden and unexpected arrhythmic cardiac arrest occurs.[15,16] Nava and colleagues[17] observed a lower mortality among family members during a mean follow-up of 8.5 years (0.08% per year) compared with AC probands. Hulot and colleagues[16] reported the long-term natural history of 130 patients with AC who were referred to a tertiary center and followed for 8.1 (±7.8) years. There were 21 deaths, which accounted for an annual mortality of 3% caused by either progressive heart failure in approximately two-thirds of patients or SCD in one-third of patients.

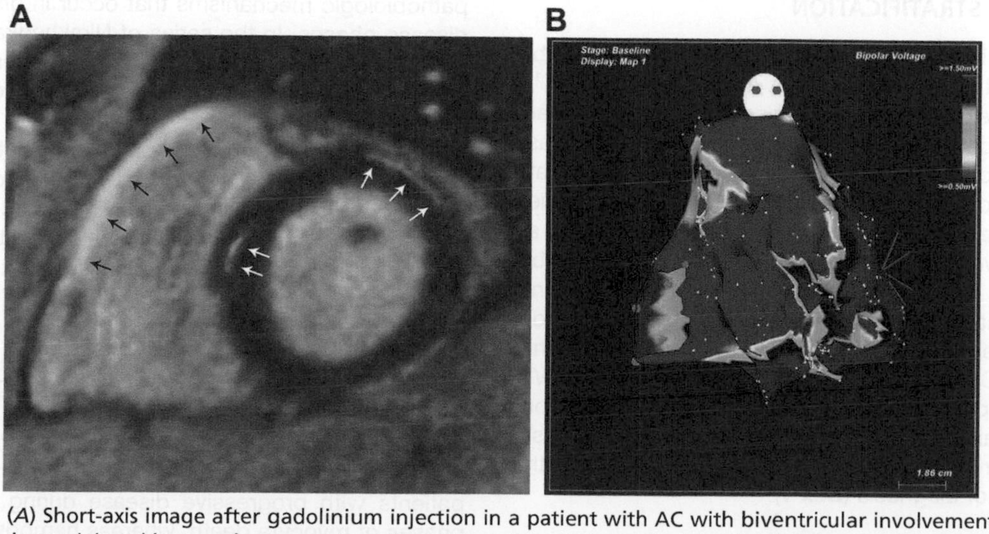

Fig. 2. (*A*) Short-axis image after gadolinium injection in a patient with AC with biventricular involvement. The image shows delayed hyperenhancement on the anteroinfundibular wall of the RV (*black arrows*), as well as on the interventricular septum and the free wall of the LV (*white arrows*). (*B*) Anteroposterior view of the RV bipolar voltage map from a patient with AC showing diffuse low-amplitude electrical activity involving anterior, lateral, inferobasal, anteroapical, and infundibular regions. (*Modified from* Corrado D, Basso C, Thiene G. Arrhythmogenic right ventricular cardiomyopathy: an update. Heart 2009;95:769, 771; with permission.)

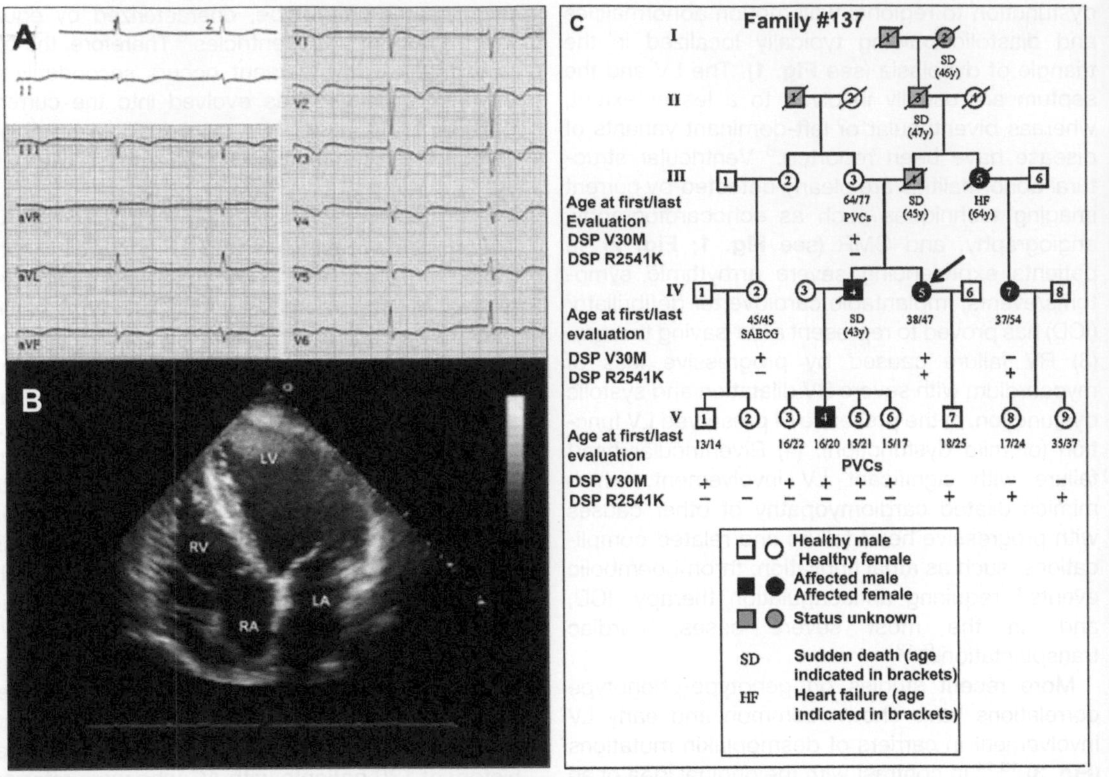

Fig. 3. Clinical findings of index case (IV,5) and pedigree of family #137 with DSP-related AC. (*A*) Twelve-lead ECG with low QRS voltages in frontal leads and T wave inversion in inferior and precordial leads. (*B*) Two-dimensional echocardiogram showing a biventricular involvement. (*C*) Family's pedigree: arrow indicates the index case; + and − denote the presence or absence of a desmosomal gene mutation. (*Modified from* Bauce B, Nava A, Beffagna G, et al. Multiple mutations in desmosomal proteins encoding genes in arrhythmogenic right ventricular cardiomyopathy/dysplasia. Heart Rhythm 2010;7:25, 26; with permission.)

RISK STRATIFICATION

SCD in patients with AC is often an unpredictable event that occurs without alarming symptoms.[1–4] This explains why there has been a trend toward indiscriminate ICD implantation once the disease was diagnosed, without an appropriate risk stratification. In recent years, several studies have tried to identify the clinical variable associated with an unfavorable arrhythmic course. The available data based on autopsy series or observational clinical investigations suggest that the most powerful predictors of SCD and worse outcome in AC include prior cardiac arrest caused by VF, unexplained syncope, VT (either sustained or nonsustained), exposure to intense physical exercise, severe RV/LV dysfunction, and young age at the time of diagnosis (**Box 1**).[18–20]

Cardiac Arrest and Malignant Tachyarrhythmias

In patients with AC, VF, and monomorphic VT are arrhythmic manifestations caused by different pathobiologic mechanisms that occur in different disease phases. In the series of Nimkhedkar and colleagues[21] concerning 10 patients undergoing surgery for life-threatening drug-refractory ventricular arrhythmias, none had a history of VF. In the series of Leclercq and Coumel,[22] only 2 out of 50 patients with VT also had a history of VF. Corrado and colleagues[19] reported that prior cardiac arrest caused by VF and hemodynamically instable VT are independent risk factors for life-saving ICD interventions in a large series of patients with AC. However, patients implanted because of VT without hemodynamic compromise had a statistically significant better outcome, with a negligible incidence of VF episodes during follow-up. These findings are in agreement with the current perspective that VF occurs in younger affected patients with progressive disease during active phases of myocyte death, whereas hemodynamically well-tolerated monomorphic VT is caused by a reentry mechanism around a stable myocardial scar as the result of a healing process that occurs in a later stage of the disease course.

Box 1
Risk factors for SCD in patients with AC

Strongest risk factors
- Prior cardiac arrest/VF
- Fast/poorly tolerated sustained VT
- Unexplained syncope
- Physical exercise/sport activity

Other recognized risk factors
- Young age at diagnosis
- Hemodynamically stable sustained VT
- Nonsustained VT
- Severe RV dysfunction
- LV involvement

Questionable risk factors
- Family history of SCD
- QRS dispersion/delayed S wave upstroke in V1/V2
- Inducibility at programmed ventricular stimulation
- Electroanatomic scar (by CARTO-system)
- Molecular genetics

Resuscitated VF is a poor prognostic factor. In the series reported by Canu and colleagues,[23] a prior history of aborted SCD from VF was documented in 2 of the 3 patients who died suddenly.

Syncope

The importance of syncope as a risk factor for SCD in AC was first reported by Marcus and colleagues[24] and was later confirmed by other groups. Turrini and colleagues[25] reported that syncope was an independent predictor of SCD with a sensitivity of 40% and a specificity of 90%. Among 15 patients with AC reported by Blomström-Lundqvist and colleagues,[26] a history of syncope was ascertained in all 3 victims of SCD versus only 2 of 12 patients who survived. Nava and colleagues[17] confirmed that syncope was the only clinical variable significantly associated with SCD in 19 AC probands, whereas it was never observed among 132 living relatives.

Syncope has been proved to be the strongest predictor of appropriate and life-saving device interventions in patients with AC who received an ICD for primary prevention (DARVIN 2). The 9% annual incidence of appropriate device discharges among patients with prior syncope is comparable with that observed in patients who underwent device implantation because of a history of cardiac arrest or sustained VT.[20]

Young individuals with genetic cardiomyopathies and/or ion channel disorders may suffer from vasovagal or, more widely, nonarrhythmic syncope, which makes differential diagnosis difficult and its prognostic value elusive. For instance, in patients with hypertrophic cardiomyopathy, several nonarrhythmic mechanisms, such as reflex-mediated change in vascular tone or heart rate, LV outflow tract obstruction, and supraventricular tachyarrhythmia, may cause syncope. In patients with AC, most episodes of syncope are secondary to ventricular tachyarrhythmias and associated with a poor prognosis similarly to sustained VT or VF.[20]

Sport Activity

AC shows a propensity for life-threatening ventricular arrhythmias during physical exercise, and participation in competitive athletics has been associated with an increased risk for SCD.[1,4,27] Identification of affected athletes by preparticipation screening has proved to result in a substantial reduction of mortality of young competitive athletes.[4] In addition, physical sport activity has been implicated as a factor promoting acceleration of the disease progression. There is experimental evidence that in heterozygous plakoglobin-deficient mice, endurance training accelerated the development of RV dysfunction and arrhythmias.[28] It has been suggested that impairment of myocyte cell-to-cell adhesion may lead to tissue and organ fragility that is sufficient to promote myocyte death, especially in conditions of mechanical stress, such as those occurring during competitive sports activity.[2] As a corollary, asymptomatic and healthy gene carriers should be advised to refrain from practicing significant physical exercise, not only for reducing the risk of ventricular arrhythmias but also to prevent disease worsening.[4,17,29] Whether prophylactic β-blocker therapy further lowers the rate of arrhythmic complications and slows down disease progression remains to be proved.

Clinical Findings

ECG and morphofunctional abnormalities

Right precordial QRS prolongation, QRS dispersion, and late potentials (LPs) on signal-averaged ECG (SAECG) have been significantly associated with an increase of the arrhythmic risk in patients with AC. These ECG abnormalities reflect a right intraventricular conduction defect caused by the fibrofatty replacement of the RV free wall, which may predispose to life-threatening ventricular arrhythmias.

Localized prolongation of QRS complex in V1 to V3 to more than 110 milliseconds has a sensitivity of 55% and a specificity of 100% for the diagnosis of the disease.[30] QRS prolongation, in the form of incomplete right bundle branch block (RBBB) or, more often, nonspecific conduction defect, is usually caused by an intraventricular myocardial delay (parietal block). Septal incomplete or complete RBBB may occasionally be the result of marked RV dilatation/dysfunction affecting the specialized right bundle branch (septal block). Right precordial QRS prolongation correlates with the arrhythmic risk, as shown by the study of Turrini and colleagues[25] in which patients who died suddenly showed a significant greater QRS prolongation (125 milliseconds) in V1 to V2/V3 compared with living patients with AC with or without VT (QRS duration = 113 milliseconds and 106 milliseconds, respectively).

Accordingly, Nasir and colleagues[31] showed that a prolonged right precordial QRS complex with a pattern of delayed S wave upstroke of 55 milliseconds or more is a significant predictor of severity and VT inducibility by programmed ventricular stimulation.

Greater prolongation of QRS in the leads exploring the RV accounts for QRS dispersion (ie, the difference in duration between the longest and the shortest QRS intervals in the surface ECG), which reflects RV regional inhomogeneity of intraventricular conduction times. Turrini and colleagues[25] showed that QRS dispersion of more than 40 milliseconds was the strongest independent predictor of SCD in AC, with a sensitivity of 90% and a specificity of 77% (**Fig. 4**).

In patients with ischemic heart disease, LPs on SAECG have been shown to be a noninvasive marker for areas of slow ventricular conduction, which is a prerequisite for reentrant arrhythmias. Several studies have investigated the clinical meaning of LPs in AC. In the original series of Marcus and colleagues,[32] among the 16 patients who underwent SAECG, 13 (81%) had LPs. Blomström-Lundqvist and colleagues[33] reported similar results with a 72% prevalence of LPs in their cohort of 18 patients with AC. In the series of Wichter and colleagues,[34] LPs were observed in 24 of 48 patients (50%), with a higher prevalence among those with a classic form of AC and more pronounced RV contraction abnormalities. Mehta and colleagues[35] showed a relationship between SAECG variables and the degree of RV enlargement. Although the SAECG seems to be a valuable test for diagnosing AC, the evidence of its usefulness for arrhythmic risk stratification is lacking. Blomström-Lundqvist and colleagues[33] found that LPs were not predictive of ventricular arrhythmia in patients with AC, as did Leclercq and Coumel[36] who showed that the prevalence of LPs was similar in patients with or without sustained VT, and that their absence did not exclude the risk of SCD. Moreover, it was reported that repeated SAECG during follow-up did not seem to be useful in predicting the susceptibility to VT.[37] Turrini and colleagues[38] showed that, although LPs were univariate predictors of

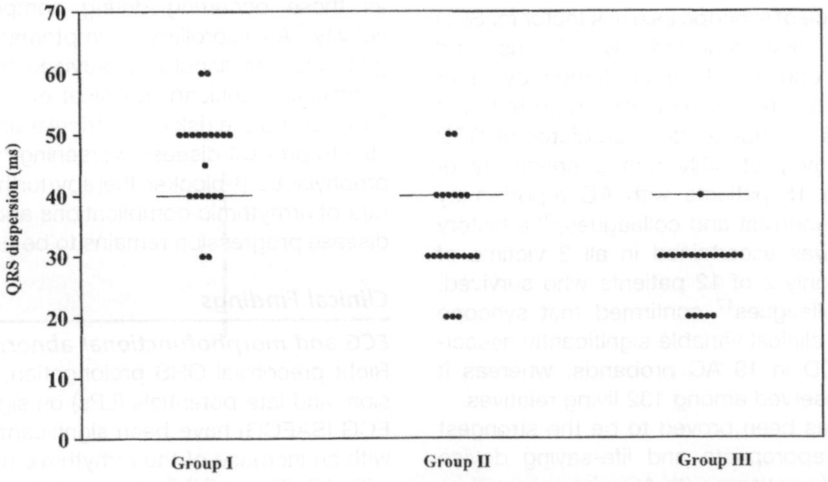

Fig. 4. Distribution of QRS dispersions in 3 AC groups: group I is composed of 20 patients who died suddenly, group II of 20 patients with sustained VT, and group III of 20 patients with no sustained ventricular tachycardia. Mean values are indicated by horizontal lines. (*Modified from* Turrini P, Corrado D, Basso C, et al. Dispersion of ventricular depolarization-repolarization: a non invasive marker for risk stratification in arrhythmogenic right ventricular cardiomyopathy. Circulation 2001;103:3078; with permission.)

sustained VT, at multivariate analysis the only independent predictor of arrhythmic events remained a decreased RV ejection fraction (**Fig. 5**). Furthermore, in patients with familial AC, an abnormal SAECG correlated with the severity of the disease, but not with ventricular electrical instability.[39] The predictive value of SAECG in this particular subgroup was low: only 44% of subjects with LPs had arrhythmias, whereas 76% of those with arrhythmias had abnormal SAECG. Likewise, the study of Nava and colleagues[40] failed to show any correlation between SAECG and the risk of life-threatening ventricular arrhythmias.

RV Dysfunction and LV Involvement

A ventricular dilatation/dysfunction is a well-established clinical marker of a worse prognosis. In the study by Hulot and colleagues[16] on the long-term follow-up of 130 patients with AC, right heart failure and LV dysfunction were identified as independent risk factors predicting cardiovascular death. Peters and colleagues[41] confirmed these results in 121 patients with AC, in whom advanced RV dilatation/dysfunction and LV involvement were major clinical variables associated with an increased risk of SCD. Turrini and colleagues[38] reported a significant association between a reduced RV ejection fraction (≤50%) and sustained ventricular arrhythmias. Several ICD studies indicated extensive RV dysfunction as an independent risk factor for appropriate device discharges.[42,43]

Inducibility at Programmed Ventricular Stimulation

The electrophysiologic study with programmed ventricular stimulation (PVS) seems to be of limited value in identifying patients with AC at risk of lethal ventricular arrhythmias because of a low predictive accuracy. The results of DARVIN studies show that the incidence of appropriate and life-saving ICD discharges did not differ among patients who were and were not inducible at PVS, regardless of their indication for ICD implant.[19,20] Moreover, the type of ventricular tachyarrhythmia inducible at the time of electrophysiologic study did not seem to predict the occurrence of VF during the follow-up. These findings are in agreement with the limitation of

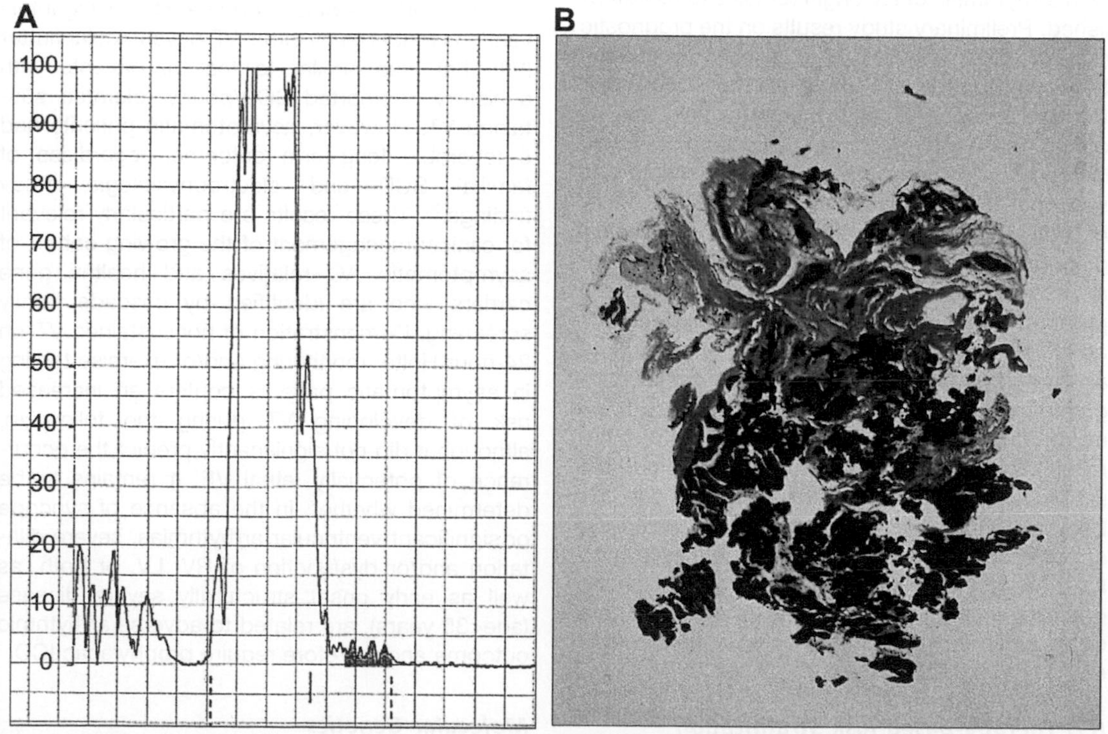

Fig. 5. Signal-averaged ECG and endomyocardial biopsy findings in a patient with AC with sustained VT and reduced RVEF (49%). (*A*) Positive LPs at 40-Hz filter (fQRS = 136 milliseconds, LAS = 77 milliseconds, RMS = 2 mV). (*B*) Severe replacement-type myocardial fibrosis (blue stain). (Trichrome Heidenhain stain × 45, reduced 34%). (*Modified from* Turrini P, Angelini A, Thiene G, et al. Late potentials and ventricular arrhythmias in arrhythmogenic right ventricular cardiomyopathy. Am J Cardiol 1999;83:1218; with permission.)

electrophysiologic studies for arrhythmic risk stratification of other nonischemic heart disease such as hypertrophic and dilated cardiomyopathy. In the study of Wichter and colleagues,[42] inducibility of VT or VF in a preimplant electrophysiologic study of AC patients with previous history of cardiac arrest or sustained VT showed just a trend toward statistical significance for subsequent appropriate device interventions. The available data do not support the routine use of PVS for assessing the risk of SCD in patients with AC, neither among patients surviving an episode of VF/VT nor among those who are asymptomatic without spontaneous clinical tachyarrhythmias.

Electroanatomic Voltage Mapping

The electroanatomic voltage mapping (EVM) by the CARTO-system allows clinicians to identify and to characterize (presence, site, and extension) electroanatomic scars (EAS), which are regions of ventricular myocardium characterized by a low electric voltage and may represent the substrate for life-threatening ventricular tachyarrhythmias. Although the technique has been shown to enhance accuracy for diagnosing AC,[7,44] its value for risk stratification of SCD in patients presenting with arrhythmias of RV origin remains to be established. Preliminary study results on the prognostic role of EVM showed a significant correlation between the presence and extent of RV-EAS and the incidence of malignant arrhythmic events during follow-up, such as SCD, cardiac arrest caused by VF, appropriate ICD intervention, and syncopal VT.[45] After adjustment for age, family history, VT, RV dilatation/dysfunction, and clinical diagnosis of AC, the presence of RV-EAS remained a statistically significant independent predictor of an adverse arrhythmic outcome.[45] In addition, patients who experienced malignant arrhythmic events over time showed a significantly greater extent of RV-EAS than those with an uneventful follow-up. In patients with RV arrhythmias, identification of a RV-EAS goes beyond the simple demonstration of RV structural damage because it provides evidence of an underlying arrhythmogenic substrate, which explains why RV-EAS seems a stronger predictor of unfavorable outcome than clinical diagnosis of AC and/or the detection of RV dilatation/dysfunction, either segmental or global.

ICD Therapy-based Risk Stratification

Implantable defibrillator is the most logical therapeutic strategy for patients with AC, whose natural history is primarily characterized by the risk of arrhythmic cardiac arrest. Several studies on either secondary or primary prevention have provided significant insights for therapy-based risk stratification of AC patients, leading to identification of clinical and electrophysiologic markers that may predict the appropriate shock against life-threatening ventricular arrhythmias.[19,20,42,43]

The DARVIN 1 study[19] yielded the following predictors of appropriate ICD interventions on potentially lethal arrhythmic events: prior cardiac arrest, VT with hemodynamic compromise, LV involvement, and younger age. A long-term follow-up study of patients with Naxos disease (an autosomal recessive variant of AC associated with palmoplantar keratoderma and woolly hair) confirmed that arrhythmic syncope, LV involvement, early onset of symptoms, and early structural progression were the stronger predictors of SCD.[46]

There is general agreement that patients who survive an episode of VF or sustained VT benefit most from ICD implantation because of their high incidence of malignant arrhythmia recurrences.[19] The life-saving role of prophylactic ICD therapy in patients with AC with no previous history of sustained tachyarrhythmias or cardiac arrest is less clear. The DARVIN 2 study showed that patients who received an ICD because of a prior syncope had an incidence of appropriate, life-saving interventions triggered by either VF or ventricular flutter (Vfl) that was similar to that of patients with a history of aborted SCD/poorly tolerated sustained VT. However, asymptomatic patients had a favorable long-term outcome, regardless of familial SCD and electrophysiologic study findings.[20] These results are particularly relevant for clinical management of the growing cohort of asymptomatic AC relatives and healthy gene carriers who are identified by cascade family screening. Demonstration of nonsustained VT on 24-hour Holter monitoring and/or exercise testing in asymptomatic patients confers an increased risk of developing VT during the follow-up, although it did not significantly predict the occurrence of potentially lethal VF. It remains to be determined whether, in the absence of syncope or significant ventricular arrhythmias, severe dilatation and/or dysfunction of RV, LV, or both, as well as early onset structurally severe disease (age<35 years), are related to adverse arrhythmic outcome and therefore require prophylactic ICD.

Molecular Genetics

At present, there is little evidence to support the use of genotyping for prediction of clinical outcome.[47] Family screening for AC mutations may determine the genetic risk of members, although it does not guarantee that disease will occur. Early identification of genetically affected individuals may raise complex management issues. A sizable proportion of gene carriers do not develop significant clinical manifestations because of the low disease penetrance. A large heterogeneity in clinical expression has been reported, as the result not only of different desmosomal gene defects but also of different mutations within the same gene and among individuals sharing the same gene mutation within the same family. According to this marked variability of AC phenotype, most relatives are likely to have a mild phenotypic expression and follow a benign course. However, patients may suffer arrhythmic events without warning symptoms and/or signs, in the setting of an unpredictable and abrupt acceleration of disease progression (hot phases).

Furthermore, studies of genotype-phenotype correlations have failed to show that genotyping is able to detect malignant AC mutations that are specifically associated with an increased susceptibility to life-threatening arrhythmic events and require prophylactic ICD therapy for sudden death prevention. An exception is the study by Merner and colleagues, which reported a malignant variant of AC linked to transmembrane TMEM43 gene mutation.[48] In other studies, no significant differences have been reported for a series of clinical, ECG, and arrhythmic variables between AC mutation carriers and noncarriers. In addition, the proportion of patients who received an ICD and the incidence of appropriate discharges during the follow-up did not differ between gene-positive and gene-negative probands, suggesting that genetic screening for AC gene mutations is unlikely to contribute significantly to arrhythmic risk assessment and stratification. These findings imply that other environmental or genetic factors, such as the presence of genetic modifiers or compound heterozygous mutations,[13] may influence the severity of clinical expression of the disease and do not support a molecular genetic approach for assessment of AC prognosis.

SUMMARY

Several clinical variables have been proposed for clinical assessment of the arrhythmic risk in AC. At present, a pragmatic approach to risk stratification entails prioritizing for ICD implantation those patients with a history of cardiac arrest, sustained and hemodynamically unstable VT, or unexplained syncope. Among the remaining asymptomatic patients, the prognostic value of individual single or combined risk factors has not been definitively established and the available evidence does not support offering prophylactic ICD therapy.

Further investigations on larger AC patient populations and for longer follow-up periods are needed to refine the assessment of the clinical profile of patients with AC carrying a higher SCD risk at preclinical/presymptomatic disease phases to optimize prevention strategies.

REFERENCES

1. Thiene G, Nava A, Corrado D, et al. Right ventricular cardiomyopathy and sudden death in young people. N Engl J Med 1988;318:129–33.
2. Basso C, Corrado D, Marcus F, et al. Arrhythmogenic right ventricular cardiomyopathy. Lancet 2009;373:1289–300.
3. Corrado D, Basso C, Thiene G. Arrhythmogenic right ventricular cardiomyopathy: an update. Heart 2009;95:766–73.
4. Corrado D, Basso C, Pavei A, et al. Trends in sudden cardiovascular death in young competitive athletes after implementation of a preparticipation screening program. JAMA 2006;296:1593–601.
5. Basso C, Ronco F, Marcus F, et al. Quantitative assessment of endomyocardial biopsy in arrhythmogenic right ventricular cardiomyopathy/dysplasia: an in vitro validation of diagnostic criteria. Eur Heart J 2008;29:2760–71.
6. Sen-Chowdhry S, Syrris P, Ward D, et al. Clinical and genetic characterization of families with arrhythmogenic right ventricular dysplasia/cardiomyopathy provides novel insights into patterns of disease expression. Circulation 2007;115:1710–20.
7. Corrado D, Basso C, Leoni L, et al. Three-dimensional electroanatomical voltage mapping and histologic evaluation of myocardial substrate in right ventricular outflow tract tachycardia. J Am Coll Cardiol 2008;51:731–9.
8. Wlodarska EK, Wozniak O, Konka M, et al. Thromboembolic complications in patients with arrhythmogenic right ventricular dysplasia/cardiomyopathy. Europace 2006;8:596–600.
9. Basso C, Thiene G, Corrado D, et al. Arrhythmogenic right ventricular cardiomyopathy: dysplasia, dystrophy or myocarditis? Circulation 1996;94:983–91.
10. Corrado D, Basso C, Thiene G, et al. Spectrum of clinicopathologic manifestations of arrhythmogenic right ventricular cardiomyopathy/dysplasia: a multicenter study. J Am Coll Cardiol 1997;30:1512–20.
11. Thiene G, Nava A, Angelini A, et al. Anatomoclinical aspects of arrhythmogenic right ventricular cardiomyopathy. In: Baroldi G, Camerini F, Goodwin JF, editors. Advances in cardiomyopathies. Milan (Italy): Springer-Verlag; 1990. p. 397–408.

12. Thiene G, Angelini A, Basso C, et al. Novel heart diseases requiring transplantation. Adv Clin Path 1998;2:65–73.
13. Bauce B, Nava A, Beffagna G, et al. Multiple mutations in desmosomal proteins encoding genes in arrhythmogenic right ventricular cardiomyopathy/dysplasia. Heart Rhythm 2010;7:22–9.
14. Norman M, Simpson M, Mogensen J, et al. Novel mutation in desmoplakin causes arrhythmogenic left ventricular cardiomyopathy. Circulation 2005;112:636–42.
15. Fontaine G, Fontaliran F, Hebert JL, et al. Arrhythmogenic right ventricular dysplasia. Annu Rev Med 1999;50:17–35.
16. Hulot JS, Jouven X, Empana JP, et al. Natural history and risk stratification of arrhythmogenic right ventricular dysplasia/cardiomyopathy. Circulation 2004;110:1879–84.
17. Nava A, Bauce B, Basso C, et al. Clinical profile and long-term follow-up of 37 families with arrhythmogenic right ventricular cardiomyopathy. J Am Coll Cardiol 2000;36:2226–33.
18. Buja G, Estes NA, Wichter T, et al. Arrhythmogenic right ventricular cardiomyopathy/dysplasia: risk stratification and therapy. Prog Cardiovasc Dis 2008;50:282–93.
19. Corrado D, Leoni L, Link MS, et al. Implantable cardioverter defibrillator therapy for prevention of sudden death in patients with arrhythmogenic right ventricular cardiomyopathy/dysplasia. Circulation 2003;108:3084–91.
20. Corrado D, Calkins H, Link M, et al. Prophylactic implantable defibrillator in patients with arrhythmogenic right ventricular cardiomyopathy/dysplasia and no prior ventricular fibrillation or sustained ventricular tachycardia. Circulation 2010;122:1144–52.
21. Nimkhedkar K, Hilton CJ, Furniss SS, et al. Surgery for ventricular tachycardia associated with right ventricular dysplasia: disarticulation of right ventricle in 9 of 10 cases. J Am Coll Cardiol 1992;19:1079–84.
22. Leclercq JF, Coumel P. Characteristics, prognosis, and treatment of the ventricular arrhythmias of right ventricular dysplasia. Eur Heart J 1989;10(Suppl D):61–7.
23. Canu G, Atallah G, Claudel JP, et al. Pronostic et évolution à long term de la dysplasie arythmogène du ventricule droit. Arch Mal Coeur Vaiss 1993;86:41–8 [in French].
24. Marcus FI, Fontaine GH, Frank R, et al. Long-term followup in patients with arrhythmogenic right ventricular disease. Eur Heart J 1989;10(Suppl D):68–73.
25. Turrini P, Corrado D, Basso C, et al. Dispersion of ventricular depolarization-repolarization: a non invasive marker for risk stratification in arrhythmogenic right ventricular cardiomyopathy. Circulation 2001;103:3075–80.
26. Blomström-Lundqvist C, Sabel KG, Olsson SB. A long term follow-up of 15 patients with arrhythmogenic right ventricular dysplasia. Br Heart J 1987;58:477–88.
27. Corrado D, Basso C, Rizzoli G, et al. Does sports activity enhance the risk of sudden death in adolescents and young adults? J Am Coll Cardiol 2003;42:1959–63.
28. Kirchhof P, Fabritz L, Zwiener M, et al. Age- and training-dependent development of arrhythmogenic right ventricular cardiomyopathy in heterozygous plakoglobin-deficient mice. Circulation 2006;114:1799–806.
29. Corrado D, Thiene G. Arrhythmogenic right ventricular cardiomyopathy/dysplasia: clinical impact of molecular genetic studies. Circulation 2006;113:1634–7.
30. Fontaine G, Umemura J, Di Donna P, et al. La durée des complexes QRS dans la dysplasie ventriculaire droite arythmogène: un noveau marqueur diagnostique non invasif. Ann Cardiol Angeiol 1993;42:399–405.
31. Nasir K, Bomma C, Tandri H, et al. Electrocardiographic features of arrhythmogenic right ventricular dysplasia/cardiomyopathy according to disease severity. Circulation 2004;110:1527–34.
32. Marcus FI, Fontaine GH, Guiraudon G, et al. Right ventricular dysplasia: a report of 24 adult cases. Circulation 1982;65:384–98.
33. Blomström-Lundqvist C, Hirsch I, Olsson SB, et al. Quantitative analysis of the signal averaged QRS in patients with arrhythmogenic right ventricular dysplasia. Eur Heart J 1988;9:301–12.
34. Wichter T, Hindricks G, Lerch H, et al. Regional myocardial sympathetic dysinnervation in arrhythmogenic right ventricular cardiomyopathy: an analysis using 123I-Meta-odobenzylguanidine Scintigraphy. Circulation 1994;89:667–83.
35. Mehta D, Goldman M, David O, et al. Value of quantitative measurements of signal averaged electrocardiographic variables in arrhythmogenic right ventricular dysplasia: correlation with echocardiographic right ventricular cavity dimensions. J Am Coll Cardiol 1996;28:713–9.
36. Leclercq JF, Coumel P. Late potentials in arrhythmogenic right ventricular dysplasia. Prevalence, diagnostic and prognostic values. Eur Heart J 1993;14:80–3.
37. Blomström-Lundqvist C, Olsson SB, Edvardsson N. Follow-up by repeated signal-averaged surface QRS in patients with the syndrome of arrhythmogenic right ventricular dysplasia. Eur Heart J 1989;10(Suppl D):54–60.
38. Turrini P, Angelini A, Thiene G, et al. Late potentials and ventricular arrhythmias in arrhythmogenic right ventricular cardiomyopathy. Am J Cardiol 1999;83:1214–9.
39. Oselladore L, Nava A, Buja G, et al. Signal-averaged electrocardiography in familial form of arrhythmogenic

right ventricular cardiomyopathy. Am J Cardiol 1995; 75(Suppl E):1038–41.
40. Nava A, Folino AF, Bauce B, et al. Signal-averaged electrocardiogram in patients with arrhythmogenic right ventricular cardiomyopathy and ventricular arrhythmias. Eur Heart J 2000;21:58–65.
41. Peters S, Peters H, Thierfelder L. Risk stratification of sudden cardiac death and malignant ventricular arrhythmias in right ventricular dysplasia-cardiomyopathy. Int J Cardiol 1999;71:243–50.
42. Wichter T, Paul M, Wollmann C, et al. Implantable cardioverter/defibrillator therapy in arrhythmogenic right ventricular cardiomyopathy: single-center experience of long-term follow-up and complications in 60 patients. Circulation 2004;109:1503–8.
43. Roguin A, Bomma CS, Nasir K, et al. Implantable cardioverter-defibrillators in patients with arrhythmogenic right ventricular dysplasia/cardiomyopathy. J Am Coll Cardiol 2004;19(43):1843–52.
44. Corrado D, Basso C, Leoni L, et al. Three-dimensional electroanatomic voltage mapping increases accuracy of diagnosing arrhythmogenic right ventricular cardiomyopathy/dysplasia. Circulation 2005;111:3042–50.
45. Migliore F, Bevilacqua M, Zorzi A, et al. The presence and extent of right ventricular electroanatomic scar (by Carto-System) predict the outcome of patients with right ventricular arrhythmias. Circulation 2010;122:A19320.
46. Protonotarios N, Tsatsopoulou A, McKenna W, et al. Genotype-phenotype assessment in autosomal recessive arrhythmogenic right ventricular cardiomyopathy/dysplasia (Naxos disease) caused by a deletion in plakoglobin. J Am Coll Cardiol 2001; 38:1477–84.
47. Corrado D, Basso C, Pilichou K, et al. Molecular biology and the clinical management of arrhythmogenic right ventricular cardiomyopathy/dysplasia. Heart 2011;97:530–9.
48. Merner ND, Hodgkinson KA, Haywood AF, et al. Arrhythmogenic right ventricular cardiomyopathy type 5 is a fully penetrant, lethal arrhythmic disorder caused by a missense mutation in the TMEM43 gene. Am J Hum Genet 2008;82:809–21.

Arrhythmogenic Cardiomyopathy: Pharmacologic Management

Mark S. Link, MD*, N.A. Mark Estes III, MD

KEYWORDS

- Antiarrhythmic agents
- Arrhythmogenic right ventricular cardiomyopathy/dysplasia
- β-Blocker • Pharmacologic management • Therapy

Pharmacologic management of disease is performed for specific reasons, which include reducing symptoms, preventing disease progression, and preventing mortality (**Fig. 1**).[1] Symptoms could include heart failure, palpitations, and syncope; disease progression can be seen with agents that prevent heart failure and remodeling in those with ischemic and nonischemic cardiomyopathies. Mortality can be sudden and arrhythmic or secondary to congestive heart failure and myocardial infarction. Occasionally, certain pharmacologic agents may perform all 3 functions.

This trio of reasons for drug use has been developed in many disease states and is particularly relevant to cardiac disease.[1] In some of the more common cardiac diseases, pharmacologic management is well advanced and based on large randomized clinical trials. Examples can be seen in coronary artery disease and congestive heart failure. In coronary disease, symptoms of angina are treated by nitrates, β-blockers, and calcium channel blockers. Progression of coronary disease is reduced by lipid lowering agents (but not by β-blockers, calcium channel blockers, or nitrates). Finally, prevention of sudden cardiac death has been seen with β-blockers, and the mortality and incidence of a myocardial infarction is decreased by aspirin. A similar pharmacologic rationale can also be seen in nonischemic cardiomyopathy and congestive heart failure. If an agent fulfills none of these 3 rationales, there is no reason to administer it.

The rationale for pharmacologic management in coronary artery disease and heart failure is based on randomized clinical trials in which there are tens of thousands of participants. Unfortunately, for the less common cardiac diseases such as arrhythmogenic cardiomyopathy (AC), there is a near-complete lack of randomized clinical trials. Thus, the rationale for management is based on case series, retrospective analysis, rare prospective registries, and inference from the more common cardiac diseases. This article discusses the role of pharmacology in AC to prevent symptoms, limit progression of disease, and prolong life. Data are, however, limited.

ANTIARRHYTHMIC AGENTS IN AC

German Series

One of the largest series of pharmacologic therapy in AC is from Germany, first published[2] in 1992 and updated[3] in 2005. In the initial series, 81 patients with highly suspected or confirmed AC and nonsustained or sustained ventricular tachycardia (VT) underwent a standardized electrophysiologic evaluation. Patients were brought to the electrophysiologic laboratory in an antiarrhythmic drug (AAD)–free state, and programmed ventricular

Cardiac Arrhythmia Center, Tufts Medical Center, Tufts University School of Medicine, 850 Washington Street, Boston, MA 02111, USA
* Corresponding author. Tufts Medical Center, Box #197, 850 Washington Street, Boston, MA 02111.
E-mail address: MLink@tuftsmedicalcenter.org

Card Electrophysiol Clin 3 (2011) 293–298
doi:10.1016/j.ccep.2011.02.005
1877-9182/11/$ – see front matter

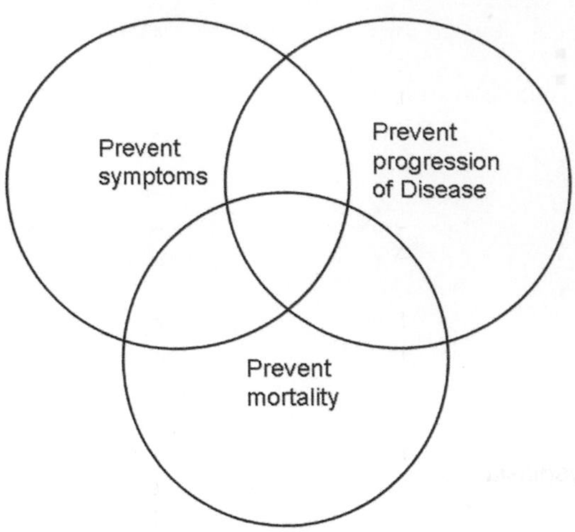

Fig. 1. Pharmacologic management of disease is performed for specific reasons, which include reducing symptoms, preventing disease progression, and preventing mortality. Some drugs may fulfill all 3 functions.

stimulation was performed. VT was inducible in 42 of these individuals and not inducible in 39. In the inducible group, the clinical arrhythmia was sustained VT in 93%, whereas 8% presented with nonsustained VT. In the noninducible group, only 20% presented with sustained VT, whereas 80% had nonsustained VT. After the initial ventricular stimulation, an AAD agent was administered. Each group underwent serial AAD testing composed of serial electrophysiologic studies in the inducible group and long-term cardiac monitoring in the noninducible group. Immediate efficacy was found in most patients, and they were discharged on the drug effective in preventing VT. Long-term follow-up was also reported with the end point of clinical tachycardia.

In the 42 inducible patients who underwent 174 drug tests, sotalol had the highest efficacy. In 26 of 38 patients given sotalol, the ventricular arrhythmia was not inducible for a success rate of 68%. Combinations of class I AAD and sotalol had an efficacy of 20% (2 of 10). Combinations of class I and amiodarone had a success rate of 50% (2 of 4). Class Ia/b (1 of 18) and class Ic (3 of 25) were rarely effective. β-Blockers alone had no efficacy (0 of 7). Amiodarone alone had a success rate of only 15% (2 of 13). Similar results were observed in the noninducible group, with sotalol being effective in 83% of patients (29 of 35) and amiodarone in 25% (1 of 4). Class Ia/b (0 of 16) and class Ic (4 of 23) were rarely effective. However, β-blockers were effective in 30% (2 of 7) of patients.

In the inducible group, 31 patients were discharged on pharmacologic therapy, including 25 with sotalol alone or sotalol in combination with type 1 AAD. In a long-term follow-up of 34 months, there were no sudden deaths in the inducible group. Of 31 patients discharged on pharmacologic therapy, 3 (10%) had nonfatal recurrences of VT. In the noninducible tachycardia group, 33 of 39 patients were discharged on pharmacologic management, including 24 with sotalol. In a follow-up of 14 months, there were no sudden deaths, and 4 of 33 patients discharged on AADs had nonfatal relapses of VT. Interestingly, in studies in patients with coronary disease, tested sotalol was also efficacious, and there have been little published data that untested sotalol in any disease state prevents arrhythmias.[1]

This group updated their experience in 2005, with 191 patients and 608 drug tests.[3] Sotalol at a dosage of 320–480 mg/d was the most effective drug resulting in a 68% overall efficacy. Combinations of amiodarone and β-blockers were also highly efficacious. Class I AADs were efficacious only in a minority of patients (18%). In a small subset of patients thought to have triggered activity or autonomic abnormal automaticity, verapamil and β-blockers had efficacy rates of 44% and 25%; however, they were not likely to be successful in reentrant tachycardias. In long-term follow-up of this group of patients, those who had success with drug testing generally did well, with a much lower recurrence rate on a drug that was effective, versus those in whom no effective drug could be found.

North American AC Registry

The next largest group of patients presented in the literature is a more recent study from the North American Registry published in 2009.[4] Of 108 patients in this registry, 95 had implantable defibrillators (ICDs). This study was a prospectively enrolled cohort, and pharmacologic therapy, including β-blockers, AADs, and ICDs, was left to the discretion of the treating physician. Fifty-eight patients (61%) received beta-adrenergic blocking agents, including atenolol, metoprolol, bisoprolol, and carvedilol. In a mean follow-up of 480 days, there were 235 clinically relevant ventricular arrhythmias observed in 32 patients. There was no clinically significant benefit of preventing VT or ventricular fibrillation with beta-blockade when compared with participants not taking AADs or β-blockers. However, there was a trend in the reduction in ICD shocks, although this result did not reach statistical significance. Atenolol potentially showed the greatest benefit in this study, although there were too few patients on the individual β-blockers class II to draw too many conclusions from this subanalysis.[4]

Thirty-eight patients were treated with sotalol, with a mean dose of 240 mg/d. In a mean of 644 days, the hazard ratios either showed no effect or favored a detrimental effect of sotalol with regards to any clinically relevant arrhythmia, any ICD shock, first clinically relevant arrhythmia, and first ICD shock. However, the mean tachycardia cycle length of those with VT was significantly greater in those taking sotalol (311 vs 292 ms) (**Fig. 2**). Patients who received the upper quartile dose of sotalol ($\geq$320 mg/d) had a worse outcome compared with individuals not in the upper quartile of sotalol.[4] Finally, in this study, 10 patients given amiodarone were followed up for a median of 545 days. When taking amiodarone, patients had a 75% lower risk of any clinically relevant ventricular arrhythmia compared with all other patients.

However, this study, as well as others with patients on AADs and β-blockers in patients with AC, should be interpreted with caution because clinical indications for β-blockers, sotalol, and amiodarone were present and it is likely that there was a selection bias that influenced outcomes. This selection bias could explain the worsened results with sotalol but not the reduction in arrhythmias with amiodarone. In addition, amiodarone is widely considered the most efficacious AAD in other disease states.

Other Clinical Series

Other data on AADs use are considerably weaker than those from the 2 prior trials. A study of 31 amiodarone refractory patients with arrhythmias, including 4 patients with AC, showed improved efficacy when beta-blockade was added to amiodarone.[5] Other data on pharmacologic therapy can be gleaned from studies on patients in ICDs. These trials may give some clues to the potential risk and benefits of β-blockers and AADs. In an early ICD AC study, sotalol slowed the VT so that it was more often pace terminated rather than shock terminated.[6] Of 132 patients with AC and ICDs, 53 patients were taking AADs in follow-up; 5 were taking amiodarone alone; 6, amiodarone plus β-blockers; 13, β-blockers; and 28, sotalol.[7] Of the 64 patients with appropriate

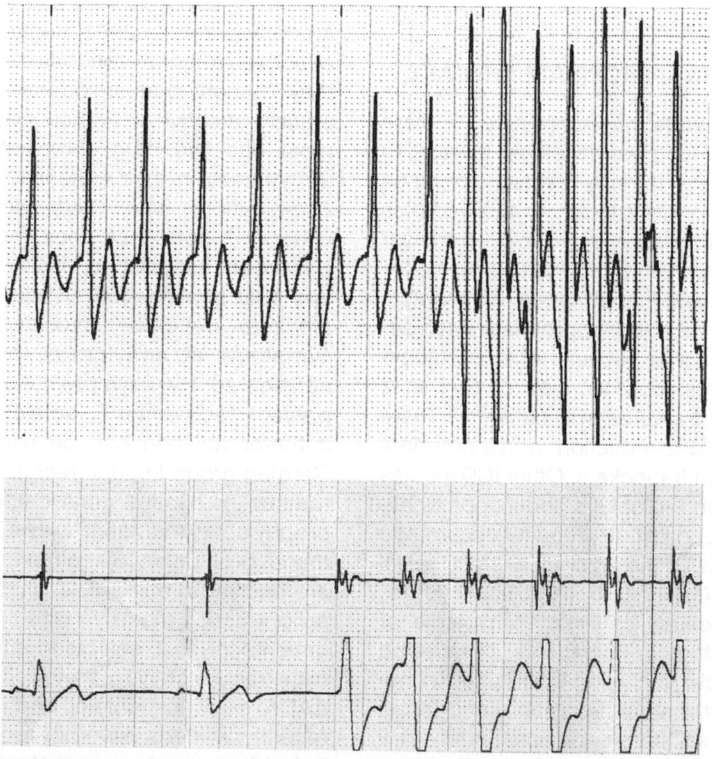

Fig. 2. ICD tracings from a patient with AC who received an ICD at age 17 years when he presented with presyncope and VT. The top panel shows the tracings obtained 1 year after the ICD was implanted; the VT had a cycle length of 220 ms and required an ICD shock for termination. The patient was then administered sotalol, and the bottom panel shows VT at 340 ms. This slower tachycardia was terminated with ATP, demonstrating that one of the potential benefits of AADs is that they may slow the VT and thus allow ATP to terminate the VT.

interventions, 53 (83%) received concomitant AAD therapy at the time of the first ICD intervention. The incidence of ICD discharges did not differ between patients who did and did not receive AAD therapy (either sotalol or any AAD), regardless of clinical presentation of cardiac arrest, VT with hemodynamic compromise, VT without hemodynamic compromise, unexplained syncope, nonsustained VT, or a family history of sudden death. Again, pharmacologic therapy was left at the discrimination of the investigator.

In another series of 43 patients with AC and ICDs, 17 received β-blockers at some point, 8 amiodarone, and 10 sotalol.[8] There was no statistically significant difference in β-blocker usage between those who did and did not have ICD treatment. However, there was a small trend toward a protective effect of β-blockers and amiodarone.

Thus, the data on AAD use in AC to prevent VT are quite limited, subject to tremendous selection bias of who should get AADs and likely swayed by the clinical presentation. There is no evidence to suggest that any β-blocker or AAD is associated with a decreased risk of sudden death; however, this hypothesis has never been completely tested.

PREVENTION OF INAPPROPRIATE THERAPY

Whereas beta-blockade may not reduce VT, there may still be a role for pharmacologic therapy to reduce inappropriate therapy because of sinus tachycardia, supraventricular tachycardias (SVTs), and atrial fibrillation with rapid ventricular response. In one study that reports on pharmacologic management and inappropriate ICD therapy, 10 of the 42 patients had inappropriate interventions. This therapy was because of sinus tachycardia in 6 patients, another type of SVT in 2 patients, and lead fractures in 2 patients.[8] There was a trend toward a reduction in inappropriate therapy for those on β-blockers. Other ICD studies do not give data on β-blockers and inappropriate therapy but do document the frequent occurrence of inappropriate ICD therapy. In a small initial series of ICDs in AC, 3 of 12 patients had inappropriate therapy because of sinus tachycardia or SVT.[6] In another study of 60 patients, 14 received inappropriate shocks, including 4 with sinus tachycardia and 3 with atrial fibrillation and rapid ventricular response.[9] In an additional study of 9 patients, inappropriate shocks were seen for sinus tachycardia (18 episodes in 3 patients) and atrial fibrillation (3 episodes in 1 patient).[10] Thus, β-blockers could be expected to slow these SVTs and prevent inappropriate therapy.

PROGRESSION OF DISEASE

With regard to the progression of disease, there are even less data. However, there is anecdotal evidence that competitive sports may increase the expression of AC.[11–13] It is thought that this effect is physiologically plausible because of the possible effect of extreme training on RV pressures and thus the increased disruption of desmosomal proteins. In mice, there are data of a training-dependent development of the expression of AC.[14] In this study of plakoglobin-deficient mice, the manifestation of the phenotype was accelerated by exercise. Such a finding would be reason to believe that drugs such as β-blockers or even ACE inhibitors may prevent the progression of disease; however, this speculation has not been studied in the population with AC. There is 1 case report of improvement in left ventricular function but not of RV function in a patient with AC and reduced ventricular function treated with carvedilol.[15]

OTHER EXPERT OPINIONS

Expert opinions of other investigators help to better interpret the aforementioned data. An international group from Italy and the United States, in an early article in 2001, suggested that the most effective drugs are amiodarone and sotalol, and they thought that amiodarone and sotalol were equally effective.[16] French experts state that the most effective drug combination for ventricular arrhythmias in their experience is amiodarone in combination with beta-adrenergic agents.[17] Others[8,18] note that once the diagnosis of AC has been established, initiation of a β-blocker and ICD implantation should be considered. β-blockers are clearly indicated for patients with symptoms of arrhythmias, but they should be considered for asymptomatic patients also. To prevent recurrent VT, sotalol, amiodarone, and catheter ablation can be used. A review by a German group in 2009 recommends that asymptomatic or healthy gene carriers do not require prophylactic treatment with ICDs but do recommend prohibition of competitive sports.[19] They are unclear in this article whether to recommend prophylactic therapy with β-blockers for all patients or just selected patients. For patients with recurrent VT, they recommend class III AADs, such as sotalol and amiodarone. More recently, experts have not recommended routine beta-blockade for asymptomatic patients. For patients with stable nonsustained or sustained VT, β-blockers alone or in combination with the class III AADs sotalol and amiodarone have been recommended.[20]

SUMMARY

There is much to be learned about the pharmacologic treatment of AC. Whether drugs prevent symptoms of VT and inappropriate therapy is simply not known. Whether drugs prevent sudden cardiac death is also not known, but seems unlikely. And finally, whether pharmacologic agents limit progression of disease is also not known. Unfortunately, the data on pharmacologic treatment will likely be slow in accumulation because of the sporadic nature of the disease in a low number of affected individuals. Yet, clinicians must make clinical decisions regarding pharmacologic therapy in the absence of robust evidence regarding risks and benefits. Given the frequent inappropriate therapies for sinus tachycardia and rapidly conducting atrial fibrillation, it would be reasonable to treat most patients with AC and an ICD with β-blockers. There is a hypothetical, but unproven, reason to use β-blockers to prevent progression of disease in individuals who are asymptomatic. At present, there is little evidence to suggest that prophylactic AADs are warranted. For treatment of ventricular arrhythmias in patients with ICDs, sotalol and amiodarone seem efficacious based on the best available evidence. However, if sotalol is to be used, it is reasonable to test for efficacy with programmed electrical stimulation or with cardiac monitoring. Amiodarone is likely the most effective AAD, and it is reasonable to use this agent using clinical end points such as VT rather than testing for efficacy with programmed stimulation. Based on the available data, amiodarone and tested sotalol are likely similar in efficacy. In patients with ICDs, β-blockers may reduce inappropriate therapy, especially in the young active population, but at present, there are no data to suggest that they reduce ventricular arrhythmias.

REFERENCES

1. Link MS, Homoud M, Foote CB, et al. Antiarrhythmic drug therapy of ventricular arrhythmias: current perspectives. J Cardiovasc Electrophysiol 1996;7:653–70.
2. Wichter T, Borggrefe M, Haverkamp W, et al. Efficacy of antiarrhythmic drugs in patients with arrhythmogenic right ventricular disease. Results in patients with inducible and noninducible ventricular tachycardia. Circulation 1992;86:29–37.
3. Wichter T, Paul TM, Eckardt L, et al. Arrhythmogenic right ventricular cardiomyopathy. Antiarrhythmic drugs, catheter ablation, or ICD? Herz 2005;30:91–101.
4. Marcus GM, Glidden DV, Polonsky B, et al. Efficacy of antiarrhythmic drugs in arrhythmogenic right ventricular cardiomyopathy: a report from the North American ARVC Registry. J Am Coll Cardiol 2009; 54:609–15.
5. Tonet J, Frank R, Fontaine G, et al. Efficacy of the combination of low doses of beta-blockers and amiodarone in the treatment of refractory ventricular tachycardia. Arch Mal Coeur Vaiss 1989;82:1511–7 [in French].
6. Link MS, Wang PJ, Haugh CJ, et al. Arrhythmogenic right ventricular dysplasia: clinical results with implantable cardioverter defibrillators. J Interv Card Electrophysiol 1997;1:41–8.
7. Corrado D, Leoni L, Link MS, et al. Implantable cardioverter-defibrillator therapy for prevention of sudden death in patients with arrhythmogenic right ventricular cardiomyopathy/dysplasia. Circulation 2003;108:3084–91.
8. Roguin A, Bomma CS, Nasir K, et al. Implantable cardioverter-defibrillators in patients with arrhythmogenic right ventricular dysplasia/cardiomyopathy. J Am Coll Cardiol 2004;43:1843–52.
9. Wichter T, Paul M, Wollmann C, et al. Implantable cardioverter/defibrillator therapy in arrhythmogenic right ventricular cardiomyopathy: single-center experience of long-term follow-up and complications in 60 patients. Circulation 2004; 109:1503–8.
10. Tavernier R, Gevaert S, De Sutter J, et al. Long term results of cardioverter-defibrillator implantation in patients with right ventricular dysplasia and malignant ventricular tachyarrhythmias. Heart 2001;85:53–6.
11. Wlodarska EK, Konka M, Zaleska T, et al. Arrhythmogenic right ventricular cardiomyopathy in two pairs of monozygotic twins. Int J Cardiol 2005;105:126–33.
12. Sen-Chowdhry S, Syrris P, Ward D, et al. Clinical and genetic characterization of families with arrhythmogenic right ventricular dysplasia/cardiomyopathy provides novel insights into patterns of disease expression. Circulation 2007;115:1710–20.
13. Marcus FI, Zareba W, Calkins H, et al. Arrhythmogenic right ventricular cardiomyopathy/dysplasia clinical presentation and diagnostic evaluation: results from the North American Multidisciplinary Study. Heart Rhythm 2009;6:984–92.
14. Kirchhof P, Fabritz L, Zwiener M, et al. Age- and training-dependent development of arrhythmogenic right ventricular cardiomyopathy in heterozygous plakoglobin-deficient mice. Circulation 2006;114: 1799–806.
15. Hiroi Y, Fujiu K, Komatsu S, et al. Carvedilol therapy improved left ventricular function in a patient with arrhythmogenic right ventricular cardiomyopathy. Jpn Heart J 2004;45:169–77.
16. Naccarella F, Naccarelli G, Fattori R, et al. Arrhythmogenic right ventricular dysplasia/cardiomyopathy: current opinions on diagnostic and therapeutic aspects. Curr Opin Cardiol 2001;16:8–16.

17. Fontaine G, Prost-Squarcioni C. Implantable cardioverter defibrillator in arrhythmogenic right ventricular cardiomyopathies. Circulation 2004;109:1445–7.
18. Calkins H. Arrhythmogenic rightventricular dysplasia/cardiomyopathy. Curr Opin Cardiol 2006;21:55–63.
19. Boldt LH, Haverkamp W. Arrhythmogenic right ventricular cardiomyopathy: diagnosis and risk stratification. Herz 2009;34:290–7.
20. Basso C, Corrado D, Marcus FI, et al. Arrhythmogenic right ventricular cardiomyopathy. Lancet 2009;373:1289–300.

Electroanatomic Mapping and Catheter Ablation of Ventricular Tachycardia in Arrhythmogenic Cardiomyopathy

Haris M. Haqqani, MBBS (Hons), PhD[a,b],
Francis E. Marchlinski, MD[c,*]

KEYWORDS

- Arrhythmogenic right ventricular cardiomyopathy/dysplasia
- Catheter ablation • Electroanatomic mapping • Therapy
- Ventricular tachycardia

Catheter ablation for scar-related ventricular tachycardia (VT) in the postinfarction setting has become an established and effective therapy.[1] The fact that the pathologic and electrophysiologic substrate for VT is uniquely subendocardial in this setting and the development of surgical subendocardial resection as a treatment that could be emulated percutaneously contributed to the modern evolution of VT ablation in ischemic cardiomyopathy.[2] In other contexts, including nonischemic dilated cardiomyopathy and arrhythmogenic cardiomyopathy (AC), the substrate for VT has been more difficult to locate, define, and ablate. In AC, the only available surgical therapy, right ventricular (RV) disconnection, could not provide definitive information regarding the mechanism of VT in these patients, and the current understanding of this has been derived largely from studies in the electrophysiology laboratory.

This article discusses the substrate underlying monomorphic VT in AC and explores the current practice of catheter ablation of VT in this condition.

CHARACTERISTICS OF MONOMORPHIC VT IN AC

As in other cardiomyopathic processes, reentrant mechanisms underlie the overwhelming majority of VT in AC, although focal ventricular arrhythmias can occur early in the course of the disease.[3] Given that most AC-related VTs arise from the free wall of the RV, most VTs display a left bundle branch block (LBBB) configuration with poor R-wave progression in the precordial leads. However, it is possible for a left ventricular (LV) VT exit or for advanced structural RV disease that distorts normal ventricular geometry within the thorax to occasionally produce a right bundle branch block (RBBB) morphology. More often, an RBBB VT morphology can be created as a result of direct LV involvement with the disease process associated with basal LV substrate abnormalities and RBBB VTs with positive R waves across all or most of the precordial leads.

Dr Haqqani is supported by a Training Fellowship from the National Health and Medical Research Council of Australia (544309). Professor Marchlinski has received research funding from Biosense Webster.
[a] School of Medicine, The University of Queensland, Brisbane, QLD, Australia
[b] Department of Cardiology, The Prince Charles Hospital, 627 Rode Road, Brisbane, QLD 4032, Australia
[c] Cardiovascular Division, Department of Medicine, University of Pennsylvania Health System, 3400 Spruce Street, Founders 9, Philadelphia, PA 19104, USA
* Corresponding author.
E-mail address: francis.marchlinski@uphs.upenn.edu

Card Electrophysiol Clin 3 (2011) 299–310
doi:10.1016/j.ccep.2011.02.009
1877-9182/11/$ – see front matter

Monomorphic VT with an LBBB configuration generally has a late precordial transition after V_4 reflecting the frequent RV free wall origin, with spread of activation away from the anterior RV and precordial leads toward the posterior LV. RV septal VT exits typically display an earlier precordial transition. Given the usual attitude of the RV and its typical axis in the thoracic cavity, leads I and aVR are useful in identifying likely exit sites. Basal sites of origin are characterized by positive forces in lead I, and more apical sites, being closer to the left side, are isoelectric or negative in lead I. Inferior exit sites in the RV display a positive vector in lead aVR, usually with a superior axis. Close attention should also be paid to the QRS morphology during VT as demonstrated in the precordial lead V_2 and inferior leads. QS complexes in these respective leads strongly suggest an epicardial exit from the mid RV free wall or inferior RV wall, respectively.[4]

Other characteristics of VT in AC are its inducibility with programmed electrical stimulation, multiple morphologies including those with a superiorly directed frontal plane axis, potential termination with overdrive pacing, and ability to be entrained with manifest or concealed fusion. These features strongly suggest a reentrant mechanism and argue against a focal VT mechanism (eg, RV outflow tract VT) as seen in structurally normal hearts.[5,6]

ELECTROPHYSIOLOGIC AND ELECTROANATOMIC SUBSTRATE UNDERLYING VT IN AC

The common underlying factor in all cardiomyopathies, ventricular scarring, promotes reentry in at least 2 ways: first, by creating anatomic and functional barriers favoring the development of unidirectional conduction block and second, by altering cell-cell coupling, leading to slowed conduction. The cause, nature, and distribution of the scarring process is unique in AC, with genetically determined desmosomopathy leading to widespread myocyte death, confluent replacement of the lost myocardium with fibrofatty tissue, and a RV free wall preponderance of this process, progressing inwards from the epicardium.[7,8] However, the electrophysiological consequences are similar to other cardiomyopathic processes, with a generalized milieu of slow and discontinuous electrical propagation that predisposes to the development of often very large macro-reentrant VT circuits. The footprints of this abnormal substrate are well recognized and can be detected with catheter recordings of bipolar electrograms.

Electrical activation through normal RV myocardium was defined in patients with no structural heart disease with the use of the CARTO electroanatomic mapping system and the Navistar catheter (Biosense Webster, Diamond Bar, CA, USA), which has a 4-mm distal tip electrode, a 2-mm ring electrode, and a 1-mm interelectrode distance. Normal RV endocardium is characterized by bipolar signals displaying 3 or fewer deflections from baseline, with peak-to-peak amplitude greater than 1.5 mV,[9] whereas areas of bipolar voltage less than 0.5 mV correspond to dense scar.[10] The definition of normal epicardial electrogram parameters is confounded by the presence of epicardial fat, which may have an insulating effect and attenuate signal amplitude. However, it has been established when sampling signals more than 1 cm away from the defined large epicardial coronary vessels that more than 95% of bipolar electrograms overlying the RV have an amplitude of greater than 1.0 mV.[11] The precision of this determination is increased by incorporating electrogram morphology as well as voltage into consideration of the extent of the epicardial substrate.

Normal ventricular electrogram morphology, as well as having fewer than 4 deflections from baseline, is characterized by sharp intrinsic deflections corresponding to rapidly progressing activation wavefronts, with total duration less than 70 ms.[12] Electrical conduction through isolated surviving bundles of myocytes enmeshed within areas of dense fibrosis is slow and serpiginous, which is reflected in long-duration, low-amplitude fractionated potentials.[13] When these bundles form isolated regions deep within confluent scar areas, local activation can occur much later than it occurs in the surrounding areas, resulting in isolated potentials (IPs) being recorded after the far field potential following an intervening isoelectric line.[14] Given the large, confluent scars seen in patients with AC, these IPs can occur well into the T wave or beyond, in which case they are sometimes referred to as very late potentials (VLPs). The prevalence and distribution of these scar-related electrograms, in addition to the bipolar signal amplitude, are important in defining the abnormal electrical substrate in AC, especially on the epicardium. In some cases, networks of VLPs have been defined by sinus rhythm activation mapping (**Fig. 1**) that mark the location of putative conducting channels anatomically constrained by dense fibrosis.[15] These channels may form critical protected diastolic isthmuses during VT as has been demonstrated in the postinfarct context.[16] Ablation of VLPs at the entrance of these channels can result in disappearance of the entire network of channels when the scar is remapped, strongly suggesting that these potentials are all linked by common conducting fibers. The electroanatomic

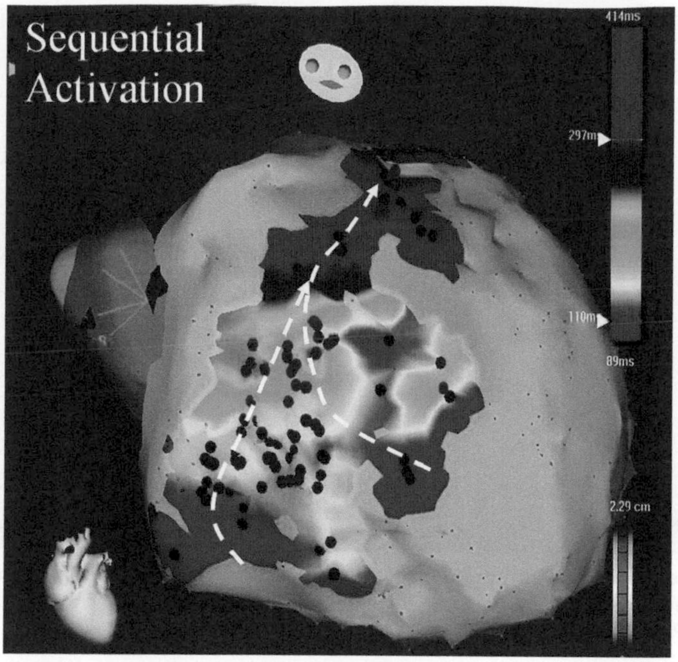

Fig. 1. Sequential pattern of isolated late potential activation in AC scar. Activation mapping of sinus rhythm epicardial isolated late potentials is shown. These networks of late potentials show patterns of linking such as those displayed here. The sequential pattern suggests that, when VT isthmuses sites are shown by entrainment to correspond to the sequential IP sites, the barriers of such VT circuits are largely anatomically determined by scar architecture. When IPs are arranged in such networks, significantly less ablation may need to be performed to eliminate them.

substrate defined as discussed has been shown to correspond to regions of myocardial loss and replacement with fibrofatty tissue.[17,18]

DISTRIBUTION OF ABNORMAL ELECTROANATOMIC SUBSTRATE

In keeping with the general pattern of perivalvular abnormalities seen in nonischemic cardiomyopathies,[19] the endocardial distribution of electroanatomic scar (confluent areas of bipolar low voltage <1.5 mV) in patients with VT in the setting of AC has been shown to extend from the tricuspid valve, the pulmonary valve, or from both over the RV free wall (**Fig. 2**).[20–23] The abnormal low voltage consistent with scar frequently extends to the septal aspects of the perivalvular regions but typically spares the apex.[20–23] The acute inferior angle of the RV, near its junction with the interventricular septum, is also characteristically included in this process. This substrate distribution has been shown to correspond to the location of VT circuits. The surface area of this region ranges from 12 to 130 cm^2 and corresponds to 34 $\pm$ 19% of the endocardial RV surface area,[20] although this value is highly variable among patients. In a significant minority of patients with AC presenting with VT, LV involvement is also seen (**Fig. 3**). When affected, the endocardium of the LV tends to display a confluent periannular area of low voltage and abnormal electrograms[20] reminiscent of the pattern seen in idiopathic nonischemic dilated cardiomyopathy.[10] Although systematic pathologic studies are not available, reports of explanted hearts studied after VT ablation in AC suggest a good correlation between fibrofatty replacement regions and abnormal areas on electroanatomic mapping.[17,20] These hearts also demonstrate that the endocardial aspect of the scarring process is often dense and confluent and displays a shoe-leather type consistency. Occasionally, there is even evidence of a regional increase in RV wall thickness along the basal aspect of the RV in proximity to the tricuspid valve, which can be identified on intracardiac echocardiographic imaging (**Fig. 4**) and endoepicardial voltage mapping (**Fig. 5**). This fact not only may decrease the likelihood of RV perforation during radiofrequency catheter ablation in these areas but also contributes to areas of surviving myocytes that participate in VT circuits being resistant to ablative therapy. It may also help explain the limited efficacy of isolated endocardial ablation alone for VT in AC.[24]

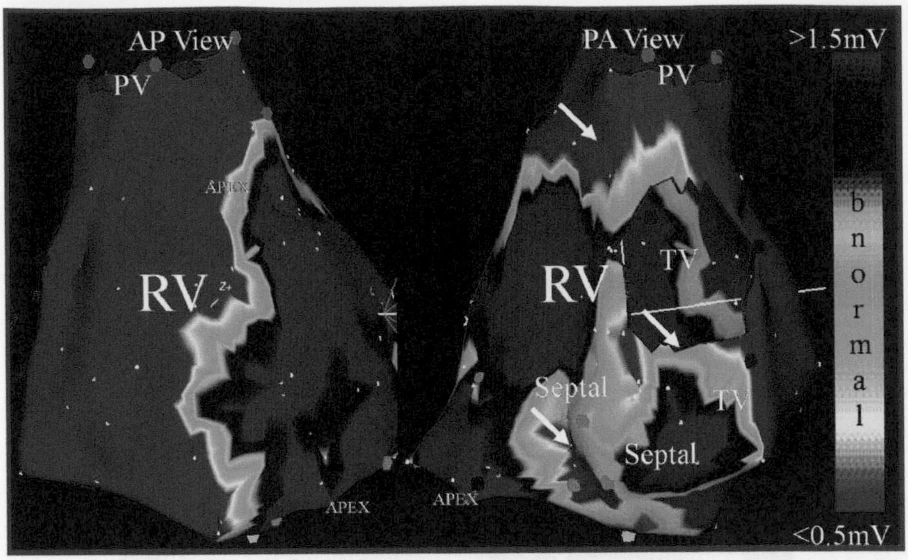

Fig. 2. Endocardial electroanatomic substrate in AC. Typical periannular distribution (*arrows*) of endocardial RV low-voltage substrate in AC with periannular involvement extending down the free wall and sparing the apex. AP, anteroposterior; PA, posteroanterior; PV, pulmonary valve; TV, tricuspid valve.

The realization in the electrophysiology laboratory of a concept long known to pathologists studying AC, namely, the beginning of the pathologic process in the epicardium and its progression inward, was a major advance in this area. By systematic percutaneous catheter mapping of the epicardium in patients with AC who had failed endocardial ablation, Garcia and colleagues[25] showed that most patients have a far more extensive electroanatomic substrate for VT here than they do on the RV endocardium (**Fig. 6**). Large confluent areas of low bipolar voltage were seen with fractionated, multicomponent, and isolated potentials dispersed throughout this zone. These findings are reflective of underlying fibrosis (rather than insulating epicardial fat) as the cause of the electrogram amplitude attenuation. On average, the area of this zone of epicardial abnormality was more than twice as large as the endocardial low-voltage substrate and displayed markedly

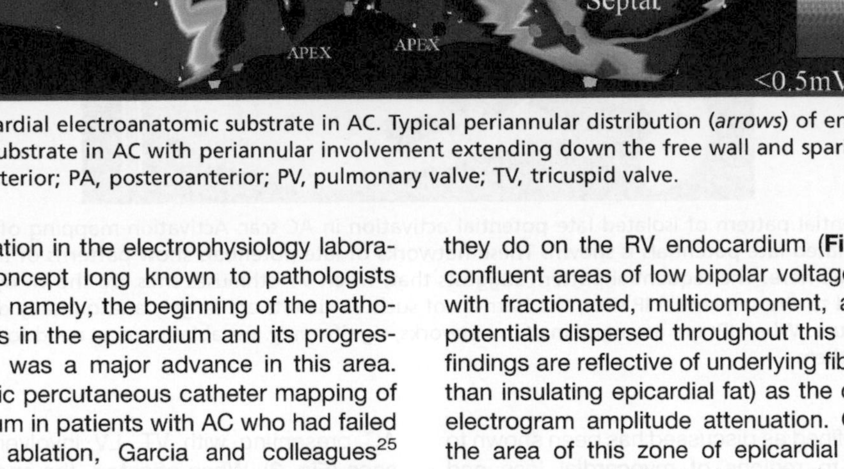

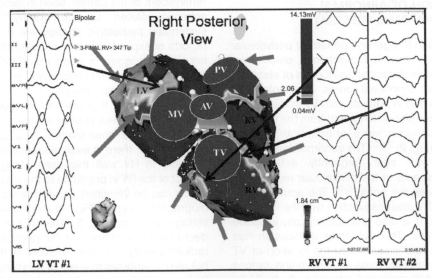

Fig. 3. Periannular RV and LV involvement in a patient with AC (*thick arrows*). When involved in AC, the LV tends to display a basal, periannular substrate distribution as shown here. In this patient, a RBBB morphology VT arose from this region, in addition to the typical LBBB morphologies exiting from the RV scar. AV, aortic valve; MV, mitral valve; PV, pulmonary valve; TV, tricuspid valve.

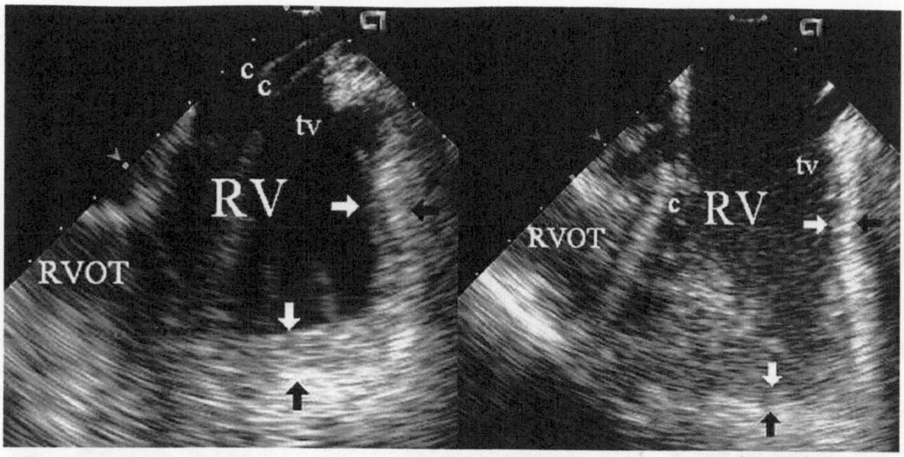

Fig. 4. Increase in RV wall thickness seen on intracardiac echocardiography (ICE). Structural changes in the RV can be seen with ICE in AC, particularly bright, echodense regions of increased wall thickness from fibrofatty infiltration. RVOT, right ventricular outflow tract.

abnormal conduction with dramatically late IPs and long stimulus to QRS times during pacing. Preliminary data suggest that it may be possible to identify patients with this more-marked epicardial VT substrate by examining the unipolar endocardial voltage maps, as unipolar electrogram amplitude, with its larger field of view, may be influenced by scar lying opposite to the endocardial recording surface (**Fig. 7**).[26]

Data have also now accumulated regarding the extent and distribution of the electroanatomic substrate in AC over time. Although the temporal progression of the disease process has long been considered inexorable and led to pessimistic views on the efficacy of catheter ablation, it is clear that this is not the case in many patients (**Fig. 8**). Riley and colleagues[27] have performed detailed serial electroanatomic mapping in 9 patients who

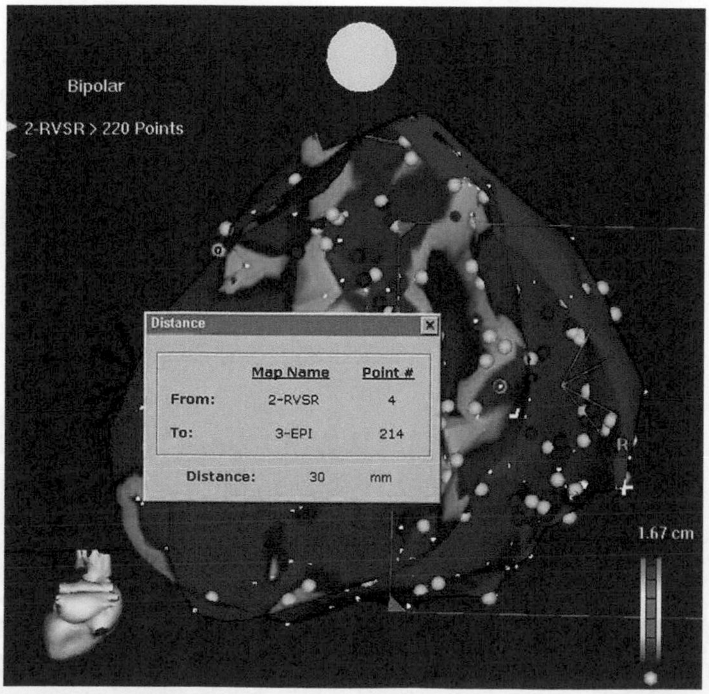

Fig. 5. Increase in RV wall thickness seen by measuring the distance between the endocardial and epicardial electroanatomic shells. These regions of longer distance between the endocardial and epicardial virtual geometries generally correspond to areas of increased wall thickness from dense scar, and hence they display confluent low-voltage substrate where mapping and ablation efforts are concentrated.

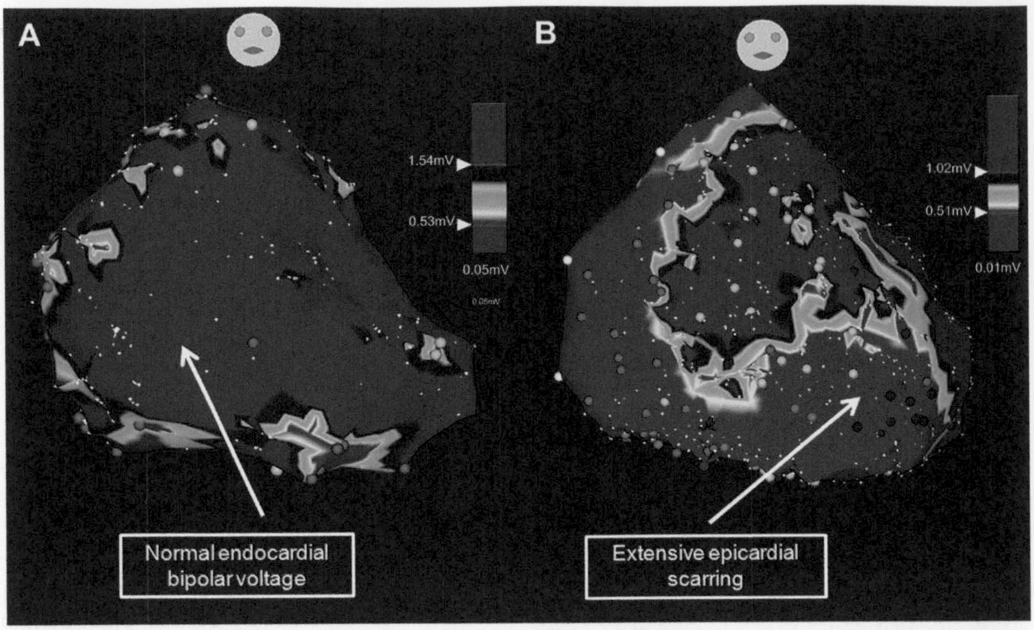

Fig. 6. Endocardial and epicardial VT substrate in AC. Electroanatomic substrate maps of a patient with AC and 8 inducible LBBB morphology VTs. Panel A displays the endocardial chamber geometry in the anteroposterior projection showing largely preserved endocardial voltages. The epicardial substrate map in panel B shows an extensive region of fractionated low-voltage potentials (bipolar peak-to-peak signal amplitude <1.0 mV as reflected in the different color scale) involving the inferior and mid RV free wall and extending from the perianular region to the apex. Seven of this patient's VTs were mapped and ablated successfully on the epicardium.

showed no change in their low-voltage, abnormal electrogram substrate over a mean of 5 years. This study suggests that aggressive efforts at VT control should not be abandoned based on an assumption that disease progression will inevitably lead to future VT recurrence.

CATHETER ABLATION: PREPROCEDURAL CONSIDERATIONS

Patients with AC-related VT represent a unique and challenging group for successful catheter ablation. Proper preparation is paramount and

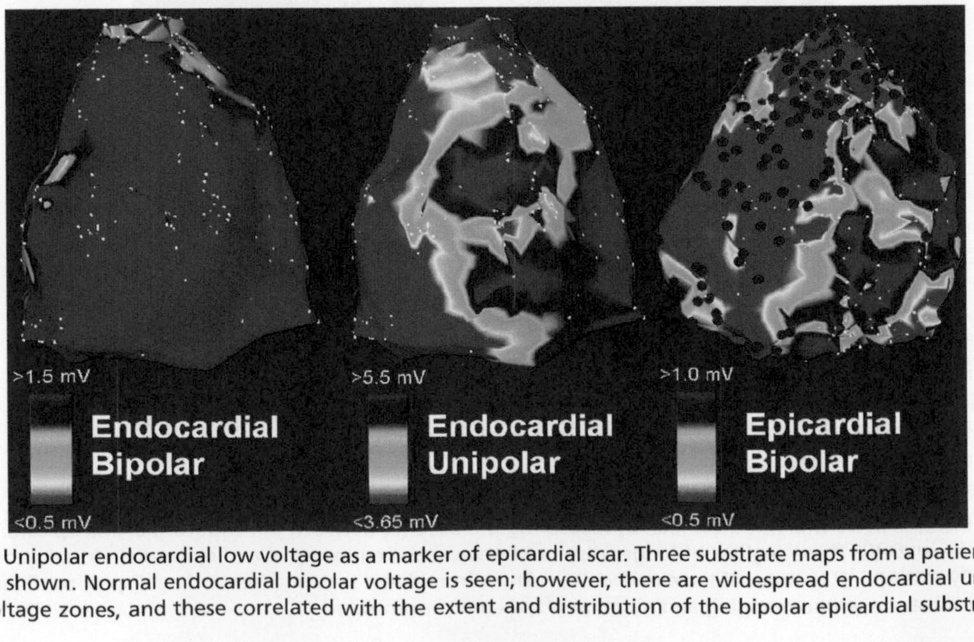

Fig. 7. Unipolar endocardial low voltage as a marker of epicardial scar. Three substrate maps from a patient with AC are shown. Normal endocardial bipolar voltage is seen; however, there are widespread endocardial unipolar low-voltage zones, and these correlated with the extent and distribution of the bipolar epicardial substrate.

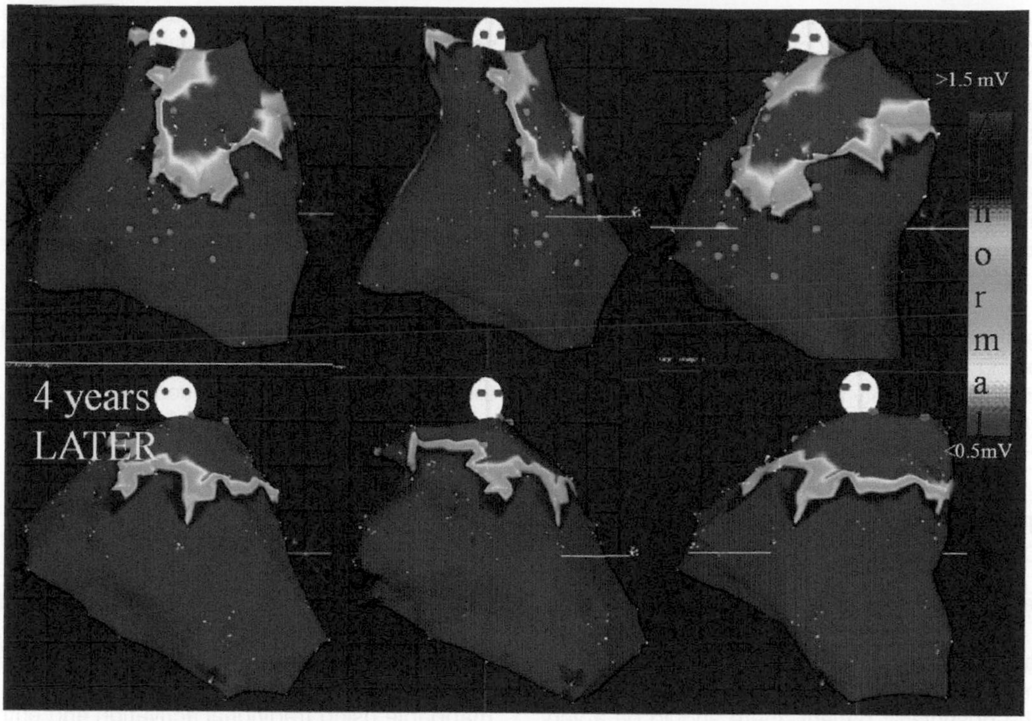

Fig. 8. Lack of progression of substrate in an patient with AC after 4 years. The endocardial substrate maps acquired 4 years apart in this patient show no significant progression in the size of the low-voltage zone.

must include, after clinical evaluation and optimization, a complete review of all VT morphologies, both surface 12-lead electrocardiogram morphologies and implantable cardioverter-defibrillator (ICD) stored electrograms. Apart from VT-related factors, there are several characteristics peculiar to these patients that considerably affect their preprocedural and intraoperative management and are worth pointing out. First, many patients presenting for catheter ablation have advanced structural RV disease with gross enlargement and severe hypokinesis, often with completely preserved LV function. In extreme cases, a Fontan-type, preload-sensitive circulatory physiology can eventuate, and periprocedural fasting and dehydration may combine with this to cause greater hemodynamic instability in VT and during sinus rhythm. Consequently, we routinely give generous intravenous fluid boluses before and during the procedure. The use of intra-aortic balloon counterpulsation has not been required in this group and is unlikely to improve hemodynamic tolerance of VT given their generally preserved LV function.

Second, a high systemic filling pressure and degree of venous stasis predispose patients to venous thromboembolism, and we routinely give low-dose heparin to help prevent this condition. Anticoagulation is completely reversed before pericardial access and reinstituted if no significant bleeding is evident in the process of gaining access. We have recently identified an association between thrombus formation on ICD leads and high pulmonary artery pressures,[28] suggestive of chronic thromboembolism potentially due to a heightened hypercoagulable state. There is concern that patients with AC commonly have elevated right-sided filling pressure and spontaneous echocardiographic contrast and may be particularly prone to right-sided lead-associated thrombotic complications related to ablation procedures or device therapy.

Third, severe anatomic distortions are often present in advanced cases of AC, and some form of periprocedural imaging can be helpful in planning access, virtual geometry creation, and substrate mapping, as well as with ablation lesion delivery. Delayed gadolinium enhancement on cardiac magnetic resonance imaging (MRI) identifies regions of scarring, where mapping efforts can be concentrated. It may also show deeper areas of intramural fibrosis when bipolar endocardial voltage maps are normal. Sagittal reconstructions are also used to ensure that there are no anatomic obstacles (such as severe RV dilation, large inferior RV aneurysms, or congestive hepatopathy) precluding safe pericardial access. In experienced hands, high-quality MRI images can be obtained with minimal artifact from ICD leads or generators, although this procedure is currently only performed in a few centers.

During ablation procedures, we routinely use intracardiac echocardiography (ICE) for real-time imaging, which assists with the definition of anatomy, manipulation of catheters, assessment of catheter contact, monitoring lesion formation, obtaining pericardial access, and online assessment for complications such as pericardial tamponade. The effort to maintain online imaging capabilities has been most important because periods of prolonged or severe hypotension during or immediately following arrhythmia induction or termination can lead to much anxiety that can be quickly assuaged by the appropriate imaging. Focused management of the hypotension can then ensue.

CATHETER ABLATION: TECHNICAL AND PROCEDURAL FACTORS

VT ablation procedures in the context of AC apply the same principles and strategy common to the ablation of all scar-related VTs. As is the situation with all nonischemic substrates, and in contrast to the postinfarct patient, there should be a very low threshold to obtain pericardial access and map the epicardium, which is particularly true when VT morphologies suggestive of epicardial exits have been positively identified or unipolar endocardial mapping suggests a more prominent epicardial substrate. The extensive epicardial substrate that is likely to exist in these patients can harbor the exits of multiple VT circuits that may become clinical in the future. The epicardium may also contain other VT circuit components such as entrance sites or midisthmus sites, even though these VTs may have an endocardial exit (see **Fig. 8**).

We generally begin these cases by acquiring a detailed endocardial electroanatomic substrate map, concentrating particularly on the periannular zones and low-voltage regions. Areas of fractionated and isolated potentials are tagged on the map, and pacing is performed from the mapping catheter to identify (1) pacemap matches of clinical VTs; (2) long stimulus-QRS sites with good pacemaps, including those showing IPs; and (3) an electrically unexcitable scar. Although an electrically unexcitable scar had been originally defined as failure of local capture with 10 mA at 2-ms pulse width,[29] more recent data suggest that capture thresholds in a dense scar may be much higher[30] and the sites that do not capture with 10 mA at 2 ms can often correspond to critical VT isthmuses. In the very large confluent scars seen in AC, unexcitable areas are defined as those with no capture at maximal stimulator output, as it is not uncommon to see sites with very high pacing thresholds deep within a dense scar. The insulating effect of large zones of dense scar prevents significant capture of the adjacent myocardium by the large virtual electrode seen at such outputs. When capture occurs at such sites, some remarkable scar physiology can be seen, including (1) extremely long stimulus to QRS intervals (>300 ms at times) and (2) extremely long and tortuous wavefront propagation within the scar before exit at remote scar borders. A characteristic example of this occurs in patients with AC and large inferior RV free wall substrate, in whom pacing at the floor of the RV, near the junction of the septum and the free wall, may still produce inferior axis QRS morphologies for VTs that use more superior RV outflow tract exits.

After substrate mapping is complete, we perform programmed ventricular stimulation and compare the surface and ICD electrogram morphology of all induced VTs with the clinical tachycardias, as well as to the pacemap morphologies acquired during substrate mapping. It is not uncommon to find many VT morphologies in patients with AC, and usually only a minority are mappable using traditional activation and entrainment mapping techniques. Any VTs that are mappable are then targeted from the endocardium in the conventional manner. As pointed out earlier, VT in AC is often caused by extremely large macroreentrant circuits and, unlike the postinfarct situation, not all circuit components may be found on the endocardium. However, any VTs that can be mapped, ablated, and terminated on the endocardium are dealt with at this stage, and their associated proven or putative arrhythmogenic machinery (including IPs, adjacent pacemap-guided exit sites, and the presumed critical VT isthmus locations) is ablated at the same time. Although in most patients endocardial ablation may be successful with the use of irrigated electrode radiofrequency energy delivery, it is a common scenario to have multiple, unmappable VTs with suboptimal endocardial pacemaps. Percutaneous epicardial access[31] is obtained early when confronted with this situation, as it is likely that an extensive epicardial substrate is found.[25] We prefer to use a posterior approach to pericardial puncture, as anatomic RV distortions in AC may increase the risks associated with an anterior needle pass. Detailed epicardial substrate mapping is then performed using a similar technique to the endocardium, with tagging of IPs and pacemapping to identify channels and potential exit sites. Close attention is also paid to sites of apparently greater separation of the endocardial and epicardial shells on the electroanatomic map, which suggest regions of increased wall thickness because of dense, confluent fibrosis, where the VT substrate may be more likely to reside.[25]

Programmed stimulation is repeated, and any stable VTs are then mapped with conventional techniques if possible. Coronary angiography is then performed to establish the proximity of the large epicardial vessels to candidate ablation sites. Of particular interest in these cases is the location of the RV marginal artery (or arteries), which usually runs diagonally down the mid–free wall of the RV, allowing for the possibility of ablating the epicardium overlying the acute inferior angle of the RV where VT exit sites and substrate are often located. Phrenic nerve proximity is not usually a consideration on the RV epicardium. Following coronary artery definition, radiofrequency energy can be delivered at candidate sites identified by entrainment mapping to terminate tolerated VT. For substrate ablation of unmappable VTs, an endocardial and epicardial lesion set is designed to incorporate as many target sites (as identified by pacemapping and electrogram morphology) within the low-voltage zone as possible, with the aim being to eliminate the critical components of all potential VT circuits. Linear lesions that cross through the entire endocardial low-voltage area, beginning at VT exit sites based on pacing at the border of the low-voltage area and terminating at the valve plane, are frequently used. On the epicardium, the tricuspid valve plane marks a region in proximity to the right coronary artery; thus, more extensive linear lesions are not used. Linear lesions, if deployed, are shorter and connect areas of pacing inexcitability and cross through good pacemap sites. More frequently, clusters of lesions target areas of late potentials, particularly those where pacing produces a long stimulus to QRS interval and a pacemap match of VT (**Fig. 9**).

For endocardial RV ablation in AC, we typically use an open-irrigated 3.5-mm electrode and commence radiofrequency applications at 30 W, with a 30-mL/min flow rate and a temperature limit of 45°C. We gradually titrate power to a 12- to 16-ohm impedance drop, depending on the starting impedance, and aim for 120-second applications. Catheter contact and lesion formation is monitored with the use of ICE,[32] and effective lesion creation is indexed by bipolar signal attenuation, increase in local pace-capture threshold, and importantly, by the loss of IPs or high-frequency late electrogram components (**Fig. 10**).[14] These end points for individual lesion delivery are often difficult to achieve in the presence of a thick RV scar, which exerts an insulating effect against radiofrequency current flow, even with irrigated-tip ablation electrodes. On the epicardium, we use similar biophysical parameters for lesion delivery, although usually with a lower irrigation flow rate (10–17 mL/min) and intermittent or continuous aspiration of fluid from the side arm of the pericardial introducer. As on the endocardium, epicardial fat and thick

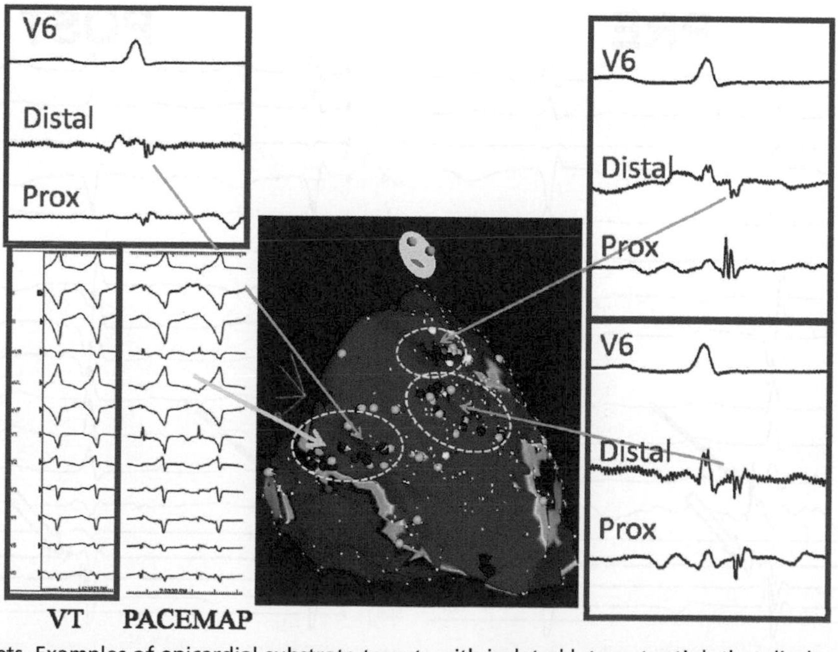

Fig. 9. IP targets. Examples of epicardial substrate targets with isolated late potentials that display slow conduction with good pacemap matches to induced VTs (*black arrow*) and attenuation of IP seen on an adjacent mapping catheter (*yellow arrow*).

fibrofatty replacement tissue can again hamper efforts to create transmural lesions.

All mappable VTs are targeted, and substrate-based ablation of all unmappable morphologies is also performed. Although a work in progress, aggressive attempts at scar homogenization on both the endocardial and epicardial aspects of the RV has become the goal. Certainly, all regions of low bipolar voltage scar associated with spontaneous or induced VT morphologies are targeted. Isolated and VLPs are comprehensively identified and targeted, particularly those clumped together in apparent networks and those displaying long stimulus to QRS times and good morphology matches while pacing. If VT with a RBBB morphology is identified, then attention is placed on the perivalvular regions of the LV.

Notwithstanding the complete elimination of IPs as an important, although sometimes difficult to achieve, aim,[14] the main procedural end point in these cases is VT noninducibility with aggressive programmed stimulation using 2 drive cycle lengths, 2 sites, and triple extrastimuli to refractoriness. Noninvasive programmed stimulation via the ICD is performed 1 to 2 days later to ensure ongoing noninducibility of all VT morphologies.

CATHETER ABLATION OF VT: OUTCOMES

The results of catheter ablation of AC-related VT have varied considerably in the single-center studies reported. Different procedural strategies and mapping techniques with variable follow-up durations and antiarrhythmic drug use account for most of the variability.[20–24,33–35] These studies trace the evolution of this challenging procedure over the last decade and more. Much has been discovered about VT substrate and mechanisms in AC over this time, and this knowledge has been appropriately reflected in changing procedural paradigms. The current strategy of abolishing all inducible VT combined with aggressive endocardial and epicardial substrate modification represents the most complete procedure yet offered to these often very sick patients. In our experience with 35 consecutive patients undergoing AC-related VT ablation, acute procedural success, in which all targeted VT was successfully ablated, was achieved in 34. The 1 patient who had failed ablation with clinical VT still inducible at the end of the case, had end-stage structural RV disease, with an endocardial RV volume of 470 mL and LV ejection fraction of 10% to 15%. For the remaining 34 patients, after a mean follow-up of 36 months from the last of what in most patients included repeat procedures, 25 of 34 patients (74%) had no further VT episodes. Seven of the remaining 9 patients had only isolated episodes, with no VT storm seen. This excellent clinical outcome in 32 of 34 patients (94%) occurred despite cessation of antiarrhythmic drugs in the majority. Nineteen patients were on

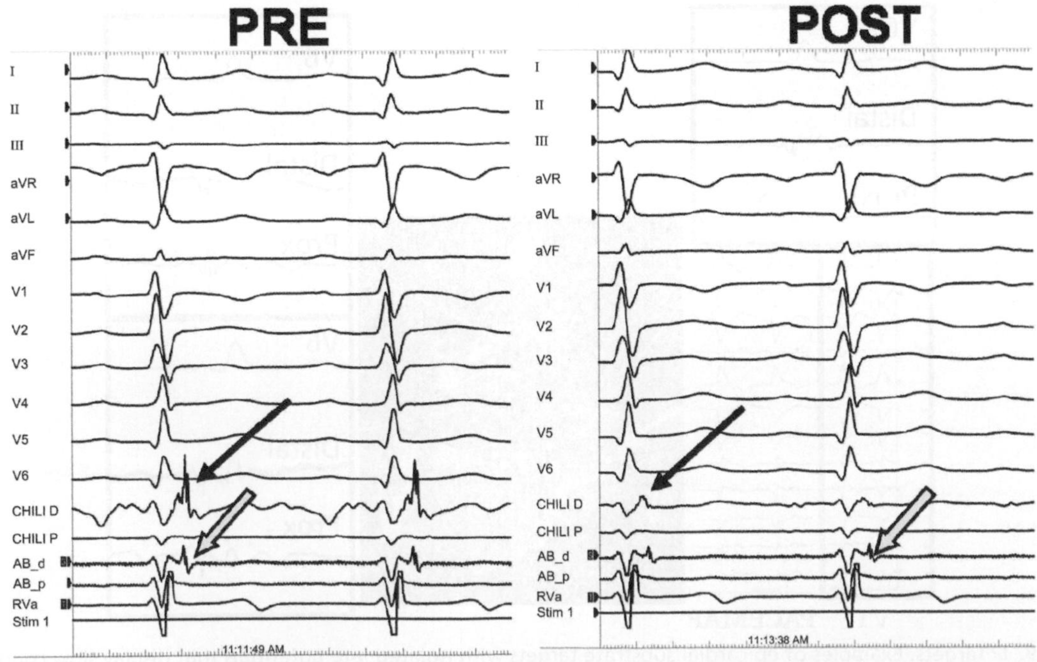

Fig. 10. Loss of IPs with radiofrequency ablation. Ideal end point of point lesion delivery, with loss of the isolated late component of the local electrogram (*black arrow*) and attenuation of IP seen on an adjacent mapping catheter (*yellow arrow*).

no antiarrhythmic drugs, and only 1 patient was still on amiodarone out of 13 patients who were initially taking this drug. These results also need to be interpreted in light of the clinical condition of these patients before being referred for catheter ablation. Most had frequent ICD shocks or VT storm, and antiarrhythmic drug intolerance was common. Some were being actively worked up for cardiac transplant for refractory VT, which was subsequently averted with successful arrhythmia control.

Despite the extensive mapping and ablation performed in this patient population, complication rates have been extremely low. There were no deaths, strokes, cardiac perforation/tamponade, or serious complications associated with gaining epicardial access, mapping, and ablation. One patient experienced a deep vein thrombosis and documented pulmonary embolism as evidenced by a ventilation/perfusion scan after the procedure.

SUMMARY

VT in AC is a difficult clinical problem to manage, with often ineffective or nontolerated antiarrhythmic drugs being the only medical defense again ICD shocks or arrhythmic storm. The understanding of the substrate and mechanisms underlying VT in this context has progressed enormously in the last decade, largely because of human studies in the electrophysiology laboratory using electroanatomic mapping. These data have informed us greatly about the central role of RV scarring in this disease and the characteristics and distribution of this arrhythmogenic substrate, particularly its extensive involvement of the epicardium. This understanding has guided the evolution of catheter ablation from a last-ditch palliative procedure in patients with end-stage AC and near incessant VT, frequent ICD shocks, and multiple antiarrhythmic drug side effects to becoming a real early option for VT management with the realistic prospect of achieving long-term drug-free arrhythmia control.

REFERENCES

1. Stevenson WG, Wilber DJ, Natale A, et al. Irrigated radiofrequency catheter ablation guided by electroanatomic mapping for recurrent ventricular tachycardia after myocardial infarction: the Multicenter Thermocool Ventricular Tachycardia Ablation Trial. Circulation 2008;118:2773–82.
2. Haqqani HM, Marchlinski FE. Electrophysiologic substrate underlying postinfarction ventricular tachycardia: characterization and role in catheter ablation. Heart Rhythm 2009;6(8 Suppl):S70–6.
3. Leclercq JF, Potenza S, Maison-Blanche P, et al. Determinants of spontaneous occurrence of sustained monomorphic ventricular tachycardia in right ventricular dysplasia. J Am Coll Cardiol 1996;28:720–4.
4. Bazan V, Bala R, Garcia FC, et al. Twelve-lead ECG features to identify ventricular tachycardia arising from the epicardial right ventricle. Heart Rhythm 2006;3:1132–9.
5. O'Donnell D, Cox D, Bourke J, et al. Clinical and electrophysiological differences between patients with arrhythmogenic right ventricular dysplasia and right ventricular outflow tract tachycardia. Eur Heart J 2003;24:801–10.
6. Joshi S, Wilber DJ. Ablation of idiopathic right ventricular outflow tract tachycardia: current perspectives. J Cardiovasc Electrophysiol 2005; 16(Suppl 1):S52–8.
7. Basso C, Thiene G, Corrado D, et al. Arrhythmogenic right ventricular cardiomyopathy. Dysplasia, dystrophy, or myocarditis? Circulation 1996;94:983–91.
8. Corrado D, Basso C, Thiene G, et al. Spectrum of clinicopathologic manifestations of arrhythmogenic right ventricular cardiomyopathy/dysplasia: a multicenter study. J Am Coll Cardiol 1997;30:1512–20.
9. Marchlinski FE, Callans DJ, Gottlieb CD, et al. Linear ablation lesions for control of unmappable ventricular tachycardia in patients with ischemic and nonischemic cardiomyopathy. Circulation 2000;101:1288–96.
10. Hsia HH, Callans DJ, Marchlinski FE. Characterization of endocardial electrophysiological substrate in patients with nonischemic cardiomyopathy and monomorphic ventricular tachycardia. Circulation 2003;108:704–10.
11. Cano O, Hutchinson M, Lin D, et al. Electroanatomic substrate and ablation outcome for suspected epicardial ventricular tachycardia in left ventricular nonischemic cardiomyopathy. J Am Coll Cardiol 2009;54:799–808.
12. Cassidy DM, Vassallo JA, Buxton AE, et al. The value of catheter mapping during sinus rhythm to localize site of origin of ventricular tachycardia. Circulation 1984;69:1103–10.
13. de Bakker JM, van Capelle FJ, Janse MJ, et al. Fractionated electrograms in dilated cardiomyopathy: origin and relation to abnormal conduction. J Am Coll Cardiol 1996;27:1071–8.
14. Nogami A, Sugiyasu A, Tada H, et al. Changes in the isolated delayed component as an endpoint of catheter ablation in arrhythmogenic right ventricular cardiomyopathy: predictor for long-term success. J Cardiovasc Electrophysiol 2008;19:681–8.
15. Lavi N, Marchlinski F. Epicardial late potentials propagation in patients with RVCM: is there a relationship or random occurrence? Heart Rhythm 2009;6:S416.
16. Arenal A, del Castillo S, Gonzalez-Torrecilla E, et al. Tachycardia-related channel in the scar tissue in patients with sustained monomorphic ventricular

tachycardias: influence of the voltage scar definition. Circulation 2004;110:2568–74.

17. Corrado D, Basso C, Leoni L, et al. Three-dimensional electroanatomic voltage mapping increases accuracy of diagnosing arrhythmogenic right ventricular cardiomyopathy/dysplasia. Circulation 2005;111:3042–50.
18. Avella A, d'Amati G, Pappalardo A, et al. Diagnostic value of endomyocardial biopsy guided by electroanatomic voltage mapping in arrhythmogenic right ventricular cardiomyopathy/dysplasia. J Cardiovasc Electrophysiol 2008;19:1127–34.
19. Marchlinski FE. Perivalvular fibrosis and monomorphic ventricular tachycardia: toward a unifying hypothesis in nonischemic cardiomyopathy. Circulation 2007;116:1998–2001.
20. Marchlinski FE, Zado E, Dixit S, et al. Electroanatomic substrate and outcome of catheter ablative therapy for ventricular tachycardia in setting of right ventricular cardiomyopathy. Circulation 2004;110:2293–8.
21. Miljoen H, State S, de Chillou C, et al. Electroanatomic mapping characteristics of ventricular tachycardia in patients with arrhythmogenic right ventricular cardiomyopathy/dysplasia. Europace 2005;7:516–24.
22. Verma A, Kilicaslan F, Schweikert RA, et al. Short- and long-term success of substrate-based mapping and ablation of ventricular tachycardia in arrhythmogenic right ventricular dysplasia. Circulation 2005; 111:3209–16.
23. Satomi K, Kurita T, Suyama K, et al. Catheter ablation of stable and unstable ventricular tachycardias in patients with arrhythmogenic right ventricular dysplasia. J Cardiovasc Electrophysiol 2006;17: 469–76.
24. Dalal D, Jain R, Tandri H, et al. Long-term efficacy of catheter ablation of ventricular tachycardia in patients with arrhythmogenic right ventricular dysplasia/cardiomyopathy. J Am Coll Cardiol 2007; 50:432–40.
25. Garcia FC, Bazan V, Zado ES, et al. Epicardial substrate and outcome with epicardial ablation of ventricular tachycardia in arrhythmogenic right ventricular cardiomyopathy/dysplasia. Circulation 2009;120:366–75.
26. Polin G, Hutchinson MD, Garcia FC, et al. Endocardial unipolar voltage mapping more accurately predicts epicardial scar than endocardial bipolar mapping in an ARVD population. Heart Rhythm 2009;6:S118.
27. Riley MP, Zado ES, Hutchinson MD, et al. Lack of uniform progression of endocardial scar in patients with arrhythmogenic right ventricular dysplasia/cardiomyopathy and ventricular tachycardia. Heart Rhythm 2008;5:S74.
28. Supple G, Ren JF, Zado ES, et al. Mobile thrombus on implantable defibrillator and pacemaker leads is associated with increased pulmonary artery pressure [abstract]. Heart Rhythm 2010;7(5S):S312.
29. Soejima K, Stevenson WG, Maisel WH, et al. Electrically unexcitable scar mapping based on pacing threshold for identification of the reentry circuit isthmus: feasibility for guiding ventricular tachycardia ablation. Circulation 2002;106:1678–83.
30. Sarrazin JF, Kuehne M, Wells D, et al. High-output pacing in mapping of postinfarction ventricular tachycardia. Heart Rhythm 2008;5:1709–14.
31. Sosa E, Scanavacca M, d'Avila A, et al. A new technique to perform epicardial mapping in the electrophysiology laboratory. J Cardiovasc Electrophysiol 1996;7:531–6.
32. Ren JF, Callans DJ, Schwartzman D, et al. Changes in local wall thickness correlate with pathologic lesion size following radiofrequency catheter ablation: an intracardiac echocardiographic imaging study. Echocardiography 2001;18:503–7.
33. Ellison KE, Friedman PL, Ganz LI, et al. Entrainment mapping and radiofrequency catheter ablation of ventricular tachycardia in right ventricular dysplasia. J Am Coll Cardiol 1998;32:724–8.
34. Reithmann C, Hahnefeld A, Remp T, et al. Electroanatomic mapping of endocardial right ventricular activation as a guide for catheter ablation in patients with arrhythmogenic right ventricular dysplasia. Pacing Clin Electrophysiol 2003;26: 1308–16.
35. Zou J, Cao K, Yang B, et al. Dynamic substrate mapping and ablation of ventricular tachycardias in right ventricular dysplasia. J Interv Card Electrophysiol 2004;11:37–45.

Implantable Cardioverter Defibrillator in Arrhythmogenic Cardiomyopathy

Domenico Corrado, MD, PhD[a,*], Maria Silvano, MD[a], Federico Migliore, MD[a], Alessio Marinelli, MD[a], Loira Leoni, MD, PhD[a], Gaetano Thiene, MD[b], Sabino Iliceto, MD[a], Gianfranco Buja, MD[a]

KEYWORDS

- Implantable cardioverter defibrillator
- Arrhythmogenic right ventricular cardiomyopathy/dysplasia
- Sudden cardiac death • Therapy Ventricular fibrillation

There is definitive clinical evidence that the implantable defibrillator (ICD) is the most effective therapy for both primary and secondary prevention of sudden cardiac death (SCD) in patients with coronary artery disease.[1–3] However, there are few available data on efficacy and safety of such a treatment in patients with nonischemic cardiomyopathies, mostly because of the relatively low disease prevalence and the relatively low event rate in affected patients. Arrhythmogenic cardiomyopathy (AC) has become an emerging indication for ICD implantation because its natural history is more strongly related to ventricular electrical instability, which can precipitate SCD mostly in young people, whereas heart failure is uncommon and occurs later during the disease course as a result of right ventricular (RV) disease progression and left ventricular (LV) involvement.[4–10] In the past, indications for ICD implantation in AC were empiric and based widely on the experience gained by different centers using analogies with coronary artery disease.[8] Because clinical variables predicting clinical outcome were undetermined, there was a tendency to implant an ICD once the disease was diagnosed, regardless of risk stratification. Although ICD confers optimal protection against SCD, economic costs, quality of life concerns including psychological repercussions, risk for inappropriate shocks, and device-related complications argue strongly against indiscriminate device implantation.

In this article the authors review the studies that have become available in the last decade on the efficacy and safety of ICD therapy in patients with AC (**Table 1**). Particular reference is reserved for DARVIN (*D*efibrillator in *A*rrhythmogenic *R*ight *V*entricular Cardiomyopathy *In*ternational Study) studies,[11,12] which have addressed the clinical impact of ICD therapy in changing the natural history of AC in a large patient population treated for both secondary and primary prevention of SCD.

DARVIN STUDIES

The DARVIN studies I and II were observational, multicenter investigations aimed to determine the efficacy and safety of ICD therapy in a large patient population with AC at high risk for SCD.[11,12]

[a] Division of Cardiology, Department of Cardiac, Thoracic and Vascular Sciences, University of Padua Medical School, Via Giustiniani, 2-35121, Padua, Italy
[b] Cardiovascular Pathology, Department of Medical-Diagnostic Sciences and Special Therapies, University of Padua Medical School, Via A. Gabelli, 35121 Padua, Italy
* Corresponding author.
E-mail address: domenico.corrado@unipd.it

Card Electrophysiol Clin 3 (2011) 311–321
doi:10.1016/j.ccep.2011.02.003

Table 1
Studies on the efficacy and safety of ICD therapy in patients with AC

Study	Year	Patients (N)	Study Design	Men (%)	Follow-Up (months)	Primary Prevention (%)	Mortality Overall (%)	Appropriate ICD Therapy (%)	Life-Saving ICD Therapy (%)	Complications (%)
Breithardt et al[19]	1994	18	SC	72	17 ± 11	0	0	59	NR	NR
Link et al[20]	1997	12	SC	58	22 ± 13	0	8	67	50	33
Tavernier et al[21]	2001	9	SC	89	32 ± 24	0	0	78	44	NR
Corrado et al[11]	2003	132	MC	70	39 ± 25	22	3	48	24	14
Wichter et al[22]	2004	60	SC	82	80 ± 43	7	13	68	40	45
Roguin et al[23]	2004	42	MC	52	42 ± 26	40	2	78	NR	14
Hodgkinson et al[24]	2005	48	MC	63	31	73	0	70	30	6
Corrado et al[12]	2010	106	MC	58	58 ± 35	100	0	24	16	14

Abbreviations: MC, multicenter; NR, data not recorded; SC, single-center.

In both studies the survival benefit of the ICD was evaluated by comparing the actual patient survival rate with projected freedom of ventricular fibrillation/flutter (VF/Vfl) (**Fig. 1**). These arrhythmias were used as surrogate for aborted SCD, based on the assumption that in all likelihood they would have been fatal without termination by the device. The end point was reached by device interrogation and review of intracardiac stored electrocardiograms (ECGs) regarding ICD interventions in response to VF/Vfl during follow-up.

DARVIN I

The DARVIN I study population consisted of 132 AC patients (93 males, 39 females; mean age 40 ± 15 years) who were recruited at 22 institutions in North Italy and at one in the United States.[11] Most of the patients (~80%) received an ICD implant because of a history of either cardiac arrest or sustained ventricular tachycardia ("secondary prevention"). During a mean follow-up of 39 ± 25 months, there were 3 deaths: one sudden, one due to infective endocarditis, and one due to congestive heart failure. Over the study period, 48% of patients (64 of 132) had at least one appropriate ICD intervention, 12% had inappropriate interventions, and 16% had ICD-related complications. Fifty-three of the 64 patients (83%) were receiving antiarrhythmic drugs at the time of the first appropriate discharges, mostly consisting of sotalol and β-blockers (alone or in association with amiodarone). The analysis of intracardiac ECG data stored by the ICD showed that 32 of 132 patients (24%) experienced VF/Vfl that in all likelihood would have been fatal in the absence of the device. The VF/Vfl-free survival rate was 72% at 36 months compared with the actual patient survival of 98% (**Fig. 2**A). Younger age, a history of cardiac arrest or hemodynamically unstable ventricular tachycardia, and LV involvement were independent clinical predictors of VF/Vfl. It is noteworthy that the ICD therapy did not improve survival in those patients implanted because of hemodynamically stable ventricular tachycardia, who had a significantly lower incidence of VF/Vfl over the follow-up (**Fig. 2**B).

Programmed ventricular stimulation (PVS) was not helpful in risk assessment of patients. More than 50% of inducible patients did not experience ICD therapy, while a similar proportion of noninducible patients had appropriate intervention during the 3.3-year follow-up period. This finding is in agreement with the limitation of electrophysiological study for arrhythmic risk stratification of other nonischemic heart diseases such as hypertrophic and dilated cardiomyopathy.[13]

Precise data on the efficacy of ICD in comparison with antiarrhythmic therapy could not be derived from this nonrandomized study. However,

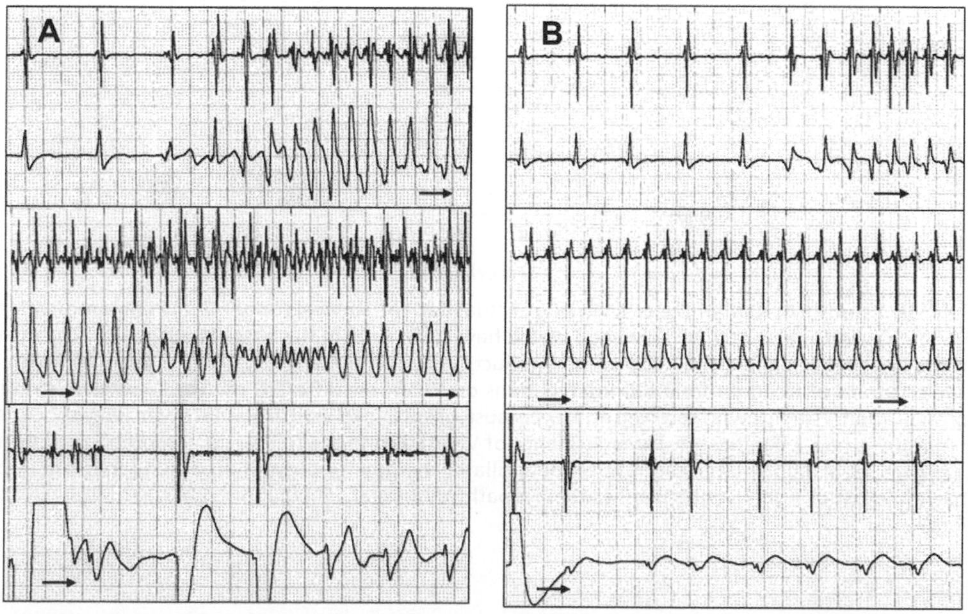

Fig. 1. Stored intracardiac ventricular electrocardiogram from AC patients who received ICD therapy. (*A*) Spontaneous onset of ventricular fibrillation is automatically terminated by a defibrillation shock, which immediately restores sinus rhythm. (*B*) Ventricular flutter at a ventricular rate of 280 beats/min, which begins abruptly after 5 beats of sinus rhythm. The ICD discharges appropriately and restores sinus rhythm. Arrows indicate tracings are continuous.

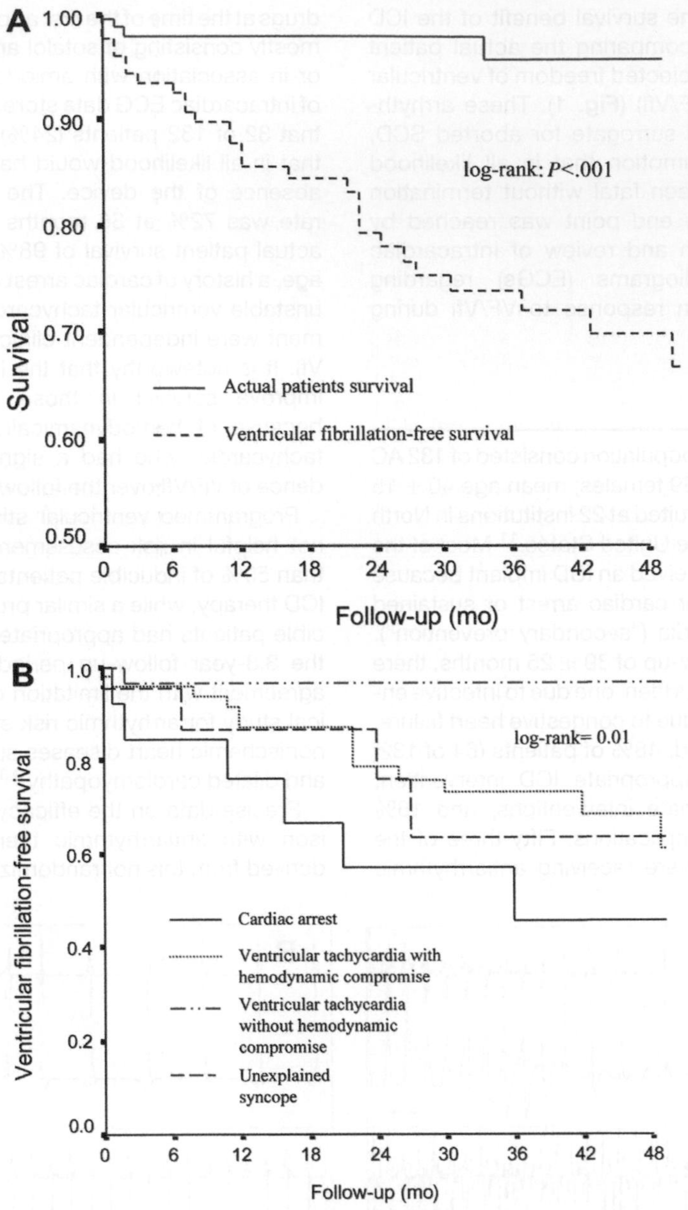

Fig. 2. DARVIN I study. (*A*) Kaplan-Meier analysis of actual patient survival (*upper line*) compared with survival free of VF/Vfl (*dashed line*) that in all likelihood would have been fatal in the absence of the ICD. The divergence between the lines reflects the estimated mortality reduction by ICD therapy of 24% at 3 years of follow-up. (*B*) Kaplan-Meier curves of freedom from ICD interventions on VF/Vfl for different patient subgroups stratified for clinical presentation. Patients who received an ICD because of sustained ventricular tachycardia without hemodynamic compromise had a significantly lower incidence of VF/Vfl during the follow-up. (*Modified from* Corrado D, Leoni L, Link MS, et al. Implantable cardioverter defibrillator therapy for prevention of sudden death in patients with arrhythmogenic right ventricular cardiomyopathy/dysplasia. Circulation 2003;108:3087, 3088; with permission.)

the majority of appropriate interventions and 53% of shocks on VF/Vfl occurred despite concomitant antiarrhythmic therapy with β-blockers and/or class III antiarrhythmic drugs. This finding highlights that the protection provided by ICD against SCD may be considerably superior. However, DARVIN I study included high-risk AC patients, not comparable with most patients with the disease who can be either not treated or treated effectively with antiarrhythmic drugs because of the low arrhythmic risk.[14–16]

DARVIN II

This international multicenter study included 106 consecutive patients (62 men and 44 women; mean age 35.6 ± 18 years), with AC and no prior VF or sustained ventricular tachycardia (VT), who received a prophylactic ICD because of one or more arrhythmic risk factors such as syncope, asymptomatic nonsustained VT, familial sudden death, and inducibility at PVS.[12] During a mean follow-up of 58 ± 35 months (4.8 years) after ICD implantation, no death occurred. Of the 106 study patients, 25 (24%) had appropriate ICD interventions, 20 (19%) had inappropriate ICD interventions, and 18 (17%) had device-related complications. In 17 of 25 patients, the arrhythmia triggering ICD discharge was VF/Vfl that may have been fatal without termination by the device. The annual rate of potentially "life-saving" shocks against VF/Vfl was 3%. At 48 months, the actual patient survival rate was 100% compared with the VF/Vfl-free survival rate of 77%. The Kaplan-Meier analysis of the incidence of ICD interventions that were triggered by VF/Vfl suggested a significant improvement in survival through the follow-up period, with an actual total patient survival rate of 100% compared with a 77% Vf/Vfl survival rate at 48 months, and an estimated benefit of ICD implantation of 23% (**Fig. 3**). The strongest predictor of an increased arrhythmic risk in the DARVIN II study population was a history of syncope. Syncope was the only independent predictor of any appropriate ICD interventions (hazard ratio [HR] = 2.94) and shock therapy on VF/Vfl (HR = 3.16) (**Fig. 4**). Patients with prior syncope had a fourfold risk for subsequent episodes of potentially fatal VF/Vfl (annual rate = 9%). Asymptomatic patients with nonsustained VT presented a trend toward an increased arrhythmic risk. These patients had an overall rate of appropriate ICD intervention of 3.7% per year and a rate of appropriate ICD intervention against VF/Vfl of 1.48% per year. Asymptomatic AC patients who received an ICD because of a family history of sudden death did not experience any appropriate ICD interventions over the follow-up. This finding is in agreement with those of previous studies showing that the majority of affected AC relatives are likely to have a benign course and that a sizable proportion of healthy gene carriers will not develop clinically significant disease owing to reduced disease penetrance.[17,18] As in the DARVIN I study, programmed ventricular stimulation had limited accuracy in predicting appropriate ICD interventions. In the DARVIN II study the positive predictive value of PVS was 30% for any appropriate ICD interventions and 35% for potentially life-saving shock against VF/Vfl. On the other hand, a negative PVS did not indicate better prognosis because approximately one-third of noninducible patients experienced appropriate ICD interventions, and approximately one-fourth experienced shock on potentially lethal arrhythmic events.

OTHER STUDIES

The first studies aimed at defining the clinical results of ICD implantation were conducted on small cohorts of AC patients.[19–21]

In 1994 Breithardt and colleagues[19] reported 18 patients with AC who received an ICD because of drug refractory VT or VF, or previous cardiac arrest without reproducible induction of VT or VF. Only the initial patient received an epicardial lead system, whereas in the subsequent 17 patients a transvenous approach was used. Among these patients, 12 received a transvenous subcutaneous system and the remaining 5 received a purely transvenous lead system. Thirteen of the devices implanted had antitachycardia pacing capabilities. Although there were no serious perioperative complications, a major problem was the placement of the transvenous lead, which required testing of 2 or more positions (range, 2–9; median, 4) in 10 of 17 patients (59%) to achieve satisfactory sensing and pacing results. During a follow-up of 17 ± 11 months, 9 of the 18 patients (50%) experienced a total of 130 episodes of appropriate ICD therapies that ranged from 1 to 40 episodes per patient (median, 11 episodes). Because of the high rate of the tachycardia or the inability of the device to perform antitachycardia pacing, 59 of these 130 episodes (45%) were terminated by shock therapy, whereas the remaining 71 episodes (55%) were effectively terminated by antitachycardia pacing.

Link and colleagues[20] reported on 12 patients with AC who were treated with ICD. The mean age was 31 ± 9 years (range, 15–48). Patients presented with presyncope syncope, or cardiac arrest (five, four and three, respectively). During programmed electrical stimulation 9 patients had sustained VT while 3 had no inducible arrhythmia. Transvenous leads were placed in 9 patients. In these patients pacing thresholds were significantly higher, R-wave amplitudes were significantly lower, and defibrillation thresholds were not significantly different from those in a cohort of patients without AC. There were no acute or chronic

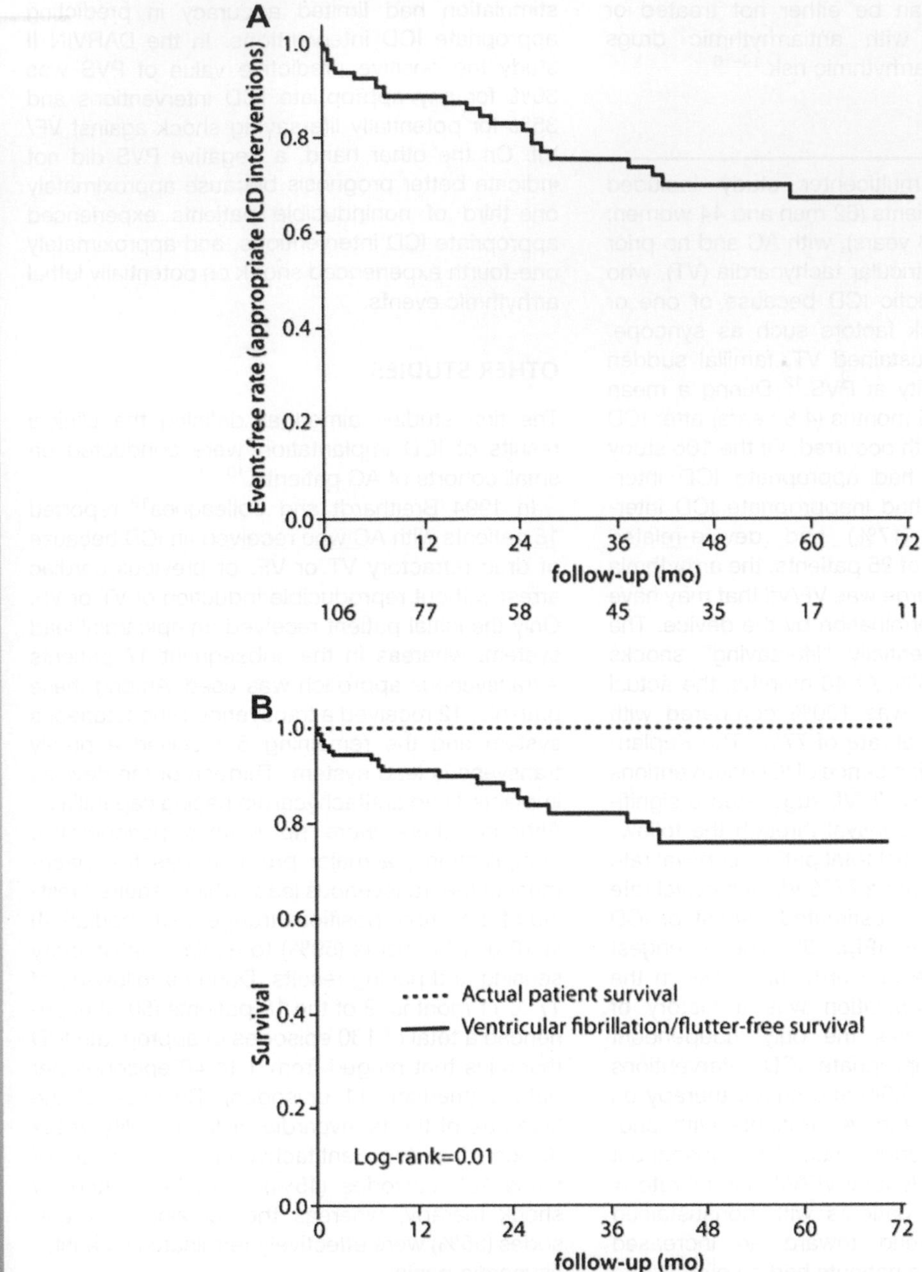

Fig. 3. DARVIN II study. (*A*) Kaplan-Meier analysis of cumulative survival from any appropriate ICD interventions. (*B*) Kaplan-Meier analysis of survival free of VF/Vfl compared with actual patient survival. The estimated mortality reduction at 48 months of follow-up is 23% (ie, the difference between the actual patient survival rate of 100% and VF/Vfl-free survival rate of 77%). (*Modified from* Corrado D, Calkins H, Link MS, et al. Prophylactic implantable defibrillator in patients with arrhythmogenic right ventricular cardiomyopathy/dysplasia and no prior ventricular fibrillation or sustained ventricular tachycardia. Circulation 2010;122:1147; with permission.)

complications of RV lead placement. Follow-up averaged 22 ± 13 months (range, 1–45). There was one sudden death at 1 month of follow-up. Of the 12 patients, 8 have had appropriate therapy delivered by the ICD. Six patients received sotalol to reduce the frequency of ICD discharges.

Tavernier and colleagues[21] described 9 consecutive patients (8 male and 1 female; mean age

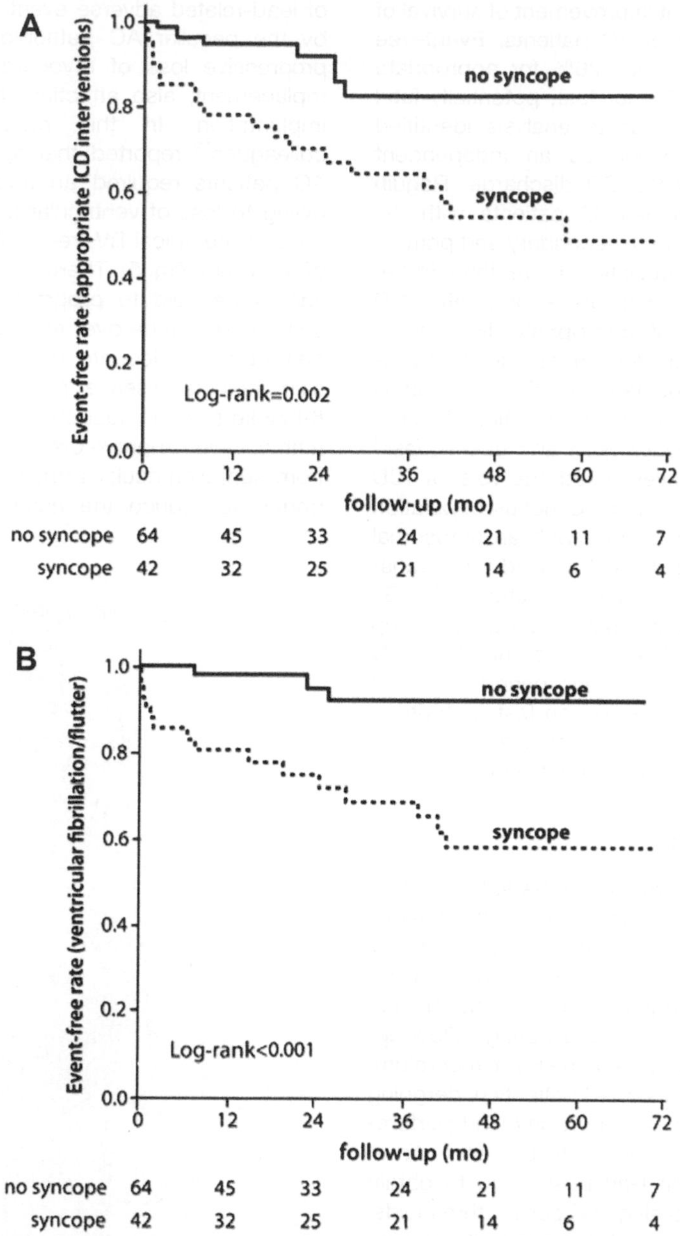

Fig. 4. DARVIN II study. Kaplan-Meier analysis of freedom from any appropriate ICD interventions (*A*) and shock therapies on VF/Vfl (*B*), stratified by syncope.

36 ± 18 years) with AC presenting with VT and hemodynamic collapse (n = 6) or VF (n = 3), treated with an ICD. After a mean follow-up of 32 ± 24 months, all patients were alive. Six patients received a median of 19 (range, 2–306) appropriate ICD interventions for events detected in the VT window; 4 received a median of 2 (range, 1–19) appropriate ICD interventions for events detected in the VF window. Inappropriate interventions were seen for sinus tachycardia (18 episodes in 3 patients), atrial fibrillation (3 episodes in 1 patient), and nonsustained polymorphic VT (1 episode in 1 patient).

In 2004, Wichter and colleagues[22] reported the largest single-center experience (60 patients) on ICD therapy in AC over a long-term follow-up period of 80 ± 43 months. The majority of patients received an ICD for secondary prevention after resuscitated cardiac arrest or sustained VT. The study results confirmed the life-saving role of ICD therapy with significant improvement of survival of this high-risk subset of AC patients. Event-free survival after 7 years was 26% for appropriate ICD therapies and 56% for fast, potentially fatal VT, respectively. Multivariate analysis identified extensive RV dysfunction as an independent predictor of appropriate ICD discharge. Roguin and colleagues[23] studied 42 patients with AC who received ICD for both secondary and primary prevention; in this population more than three-quarters (78%) received an appropriate ICD therapy. Predictors of appropriate firing were induction of ventricular tachycardia during electrophysiologic study, spontaneous VT, male versus female gender, and severe RV dilatation. Another relevant study by Hodgkinson and colleagues[24] published in 2005 investigated the role of ICD therapy in a genetically homogeneous population of 11 Newfoundland families with an autosomal dominant form of familial AC caused by a transmembrane TMEM43 gene mutation.[25] By comparing an ICD-treated patient subgroup group with a matched historical control group, the study showed that during a 5-year period, 30% of patients had ICD intervention on fast, potentially life-threatening VT with an estimated mortality reduction of 28% at 5 years of follow-up.

SAFETY OF ICD THERAPY

Concerns have been raised on the safety of ICD therapy in AC patients because of the risk of perforation due to the lead implantation into a thin RV free wall, as well as on the difficulty in obtaining and maintaining adequate sensing and pacing thresholds at implantation and during follow-up, due to the progressive loss of the RV myocardium.

The referenced series of AC patients undergoing ICD implantation did not report any lead perforation. However, a more difficult and time-consuming ventricular lead positioning to obtain adequate R-wave sensing and pacing thresholds, because of the RV myocardial atrophy with ensuing reduced electrical activity, has been reported. The study of Wichter and colleagues[22] demonstrated a high rate of device-related complications over a long-term follow-up. Thirty-seven of 60 patients (62%) had a total of 53 serious adverse events, 10 occurring during the perioperative phase and 43 during the follow-up. There were 31 lead-related adverse events in 21 patients (35%); insulation failure/oversensing in 10, undersensing in 8, lead fracture in 5, lead dislodgment in 2, lead thrombosis in 2, and subcutaneous lead fracture in 1. Surgical revision or implantation of an additional pace/sense lead was required in 26 of 31 lead-related complications (84%). This high rate of lead-related adverse events may be explained by the peculiar AC pathobiology that leads to progressive loss of myocardium with fibrofatty replacement, also affecting the site of RV lead implantation. In this regard, Corrado and colleagues[12] reported that approximately 4% of AC patients required an additional septal lead owing to loss of ventricular sensing/pacing functions at the apical RV free wall during a follow-up of 3.3 years (**Fig. 5**). Therefore, particular attention should be paid to progressive loss of R-wave sensing amplitude over time, which may not only compromise adequate device function but may also indicate disease progression. The use of β-blockers and dual-chamber detection algorithms, which improve discrimination of ventricular from supraventricular arrhythmias, have been reported to reduce the number of inappropriate

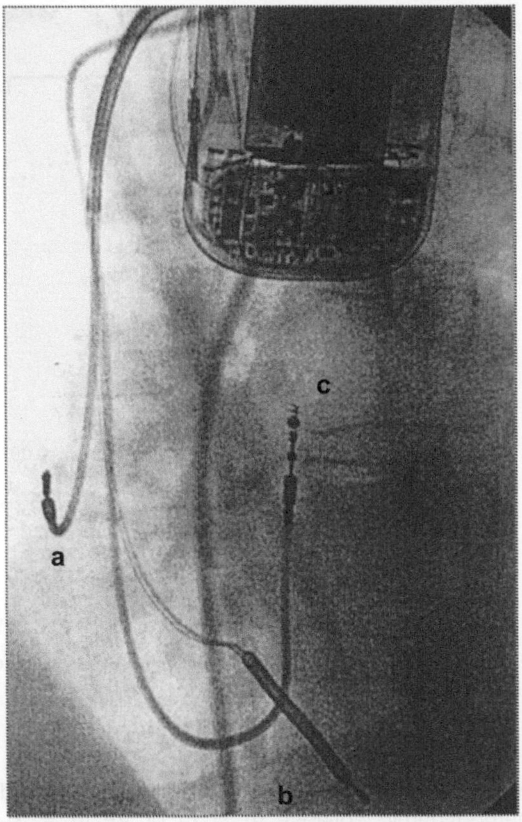

Fig. 5. Chest radiograph (60° left anterior oblique) of an AC patient who received an ICD for prevention of sudden death. Besides the original atrial lead (a) and the double-coil ventricular lead for cardioversion (b), a third ventricular lead (c) was subsequently added and screwed onto the mid septum (spared of the disease) to assure a reliable sensing and pacing function, which had progressively decreased after the device implantation.

interventions in young AC patients. However, limitation of the number of implanted leads may be a favorable approach, mostly in the young patient subgroup, because of the substantial incidence of lead failure over time (cumulatively 37% at 7 years in the Wichter study[22]), which includes not only compromise in pacing/sensing or defibrillation function by the mechanisms previously described but also mechanical lead complications (lead insulation failure or fracture) which, in turn, may contribute to inappropriate or inadequate ICD discharges.

INDICATIONS FOR ICD IMPLANTATION

The available data demonstrate that ICD therapy improves long-term prognosis and survival when applied to AC patients at high risk for SCD. Although ICD confers optimal protection against sudden death, the significant rate of inappropriate interventions and complications, as well as the psychological repercussions mostly in the younger age group, strongly suggest the need to accurately stratify the patient arrhythmic risk before device implantation. **Fig. 6** shows the pyramid of arrhythmic risk stratification and the current indications to ICD implantation in AC patients, based on the annual rate of appropriate ICD interventions against life-threatening ventricular arrhythmias (ie, episodes of VF/Vfl) derived from observational studies. The best candidates for ICD therapy are patients with prior cardiac arrest and those with VT with hemodynamically unstable VT (ie, associated with syncope or shock); syncope that remains unexplained after exclusion of noncardiac causes and vasovagal mechanisms is also considered a valuable predictor of sudden death and represents an indication for ICD implantation per se. In this high-risk group of patients, the rate of appropriate ICD intervention against life-threatening ventricular tachyarrhythmias (that in all likelihood would have been fatal in the absence of shock therapy) is approximately 8% to 10% per year and the estimated mortality reduction at 36 months of follow-up ranges from 24% to 35%.[11,22] By contrast, ICD implantation for primary prevention in the general AC population seems to be unjustified. As indicated by the DARVIN II study on prophylactic device implantation in AC patients with no sustained VT or VF, asymptomatic probands and relatives do not benefit from ICD

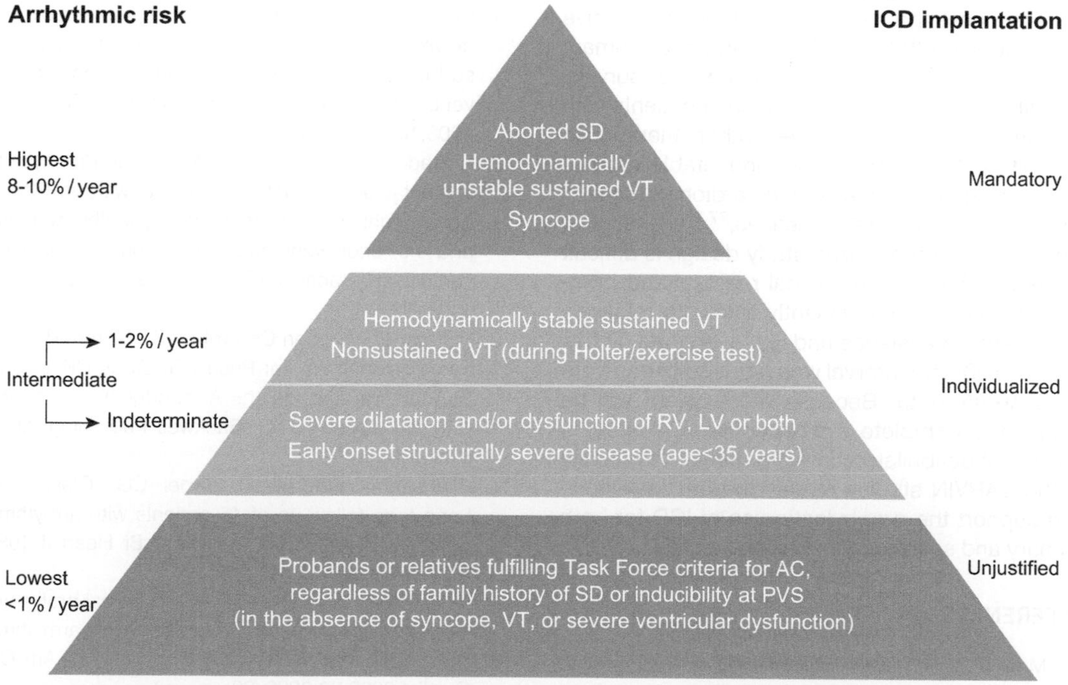

Fig. 6. Pyramid of arrhythmic risk stratification and current indications to ICD implantation in AC patients, based on the annual rate of appropriate ICD interventions against life-threatening ventricular arrhythmias (ie, episodes of VF/Vfl) derived from observational studies. PVS, programmed ventricular stimulation; SD, sudden death. (*Adapted from* Corrado D, Basso C, Pilichou K, et al. Molecular biology and the clinical management of arrhythmogenic right ventricular cardiomyopathy/dysplasia. Heart 2011;97:530–9; with permission.)

therapy, regardless of familial sudden death or inducibility at PVS.[12] This patient cohort carries a low arrhythmic risk over a long-term follow-up (ICD intervention rate <1 per year), in addition to a significant rate of device-related complications and inappropriate discharges. Patients with well-tolerated sustained VT or nonsustained VT on Holter or exercise testing have an intermediate arrhythmic risk (ICD intervention rate ~1%–2% per year). In this patient subgroup, the decision for ICD implantation needs to be individualized; antiarrhythmic drug therapy (including β-blockers) and/or catheter ablation seem to be a reasonable first-line therapy. In the absence of syncope or significant ventricular arrhythmias, whether severe dilatation and/or dysfunction of right ventricle, left ventricle, or both, as well as early-onset structurally severe disease (age <35 years) require prophylactic ICD remains to be determined.

SUMMARY

There is compelling evidence that ICD provides life-saving protection by effectively terminating VT and fibrillation in high-risk patients with AC.

The design of both DARVIN studies was that of a retrospective international multicenter survey with possible limitations in patient selection. Such limits suggest the need for a future prospective and controlled study, with total mortality as primary end point, to conclusively define the survival benefit of defibrillator implantation in patients with AC and its superiority over other therapeutic modalities. However, for any inheritable cardiac diseases such as hypertrophic cardiomyopathy,[26] cardiac ion channel diseases,[27,28] and AC, a prospective randomized study design is difficult to perform because of ethical reasons and practical limitations predominantly linked to relatively low disease prevalence and low event rate. In this regard, a 20-year interval was required to generate the DARVIN data. Because many years will be required to complete a prospective evaluation in the use of defibrillators in AC patients, the results of the DARVIN studies remain the best available, and support the prophylactic use of ICD for both primary and secondary prevention of SCD.

REFERENCES

1. Moss AJ, Hall WJ, Cannom DS, et al. Improved survival with an implanted defibrillator in patients with coronary disease at high risk for ventricular arrhythmia. N Engl J Med 1996;335:1933–40.
2. The Antiarrhythmics versus Implantable Defibrillators (AVID) Investigators. A comparison of antiarrhythmic-drug therapy with implantable defibrillators in patients resuscitated from near-fatal ventricular arrhythmias. N Engl J Med 1997;337:1576–83.
3. Buxton AE, Lee KL, Fisher JD, et al. A randomized study of the prevention of sudden death in patients with coronary artery disease. N Engl J Med 1999; 341:1882–90.
4. Marcus FI, Fontaine G, Guiraudon G, et al. Right ventricular dysplasia. A report of 24 adult cases. Circulation 1982;65:384–98.
5. Thiene G, Nava A, Corrado D, et al. Right ventricular cardiomyopathy and sudden death in young people. N Engl J Med 1988;318:129–33.
6. Basso C, Thiene G, Corrado D, et al. Arrhythmogenic right ventricular cardiomyopathy. Dysplasia, dystrophy, or myocarditis? Circulation 1996;94:983–91.
7. Corrado D, Basso C, Thiene G, et al. Spectrum of clinicopathologic manifestations of arrhythmogenic right ventricular cardiomyopathy/dysplasia: a multicenter study. J Am Coll Cardiol 1997;30:1512–20.
8. Corrado D, Basso C, Thiene G. Arrhythmogenic right ventricular cardiomyopathy: diagnosis, prognosis, and treatment. Heart 2000;83:588–95.
9. Basso C, Corrado D, Marcus FI, et al. Arrhythmogenic right ventricular cardiomyopathy. Lancet 2009;373:1289–300.
10. Corrado D, Basso C, Thiene G. Arrhythmogenic right ventricular cardiomyopathy: an update. Heart 2009;95:766–73.
11. Corrado D, Leoni L, Link MS, et al. Implantable cardioverter defibrillator therapy for prevention of sudden death in patients with arrhythmogenic right ventricular cardiomyopathy/dysplasia. Circulation 2003;108:3084–91.
12. Corrado D, Calkins H, Link MS, et al. Prophylactic implantable defibrillator in patients with arrhythmogenic right ventricular cardiomyopathy/dysplasia and no prior ventricular fibrillation or sustained ventricular tachycardia. Circulation 2010;122: 1144–52.
13. McKenna WJ, Sen-Chowdhry S, Maron BJ. The cardiomyopathies. In: Priori SG, Zipes DP, editors. Sudden cardiac death. A handbook for clinical practice. Oxford (UK): Backwell Publishing; 2006. p. 109–31.
14. Blomstrom-Lundqvist C, Sabel CG, Olsson SB. Long term follow-up of 15 patients with arrhythmogenic right ventricular dysplasia. Br Heart J 1987; 58:477–88.
15. Nava A, Bauce B, Basso C, et al. Clinical profile and long-term follow-up of 37 families with arrhythmogenic right ventricular cardiomyopathy. J Am Coll Cardiol 2000;36:2226–33.
16. Hulot JS, Jouven X, Empana JP, et al. Natural history and risk stratification of arrhythmogenic right ventricular dysplasia/cardiomyopathy. Circulation 2004; 110:1879–84.

17. Corrado D, Thiene G. Arrhythmogenic right ventricular cardiomyopathy/dysplasia: clinical impact of molecular genetic studies. Circulation 2006;113:1634–7.
18. Corrado D, Basso C, Pilichou K, et al. Molecular biology and the clinical management of arrhythmogenic right ventricular cardiomyopathy/dysplasia. Heart 2011;97:530–9.
19. Breithardt G, Wichter T, Haverkamp W, et al. Implantable cardioverter defibrillator therapy in patients with arrhythmogenic right ventricular cardiomyopathy, long QT syndrome, or no structural heart disease. Am Heart J 1994;127:1151–8.
20. Link M, Wang PJ, Haugh CJ, et al. Arrhythmogenic right ventricular dysplasia: clinical results with implantable cardioverter defibrillator. J Intervent Card Electrophysiol 1997;1:41–8.
21. Tavernier R, Gevaert S, de Sutter J, et al. Long term results of cardioverter defibrillator implantation in patients with right ventricular dysplasia and malignant ventricular tachyarrhythmias. Heart 2001;85:53–6.
22. Wichter T, Paul M, Wollmann C, et al. Implantable cardioverter/defibrillator therapy in arrhythmogenic right ventricular cardiomyopathy: single-center experience of long-term follow-up and complications in 60 patients. Circulation 2004;109:1503–8.
23. Roguin A, Bomma CS, Nasir K, et al. Implantable cardioverter defibrillators in patients with arrhythmogenic right ventricular dysplasia/cardiomyopathy. J Am Coll Cardiol 2004;43:1843–52.
24. Hodgkinson KA, Parfrey PS, Basset AS, et al. The impact of implantable cardioverter-defibrillator therapy on survival in autosomal-dominant arrhythmogenic right ventricular cardiomyopathy (ARVD5). J Am Coll Cardiol 2005;45:400–8.
25. Merner ND, Hodgkinson KA, Haywood AF, et al. Arrhythmogenic right ventricular cardiomyopathy type 5 is a fully penetrant, lethal arrhythmic disorder caused by a missense mutation in the TMEM43 gene. Am J Hum Genet 2008;82:809–21.
26. Maron BJ, Shen WK, Link MS, et al. Efficacy of implantable cardioverter-ICDs for the prevention of sudden death in patients with hypertrophic cardiomyopathy. N Engl J Med 2000;342:365–73.
27. Brugada J, Brugada R, Antzelevitch C, et al. Long-term follow-up of individuals with the electrocardiographic pattern of right bundle-branch block and ST-segment elevation in precordial leads V1 to V3. Circulation 2002;105:73–8.
28. Schwartz PJ, Spazzolini C, Priori SG, et al. Who are the long-QT syndrome patients who receive an implantable cardioverter-defibrillator and what happens to them?: data from the European Long-QT Syndrome Implantable Cardioverter-Defibrillator (LQTS ICD) Registry. Circulation 2010;122:1272–82.

Arrhythmogenic Cardiomyopathy and Sports-Related Sudden Death

Maurizio Schiavon, MD[a], Alessandro Zorzi, MD[b], Cristina Basso, MD, PhD[c], Antonio Pelliccia, MD[d], Gaetano Thiene, MD[c], Domenico Corrado, MD, PhD[b,*]

KEYWORDS

- Arrhythmogenic right ventricular cardiomyopathy/dysplasia
- Competitive athletes • Sports activity • Sudden death

Arrhythmogenic cardiomyopathy (AC) is an inherited heart muscle disease characterized pathologically by right ventricular (RV) fibrofatty myocardial replacement and clinically by ventricular electric instability, which may lead to cardiac arrest from ventricular fibrillation (VF), mostly in young people and athletes.[1–5] AC shows a propensity for life-threatening ventricular arrhythmias during physical exercise, and participation in competitive athletics has been associated with an increased risk for sudden cardiac death (SCD).[6–10] In addition, physical sport activity has been implicated as a factor promoting acceleration of disease progression. Identification of affected athletes by preparticipation screening has proved to result in mortality reduction during sports activity.[11]

This article examines the role of AC in causing SCD in young competitive athletes and addresses prevention strategy based on identification of affected athletes at preparticipation screening.

SCD DURING SPORTS

Although sudden death during sport is a rare event, it has a devastating effect on the community because it occurs in apparently healthy individuals and assumes great visibility through the news media because of the high public profile of competitive athletes.[7,8,12] The frequency of sudden death in young athletes during organized competitive sports varies in the different series reported in the literature. A retrospective analysis in the United States has estimated the prevalence of fatal events in high school and college athletes (aged 12–24 years) to be less than 1 in 100,000 per year,[13,14] whereas a prospective population-based study in Italy reported a 3 times greater incidence among competitive athletes aged 12 to 35 years.[10]

The vast majority of athletes who die suddenly have underlying structural heart diseases, which provide a substrate for VF. SCD is usually the result of an interaction between transient acute abnormalities (trigger) and structural cardiovascular abnormalities (substrate). Triggers of SCD in young competitive athletes include exercise-related sympathetic stimulation, abrupt hemodynamic changes, and acute myocardial ischemia leading to life-threatening ventricular arrhythmias.[7,12,15,16] The causes of SCD reflect the age of the participants. Although atherosclerotic

[a] Department of Social Health, Center for Sports Medicine and Physical Activity, ULSS 16, Padua, Italy
[b] Division of Cardiology, Department of Cardiac, Thoracic and Vascular Sciences, University of Padua Medical School, Via Giustiniani, 2-35121 Padua, Italy
[c] Cardiovascular Pathology, Department of Medical-Diagnostic Sciences and Special Therapies, University of Padua Medical School, Via A. Gabelli, 35121 Padua, Italy
[d] Institute of Sports Medicine and Science, Rome, Italy
* Corresponding author.
E-mail address: domenico.corrado@unipd.it

Card Electrophysiol Clin 3 (2011) 323–331
doi:10.1016/j.ccep.2011.02.010

coronary artery disease accounts for the vast majority of fatalities in adults (aged $\geq$35 years),[17–19] in younger athletes there is a broad spectrum of cardiovascular substrates (including congenital and inherited heart disorders) (**Box 1**).[6–12,20–25] Cardiomyopathies have been consistently implicated as the leading cause of sports-related cardiac arrest in the young, with hypertrophic cardiomyopathy accounting for more than one-third of fatal cases in the United States[8] and AC for approximately one-fourth in the Veneto region of Italy.[9]

About 6% to 10% of sudden death victims have no evidence of structural heart disease. The cause of their sudden death is probably related to a primary electric heart disorder such as inherited cardiac ion channel defects (channelopathies), including long and short QT syndromes, catecholaminergic polymorphic ventricular tachycardia, and Brugada syndrome.[25–28] Finally, sudden death during sport can also be the result of a nonpenetrating blow to the chest wall (commotio cordis), which can trigger an abrupt VF in the absence of any cardiac structural lesions.[29]

SCD FROM AC IN YOUNG COMPETITIVE ATHLETES

Systematic monitoring and pathologic investigation of sudden death in young people and athletes of the Veneto region of Italy showed that AC is the most common pathologic substrate accounting for nearly one-forth of athletic field fatal events.[9,10] The incidence of sudden death from AC in athletes was estimated to be 0.5 per 100,000 persons per year (**Fig. 1**). Sudden death victims with AC were all men with a mean age of 22.6 $\pm$ 4 years.[10] At postmortem, the hallmark lesion of the disease was the transmural replacement of the RV myocardium by fibrofatty tissue (**Fig. 2**).[1–3] Hearts demonstrated massive regional or diffuse fibrofatty infiltration, parchmentlike translucence of the RV free wall, and mild to moderate RV dilatation, together with aneurysmal dilatations of the posterobasal, apical, and outflow tract regions. These RV pathologic features allowed differential diagnosis with training-induced RV adaptation (athlete's heart), usually consisting of global RV enlargement without regional dilatation/dysfunction. Histologically, fibrofatty infiltration is usually associated with focal myocardial necrosis and patchy inflammatory infiltrates. Fibrofatty scar and aneurysms are potential sources of life-threatening ventricular arrhythmias. The histopathologic arrangement of the surviving myocardium embedded in the replacing fibrofatty tissue may lead to inhomogeneous intraventricular conduction predisposing to reentrant mechanisms. Life-threatening ventricular arrhythmias may occur either during the hot phase of myocyte death as abrupt VF or later in the form of scar-related macroreentrant ventricular tachycardia.[30]

The risk of sudden death from AC has been estimated to be 5.4 times greater during competitive sports than during sedentary activity (see **Fig. 1**). Several reasons may explain such a propensity of AC to precipitate effort-dependent sudden cardiac arrest. Physical exercise acutely increases the RV afterload and causes cavity enlargement, which in turn may elicit ventricular arrhythmias by stretching the diseased RV myocardium.[31] The advent of molecular genetic era has provided new insights in understanding the pathogenesis of AC, showing that it is a desmosomal disease resulting from defective cell adhesion proteins such as plakoglobin, desmoplakin, plakophilin-2, desmoglein-2, and desmocollin-2.[4,5] It has been advanced that impairment of myocyte cell-to-cell adhesion may lead to tissue and organ fragility that is sufficient to promote myocyte death and subsequent fibrofatty repair, especially under conditions of mechanical stress, such as that occurring during competitive sports activity.[4,5,32–34] The adverse effect of exercise on the phenotypic expression of AC was recently confirmed by Kirchhof and colleagues[35] in an experimental study on heterozygous plakoglobin-deficient mice. When compared with wild-type controls, the mutant mice had increased RV volume, reduced RV function, and

Box 1
Cardiovascular causes of sudden death associated with sports

Athletes aged 35 years or older

- Atherosclerotic coronary artery disease

Athletes younger than 35 years

- Hypertrophic cardiomyopathy
- Arrhythmogenic cardiomyopathy
- Premature coronary atherosclerosis
- Congenital anomalies of coronary arteries
- Myocarditis
- Aortic rupture
- Valvular disease
- Preexcitation syndromes and conduction diseases
- Ion channel diseases
- Congenital heart disease, operated or unoperated

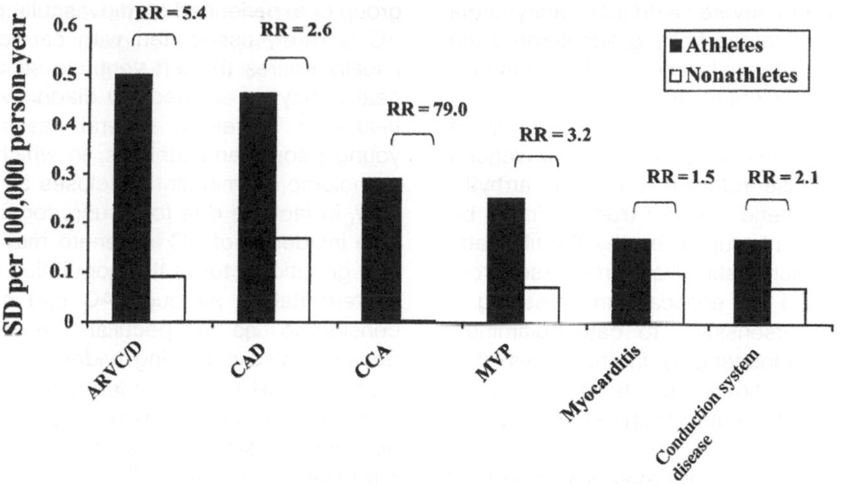

Fig. 1. Incidence and relative risk (RR) of sudden death from major cardiovascular causes among young athletes and nonathletes. ARVC/D, arrhythmogenic cardiomyopathy; CAD, coronary artery disease; CCA, congenital coronary artery anomalies; MVP, mitral valve prolapse. (*Modified from* Corrado D, Basso C, Rizzoli G, et al. Does sports activity enhance the risk of sudden death in adolescents and young adults? J Am Coll Cardiol 2003;42:1961; with permission.)

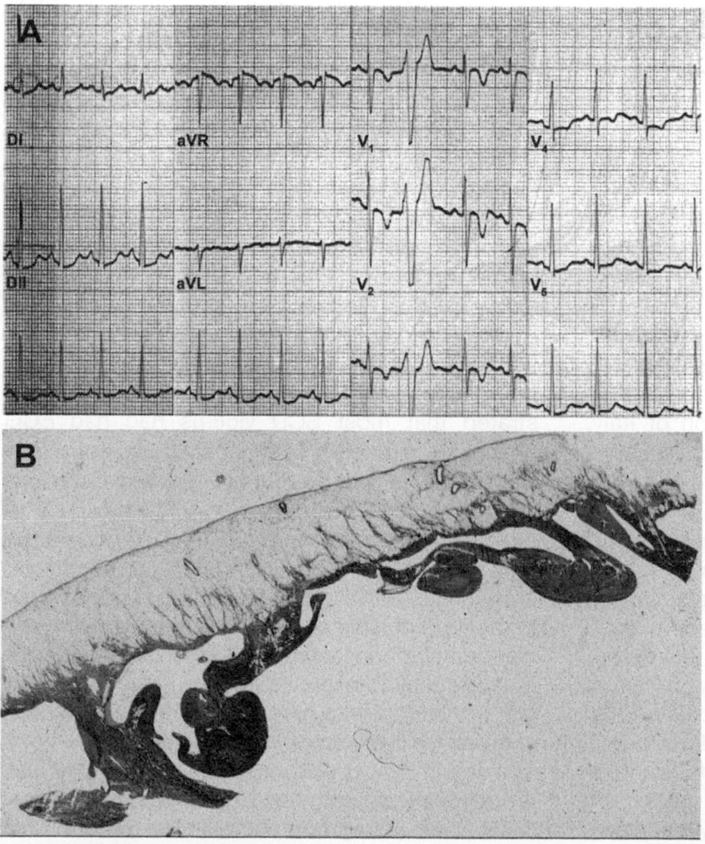

Fig. 2. Electrocardiographic and pathologic features in a 19-year-old soccer player who died suddenly of AC. (*A*) The 12-lead ECG obtained at preparticipation screening shows inverted T waves from V_1 to V_4 and premature ventricular beats with a left bundle branch block morphology. (*B*) Panoramic histologic view of the RV free wall showing transmural fibrofatty myocardial replacement (Heidenhain trichrome, original magnification ×25). (*From* Corrado D, Basso C, Thiene G. Sudden Death in young athletes. In: Marcus FI, Nava A, Thiene G, editors. Arrhythmogenic RV Cardiomyopathy/Dysplasia: Recent Advances. Milan, New York: Springer; 2007. p. 205–211; with permission.)

more frequent and severe ventricular tachycardia of RV origin. Endurance training accelerated the development of RV dysfunction and arrhythmias in plakoglobin-deficient mice.

Alternatively, denervation supersensitivity of the RV to catecholamines has been advanced to explain exercise-induced ventricular arrhythmias.[36] Sympathetic nerve trunks may be damaged and/or interrupted by the RV fibrofatty replacement, which distinctively progresses from the epicardium to the endocardium, resulting in denervation supersensitivity to catecholamines. Arrhythmogenic mechanisms in the denervated supersensitive myofibers include dispersion of refractoriness and reentry, triggered activity, or both.

Finally, in a subgroup of patients with familial AC, a cardiac ryanodine receptor (RYR2) missense mutation leading to abnormal calcium release from the sarcoplasmic reticulum has been identified.[37] Wall mechanical stress, such as that induced by RV volume overload during exercise, is expected to exacerbate the cardiac ryanodine channel dysfunction.[37] Therefore, a potential arrhythmogenic mechanism of sport-related cardiac arrest in patients with AC is triggered activity due to late afterdepolarizations, which are provoked by intracellular calcium overload and enhanced by adrenergic stimulation.[38]

CAUSES OF SCD IN YOUNG ATHLETES: ITALIAN VERSUS US EXPERIENCE

Although AC has been demonstrated to be the leading cause of SCD in athletes of Veneto, Italy, previous studies in the United States showed a higher prevalence of other pathologic substrates such as hypertrophic cardiomyopathy, anomalous coronary arteries, and myocarditis.[1–12]

This discrepancy may be explained by several factors. There have been no previous investigations, such as the Juvenile Sudden Death Research Project in the Veneto region of Italy, that have prospectively investigated a consecutive series of sudden death in young people occurring in a well-defined geographic area with a homogeneous ethnic group.[9,11] Therefore, the previously reported causes in the United States may have been influenced by the unavoidable limitations in patient selection because of retrospective analysis. Moreover, in other large studies, the autopsies were usually performed by different examiners, including local pathologists and medical examiners.[13] In the Italian study, to obtain a higher level of confidence in the results, morphologic examination of all hearts was performed according to a standard protocol by the same group of experienced cardiovascular pathologists. AC is rarely associated with cardiomegaly and usually spares the left ventricle so that affected hearts may be erroneously diagnosed as normal hearts.[1–3] Therefore, several cases of SCD in young people and athletes, in which the routine pathologic examination discloses a normal heart, may, in fact, be due to an unrecognized AC. The high incidence of AC in Veneto may be because of a genetic factor in the population of the northeastern Italy,[32] although AC can no longer be considered as a peculiar Venetian disease because there is growing evidence that it is ubiquitous, it is still largely underdiagnosed both clinically and at postmortem investigation, and it accounts for significant arrhythmic morbidity and mortality worldwide.[3,39,40]

CLINICAL PROFILE OF ATHLETES DYING SUDDENLY FROM AC

Early identification of athletes with AC plays a crucial role in the prevention of SCD during sport. The most frequent clinical manifestations of the disease consist of electrocardiographic (ECG) depolarization/repolarization changes mostly localized to right precordial leads, global and/or regional morphologic and functional alterations of the RV, and arrhythmias of RV origin (**Fig. 3**).[1–5,39–42] The disease should be suspected even in asymptomatic individuals on the basis of ECG abnormalities and ventricular arrhythmias.[1,6,9] Ultimately, the diagnosis relies on visualization of morphofunctional RV abnormalities by imaging techniques (such as echocardiography, angiography, and cardiac magnetic resonance) and, in selected cases, by histopathologic demonstration of fibrofatty substitution at endomyocardial biopsy.[4,5]

By reviewing clinical and ECG findings of 22 young competitive athletes who died suddenly from AC proven at autopsy, it has been demonstrated that most SCD victims had had ECG changes, ventricular arrhythmias, or both (see **Fig. 2**).[15,43] Right precordial T wave inversion (beyond lead V_1) had been recorded in 88% of athletes, right precordial QRS duration greater than 110 millisecond in 76%, and ventricular arrhythmias with a left bundle branch block pattern in the form of isolated/coupled premature ventricular beats or nonsustained ventricular tachycardia in 76%. Limited exercise testing–induced ventricular arrhythmia was recorded in 50%. Of interest, submaximal exercise testing, available in 5 athletes, showed pseudonormalization of right precordial repolarization abnormalities in all athletes. Thus, most young competitive athletes who died

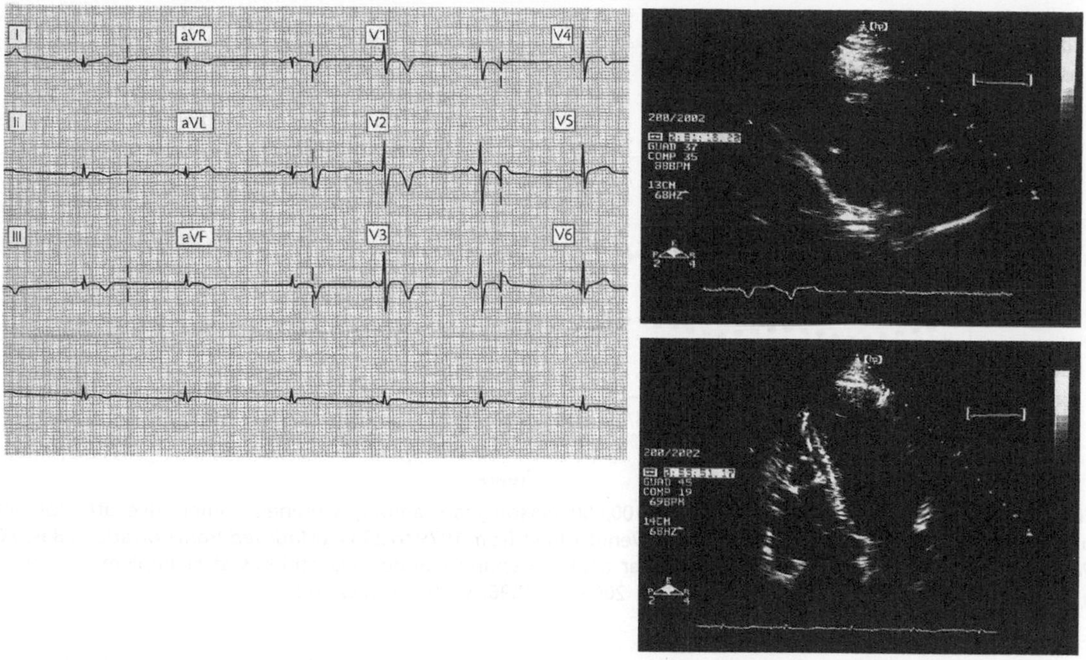

Fig. 3. ECG and echocardiographic findings in an asymptomatic athlete diagnosed with AC. The athlete was referred for further evaluation because of ECG abnormalities found at preparticipation evaluation, which consisted of inverted T waves in the inferior and anteroseptal leads and low QRS voltages in the peripheral leads (*A*). AC was suspected at echocardiographic examination, showing mild RV dilatation, basal and apical wall motion abnormalities with diastolic bulging of the RV inflow tract, and trabecular disarrangement. (*B*) The RV long-axis view. (*C*) The 4-chamber view. Final diagnosis was achieved by cardiac magnetic resonance (not shown). (*Modified from* Corrado D, Basso C, Pelliccia A, et al. Sports and heart disease. In: Camm J, Luscher TF, Serruys PW, editors. The ESC textbook of cardiovascular medicine. New York: Oxford University Press; 2009. p. 1215–37; with permission.)

suddenly from AC showed ECG abnormalities that could raise the suspicion of the underlying cardiovascular disease at preparticipation evaluation and lead to further testing for a definitive diagnosis.

PREPARTICIPATION SCREENING AND PREVENTION OF SCD

For more than 20 years, a systematic preparticipation screening, based on 12-lead ECG, in addition to history and physical examination, has been the practice in Italy.[9,11,12,43,44] This screening strategy has been proved to be effective in the identification of athletes with previously undiagnosed hypertrophic cardiomyopathy, thanks to the high sensitivity (up to 95%) of 12-lead ECG for suspicion/detection of this condition in otherwise asymptomatic athletes. Moreover, during long-term follow-up, no deaths were recorded among these disqualified athletes with hypertrophic cardiomyopathy, suggesting that restriction from competition may reduce the risk of sudden death.[9]

A time trend analysis of the incidence of SCD in young competitive athletes aged 12 to 35 years in the Veneto region of Italy between 1979 and 2004 has provided compelling evidence that ECG screening is a lifesaving strategy.[11] The long-term effect of the Italian screening program on prevention of SCD in athletes was assessed by comparing temporal trends in SCD among screened athletes and unscreened nonathletes. The assessed intervals were prescreening (1979–1981), early screening (1982–1992), and late screening (1993–2004). The analysis demonstrated a sharp decline of SCD in athletes after the introduction of the nationwide screening program in 1982 (**Fig. 4**). There were 55 cases of SCD in screened athletes (1.9 deaths per 100,000 person-years) and 265 deaths in unscreened nonathletes (0.79 deaths per 100,000 person-years). The annual incidence of SCD in athletes decreased by 89%, from 3.6 per 100,000 person-years during the prescreening period to 0.4 per 100,000 person-years during the late screening period. By comparison, the incidence of SCD in the unscreened nonathletic population of the same age did not change significantly over that time. Most of the mortality

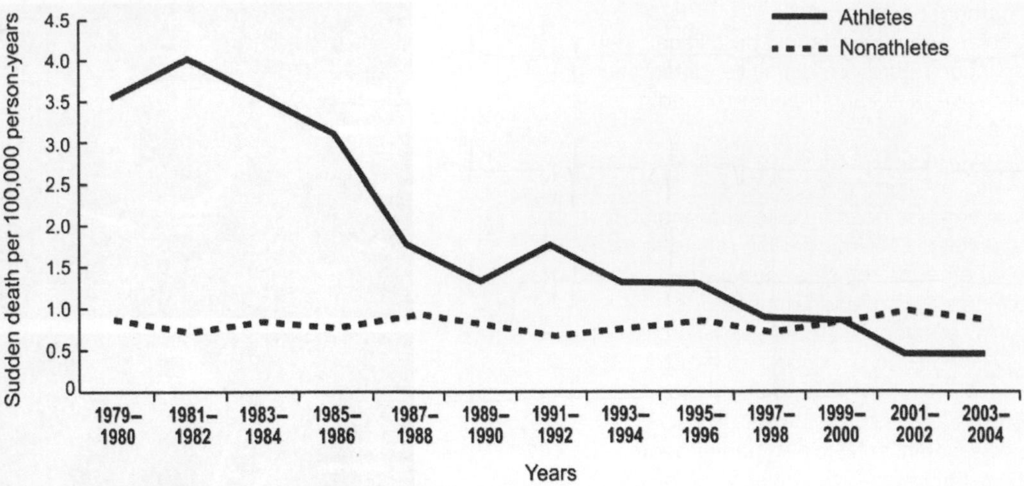

Fig. 4. Annual incidence rates of SCD per 100,000 person-years among screened competitive athletes and unscreened nonathletes aged 12 to 35 years in Veneto, Italy, from 1979 to 2004. (*Modified from* Corrado D, Basso C, Pavei A, et al. Trends in sudden cardiovascular death in young competitive athletes after implementation of a preparticipation screening program. JAMA 2006;296:1596; with permission.)

reduction was attributable to fewer deaths from hypertrophic cardiomyopathy and AC (**Fig. 5**). A parallel analysis of the causes of disqualifications from competitive sports at the Center for Sports Medicine in the Padua country area showed that the proportion of athletes identified and disqualified for cardiomyopathies doubled from the early to the late screening period. This observation indicates that mortality reduction was a reflection of a lower incidence of SCD from cardiomyopathies, as a result of increasing identification over time of affected athletes at preparticipation screening.

ATHLETIC PARTICIPATION

The ultimate diagnosis of cardiomyopathy in a young competitive athlete may be problematic because of the presence of physiologic (and reversible) structural and electric adaptations of the cardiovascular system to long-term athletic training. This condition known as athlete's heart is characterized by an increase in ventricular cavity dimension and wall thickness, which overlaps with cardiomyopathies.[45] An accurate differential diagnosis is crucial because of the potentially adverse outcome associated with cardiomyopathy in an athlete and, on the other hand, the possibility of misdiagnosis of pathologic conditions requiring unnecessary disqualifications from sport, with financial and psychological consequences.

A sizeable proportion of highly trained athletes have an increase in RV cavity dimensions, which raises the question of AC. Morphologic criteria in favor of a physiologic RV enlargement consist of preserved global and regional ventricular function, without evidence of wall motion abnormalities such as dyskinetic regions and/or diastolic bulgings.

During the last 2 decades, the advances in molecular genetics have allowed identification of a growing number of defective genes involved in

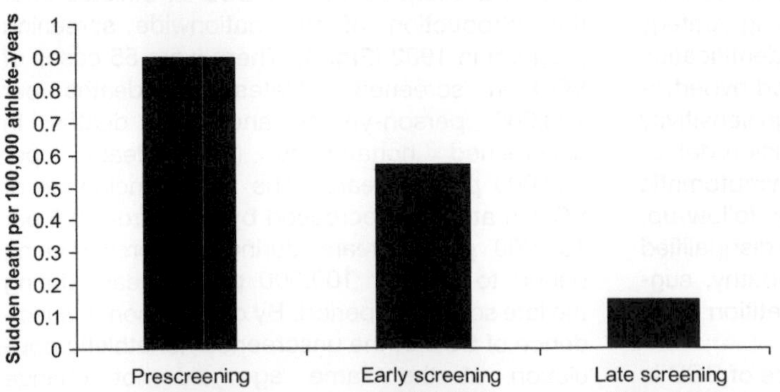

Fig. 5. Average annual incidence rates of SCD from AC among young competitive athletes of the Veneto, Italy, before and after implementation of systematic preparticipation screening. Death rates from AC declined from 0.90 per 100,000 person-years in the prescreening period (1979–1981) to 0.15 per 100,000 in the late screening period (1993–2004) (relative risk, 0.16; 95% confidence interval, 0.03–1.41; $P = .02$).

the pathogenesis of AC.[4,5,46] It is hoped that molecular genetic tests will be clinically available in the near future for definitive differential diagnosis between AC and training-related physiologic RV changes.

A high prevalence of RV arrhythmias in association with a slight but consistent RV dilatation/dysfunction has been reported among elite endurance athletes.[47,48] This finding raised the question as to whether the long-term extreme RV pressure and volume load of endurance sports may account for an AC phenocopy, that is, an exercise-induced AC-like syndrome. This concept was recently reinforced by the finding that the proportion of genotype-positive athletes with an AC-like phenotype was significantly lower than expected (12.5% vs 27%–55%) for the typical form of genetically determined AC.[49] Although strenuous physical exercise may itself cause an acquired form of AC, affected athletes may have unrecognized genes and/or polymorphisms that predispose them to develop an AC-like phenotype as a result of their heart exposure to intense endurance sports.

According to US and European recommendations for sports eligibility,[50,51] athletes with a clinical diagnosis of AC should be excluded from all competitive sports. This recommendation is independent of age, gender, and phenotypic appearance and does not differ for athletes without symptoms, receiving treatment with drugs, or undergoing, catheter ablation and/or, implantable defibrillator. The presence of a freestanding automated external defibrillator at sporting events should neither be considered absolute protection against SCD[52] nor justification for participation in competitive sports in athletes with previously diagnosed AC.

SUMMARY

AC shows a propensity for life-threatening ventricular arrhythmias during physical exercise, and participation in competitive athletics has been associated with an increased risk for SCD. In addition, physical sport activity has been implicated as a factor promoting acceleration of disease progression. Prevention strategies are based on identification of affected athletes at preparticipation screening based on 12-lead ECG, in addition to history and physical examination. According to US and European recommendations for sports eligibility, athletes with a clinical diagnosis of AC should be excluded from all competitive sports. Identification of affected athletes by preparticipation screening with consequent disqualification has proved to result in mortality reduction during sports activity.

REFERENCES

1. Thiene G, Nava A, Corrado D, et al. Right ventricular cardiomyopathy and sudden death in young people. N Engl J Med 1988;318:129–33.
2. Basso C, Thiene G, Corrado D, et al. Arrhythmogenic right ventricular cardiomyopathy. Dysplasia, dystrophy, or myocarditis? Circulation 1996;94:983–91.
3. Corrado D, Basso C, Thiene G, et al. Spectrum of clinicopathologic manifestations of arrhythmogenic right ventricular cardiomyopathy/dysplasia: a multicenter study. J Am Coll Cardiol 1997;30:1512–20.
4. Basso C, Corrado D, Marcus F, et al. Arrhythmogenic right ventricular cardiomyopathy. Lancet 2009;373:1289–300.
5. Corrado D, Basso C, Thiene G. Arrhythmogenic right ventricular cardiomyopathy: an update. Heart 2009;95:766–73.
6. Corrado D, Thiene G, Nava A, et al. Sudden death in young competitive athletes: clinico-pathologic correlations in 22 cases. Am J Med 1990;89:588–96.
7. Corrado D, Basso C, Thiene G. Sudden death in young athletes. Lancet 2005;366(Suppl 1):S47–8.
8. Maron BJ. Sudden death in young athletes. N Engl J Med 2003;349:1064–75.
9. Corrado D, Basso C, Schiavon M, et al. Screening for hypertrophic cardiomyopathy in young athletes. N Engl J Med 1998;339:364–9.
10. Corrado D, Basso C, Rizzoli G, et al. Does sports activity enhance the risk of sudden death in adolescents and young adults? J Am Coll Cardiol 2003;42:1959–63.
11. Corrado D, Basso C, Pavei A, et al. Trends in sudden cardiovascular death in young competitive athletes after implementation of a preparticipation screening program. JAMA 2006;296:1593–601.
12. Corrado D, Basso C, Schiavon M, et al. Pre-participation screening of young competitive athletes for prevention of sudden cardiac death. J Am Coll Cardiol 2008;52:1981–9.
13. Van Camp SP, Bloor CM, Mueller FO, et al. Non-traumatic sports death in high school and college athletes. Med Sci Sports Exerc 1995;27:641–7.
14. Maron BJ, Gohman TE, Aeppli D. Prevalence of sudden cardiac death during competitive sports activities in Minnesota high school athletes. J Am Coll Cardiol 1998;32:1881–4.
15. Corrado D, Basso C, Thiene G. Sudden death in young athletes. In: Marcus FI, Nava A, Thiene G, editors. Arrhythmogenic RV cardiomyopathy/dysplasia: recent advances. Milan, New York: Springer; 2007. p. 205–11.
16. Corrado D, Migliore F, Bevilacqua M, et al. Sudden cardiac death in athletes: can it be prevented by screening? Herz 2009;34:259–66.

17. Thompson PD, Funk EJ, Carleton RA, et al. Incidence of death during jogging in Rhode Island from 1975 through 1980. JAMA 1982;247:2535–8.
18. Burke AP, Farb A, Malcom GT, et al. Plaque rupture and sudden death related to exertion in men with coronary artery disease. JAMA 1999;281:921–6.
19. Giri S, Thompson PD, Kiernan FJ, et al. Clinical and angiographic characteristics of exertion-related acute myocardial infarction. JAMA 1999;282:1731–6.
20. Corrado D, Basso C, Poletti A, et al. Sudden death in the young: is coronary thrombosis the major precipitating factor? Circulation 1994;90:2315–23.
21. Burke AP, Farb A, Virmani R, et al. Sports-related and non-sports-related sudden cardiac death in young adults. Am Heart J 1991;121:568–75.
22. Basso C, Maron BJ, Corrado D, et al. Clinical profile of congenital coronary artery anomalies with origin from the wrong aortic sinus leading to sudden death in young competitive athletes. J Am Coll Cardiol 2000;35:1493–501.
23. Basso C, Thiene G, Corrado D, et al. Hypertrophic cardiomyopathy: pathologic evidence of ischemic damage in young sudden death victims. Hum Pathol 2000;31:988–98.
24. Basso C, Corrado D, Rossi L, et al. Ventricular preexcitation in children and young adults: atrial myocarditis as a possible trigger of sudden death. Circulation 2001;103:269–75.
25. Corrado D, Basso C, Buja G, et al. Right bundle branch block, right precordial ST-segment elevation, and sudden death in young people. Circulation 2001;103:710–7.
26. Corrado D, Basso C, Thiene G. Sudden cardiac death in young people with apparently normal heart. Cardiovasc Res 2001;50:399–408.
27. Wilde AA, Antzelevitch C, Borggrefe M, et al, Study Group on the Molecular Basis of Arrhythmias of the European Society of Cardiology. Proposed diagnostic criteria for the Brugada syndrome: consensus report. Circulation 2002;106:2514–9.
28. Corrado D, Pelliccia A, Antzelevitch C, et al. ST segment elevation and sudden death in the athlete. Blackwell Futura. In: Antzelevitch C, Brugada P, editors. The Brugada syndrome: from bench to bedside. Oxford (UK): Blackwell Publishing; 2005. p. 119–29.
29. Maron BJ, Gohman TE, Kyle SB, et al. Clinical profile and spectrum of commotio cordis. JAMA 2002;287:1142–6.
30. Corrado D, Leoni L, Link MS, et al. Implantable cardioverter-defibrillator therapy for prevention of sudden death in patients with arrhythmogenic right ventricular cardiomyopathy/dysplasia. Circulation 2003;108:3084–91.
31. Douglas PS, O'Toole ML, Hiller WDB, et al. Different effects of prolonged exercise on the right and left ventricles. J Am Coll Cardiol 1990;15:64–9.
32. Corrado D, Thiene G. Arrhythmogenic right ventricular cardiomyopathy/dysplasia: clinical impact of molecular genetic studies. Circulation 2006;113:1634–7.
33. Gerull B, Heuser A, Wichter T, et al. Mutations in the desmosomal protein plakophilin-2 are common in arrhythmogenic right ventricular cardiomyopathy. Nat Genet 2004;36:1162–4.
34. Basso C, Czarnowska E, Della Barbera M, et al. Ultrastructural evidence of intercalated disc remodelling in arrhythmogenic right ventricular cardiomyopathy: an electron microscopy investigation on endomyocardial biopsies. Eur Heart J 2006;27:1847–54.
35. Kirchhof P, Fabritz L, Zwiener M, et al. Age- and training-dependent development of arrhythmogenic right ventricular cardiomyopathy in heterozygous plakoglobin-deficient mice. Circulation 2006;114:1799–806.
36. Wichter T, Hindricks G, Lerch H, et al. Regional myocardial sympathetic dysinnervation in arrhythmogenic right ventricular cardiomyopathy. Circulation 1994;89:667–83.
37. Tiso N, Stephan DA, Nava A, et al. Identification of mutations in the cardiac ryanodine receptor gene in families affected with arrhythmogenic right ventricular cardiomyopathy type 2 (ARVD2). Hum Mol Genet 2001;10:189–94.
38. Priori SG, Napolitano C, Tiso N, et al. Mutations in the cardiac ryanodine receptor gene (hryr2) underlie catecholaminergic polymorphic ventricular tachycardia. Circulation 2000;103:196–200.
39. Marcus F, Fontaine G, Guiraudon G, et al. Right ventricular dysplasia: a report of 24 adult cases. Circulation 1982;65:384–98.
40. Corrado D, Fontaine G, Marcus FI, et al. Arrhythmogenic right ventricular dysplasia/cardiomyopathy: need for an international registry. Study Group on Arrhythmogenic Right Ventricular Dysplasia/Cardiomyopathy of the Working Groups on Myocardial and Pericardial Disease and Arrhythmias of the European Society of Cardiology and of the Scientific Council on Cardiomyopathies of the World Heart Federation. Circulation 2000;101:101–6.
41. Corrado D, Basso C, Thiene G. Arrhythmogenic right ventricular cardiomyopathy: diagnosis, prognosis, and treatment. Heart 2000;83:588–95.
42. Turrini P, Corrado D, Basso C, et al. Dispersion of ventricular depolarization-repolarization a noninvasive marker for risk stratification in arrhythmogenic right ventricular cardiomyopathy. Circulation 2001;103:3075–80.
43. Corrado D, Basso C, Pelliccia A, et al. Sports and heart disease. In: Camm J, Luscher TF, Serruys PW, editors. The ESC textbook of cardiovascular medicine. New York: Oxford University Press; 2009. p. 1215–37.

44. Corrado D, Pelliccia A, Bjornstad HH, et al. Cardiovascular pre-participation screening of young competitive athletes for prevention of sudden death: proposal for a common European protocol. Consensus Statement of the Study Group of Sport Cardiology of the Working Group of Cardiac Rehabilitation and Exercise Physiology and the Working Group of Myocardial and Pericardial Diseases of the European Society of Cardiology. Eur Heart J 2005;26:516–24.
45. Maron BJ, Pelliccia A, Spirito P. Cardiac disease in young trained athletes. Insights into methods for distinguishing athlete's heart from structural heart disease, with particular emphasis on hypertrophic cardiomyopathy. Circulation 1995;91:1596–601.
46. Corrado D, Basso C, Pilichou K, et al. Molecular biology and the clinical management of arrhythmogenic right ventricular cardiomyopathy/dysplasia. Heart 2011;97:530–9.
47. Heidbüchel H, Hoogsteen J, Fagard R, et al. High prevalence of right ventricular involvement in endurance athletes with ventricular arrhythmias. Role of an electrophysiologic study in risk stratification. Eur Heart J 2003;24:1473–80.
48. Ector J, Ganame J, van der Merwe N, et al. Reduced right ventricular ejection fraction in endurance athletes presenting with ventricular arrhythmias: a quantitative angiographic assessment. Eur Heart J 2007;28:345–53.
49. La Gerche A, Robberecht C, Kuiperi C, et al. Lower than expected desmosomal gene mutation prevalence in endurance athletes with complex ventricular arrhythmias of right ventricular origin. Heart 2010;96: 1268–74.
50. Maron BJ, Zipes DP. 36th Bethesda conference: recommendations for determining eligibility for competition in athletes with cardiovascular abnormalities. J Am Coll Cardiol 2005;45:1373–5.
51. Pelliccia A, Fagard R, Bjornstad HH, et al. Recommendations for competitive sports participation in athletes with cardiovascular disease: a consensus document from the Study Group of Sports Cardiology of the Working Group of Cardiac Rehabilitation and Exercise Physiology and the Working Group of Myocardial and Pericardial Diseases of the European Society of Cardiology. Eur Heart J 2005;26: 1422–45.
52. Drezner JA, Rogers KJ. Sudden cardiac arrest in intercollegiate athletes: detailed analysis and outcomes of resuscitation in nine cases. Heart Rhythm 2006;3:755–9.

Index

Note: Page numbers of article titles are in **boldface** type.

Card Electrophysiol Clin 3 (2011) 333–337
doi:10.1016/S1877-9182(11)00029-3
1877-9182/11/$ – see front matter

G

H

I

L

M

N

O

P

W

Printed and bound by CPI Group (UK) Ltd, Croydon, CR0 4YY
03/10/2024
01040350-0017